Understanding the Lived Experiences of Persons with Disabilities in Nine Countries

Over the last three decades, a number of reforms have taken place in European social policy with an impact on the opportunities for persons with disabilities to be full and active members of society. The policy reforms have aimed to change the balance between citizens' rights and duties and the opportunities to enjoy choice and autonomy, live in the community and participate in political decision-making processes of importance for one's life.

How do the reforms influence the opportunities to exercise Active Citizenship? This volume presents the findings from the first cross-national comparison of how persons with disabilities reflexively make their way through the world, pursuing their own interests and values. The volume considers how their experiences, views and aspirations regarding participation vary across Europe.

Based on retrospective life-course interviews, the volume examines the scope for agency on the part of persons with disabilities, i.e. the extent to which men and women with disabilities are able to make choices and pursue lives they have reasons to value. Drawing on structuration theory and the capability approach, the volume investigates the opportunities for exercising Active Citizenship among men and women in nine European countries.

The volume identifies the policy implications of a process-oriented and multi-dimensional approach to Active Citizenship in European disability policy. It will appeal to policymakers and policy officials, as well as to researchers and students of disability studies, comparative social policy, international disability law and qualitative research methods.

Julie Beadle-Brown is Professor in Intellectual and Developmental Disabilities at the Tizard Centre, University of Kent, UK and Professor in Disability Studies at the Living with Disability Research Centre, La Trobe University, Australia. Her research, teaching and consultancy has particularly focused on deinstitutionalisation and the development of community-based services and on the implementation of person-centred approaches such as person-centred active support to improve quality of life.

Mario Biggeri is Associate Professor of Development Economics at the University of Florence and Director of the Degree of Economic Development, International

Social and Health Cooperation and Conflict Resolution. He is the scientific director of the research centre ARCO – Action Research for CO-Development – and Fellow of the Human Development and Capability Association.

Rune Halvorsen is Associate Professor in Social Policy in the Department of Social Work, Child Welfare and Social Policy, Oslo and Akershus University College, Norway. His research focuses on comparative and international social policies, social citizenship and social movements.

Bjørn Hvinden is Professor in Sociology and Head of Research at Norwegian Social Research (NOVA), an institution in the Oslo and Akershus University College, Norway. His main research interests are comparative and European social policies, social citizenship, climate change and welfare, disability, poverty and youth job insecurity.

Jan Tøssebro is Professor of Social Work and Director of NTNU Social Research, Trondheim, Norway. His primary research interests are disability policy, notably deinstitutionalisation, inclusive education, families with disabled children, standards of living and working life experience.

Anne Waldschmidt is Professor of Sociology, Politics of Rehabilitation and Disability Studies and the Director of the International Research Unit in Disability Studies at the University of Cologne, Germany. Her research focuses on the cultural and political sociologies of 'dis/ability', body sociology, contemporary disability history, the political participation of persons with disabilities and transnational disability policies.

Routledge Advances in Disability Studies

www.routledge.com/Routledge-Advances-in-Disability-Studies/book-series/RADS

Towards a Contextual Psychology of Disablism
Brian Watermeyer

Disability, Hate Crime and Violence
Edited by Alan Roulstone and Hannah Mason-Bish

Branding and Designing Disability
Reconceptualising Disability Studies
Elizabeth DePoy and Stephen Gilson

Crises, Conflict and Disability
Ensuring Equality
Edited by David Mitchell and Valerie Karr

Disability, Spaces and Places of Policy Exclusion
Edited by Karen Soldatic, Hannah Morgan and Alan Roulstone

Changing Social Attitudes Toward Disability
Perspectives from Historical, Cultural, and Educational Studies
Edited by David Bolt

Disability, Avoidance and the Academy
Challenging Resistance
Edited by David Bolt and Claire Penketh

Autism in a De-centered World
Alice Wexler

Disabled Childhoods
Monitoring Differences and Emerging Identities
Janice McLaughlin, Edmund Coleman-Fountain and Emma Clavering

Intellectual Disability and Being Human
A Care Ethics Model
Chrissie Rogers

The Changing Disability Policy System
Active Citizenship and Disability in Europe Volume 1
Edited by Rune Halvorsen, Bjørn Hvinden, Jerome Bickenbach, Delia Ferri and Ana Marta Guillén Rodriguez

Understanding the Lived Experiences of Persons with Disabilities in Nine Countries
Active Citizenship and Disability in Europe Volume 2
Edited by Rune Halvorsen, Bjørn Hvinden, Julie Beadle-Brown, Mario Biggeri, Jan Tøssebro and Anne Waldschmidt

Intellectual Disability and the Right to a Sexual Life
A Continuation of the Autonomy/Paternalism Debate
Simon Foley

Intellectual Disability Politics in the Era of 'Post-Institutionalism'
Niklas Altermark

Understanding the Lived Experiences of Persons with Disabilities in Nine Countries

Active Citizenship and Disability in Europe Volume 2

Edited by Rune Halvorsen, Bjørn Hvinden, Julie Beadle-Brown, Mario Biggeri, Jan Tøssebro and Anne Waldschmidt

Routledge
Taylor & Francis Group
LONDON AND NEW YORK

First published 2018
by Routledge
2 Park Square, Milton Park, Abingdon, Oxon OX14 4RN

and by Routledge
711 Third Avenue, New York, NY 10017

Routledge is an imprint of the Taylor & Francis Group, an informa business

British Library Cataloguing in Publication Data
A catalogue record for this book is available from the British Library

Library of Congress Cataloging in Publication Data
A catalog record for this book has been requested

ISBN: 978-1-138-65292-7 (hbk)
ISBN: 978-1-315-62392-4 (ebk)

Typeset in Times New Roman
by Wearset Ltd, Boldon, Tyne and Wear

Contents

Figures

Tables

Contributors

Caterina Arciprete is a researcher at the research centre ARCO – Action Research for CO-Development. She has a PhD in Development Economics from the University of Florence. Her research focuses on disability, gender issues and child poverty.

Rita Barbuto is the Regional Development Officer for the European Region of Disabled Peoples' International and Director of DPI Italia ONLUS. She is an expert in human rights and disability, bioethics and disability, and gender and disability issues. She is widely consulted as a peer counsellor, and provides training to faculty and students at several Italian universities.

Julie Beadle-Brown is Professor in Intellectual and Developmental Disabilities at the Tizard Centre, University of Kent, UK and Professor in Disability Studies at the Living with Disability Research Centre, La Trobe University, Australia. Her research, teaching and consultancy has particularly focused on deinstitutionalisation and the development of community-based services and on the implementation of person-centred approaches such as person-centred active support to improve quality of life.

Mario Biggeri is Associate Professor of Development Economics at the University of Florence and Director of the Degree of Economic Development, International Social and Health Cooperation and Conflict Resolution. He is the scientific director of the research centre ARCO – Action Research for CO-Development – and Fellow of the Human Development and Capability Association.

Kjetil Klette Bøhler is Senior Researcher at Norwegian Social Research (NOVA), an institution in the Oslo and Akershus University College of Applied Sciences, Norway. Recently he has worked with research on Active Citizenship for persons with disabilities and research on the consequences of unemployment among young adults in Europe. In addition, Bøhler works with research dealing with the intersection between aesthetics and politics, and in particular the relationship between music and politics in a changing Latin America.

Federico Ciani is the Coordinator of the Inclusive Development Unit of the research centre ARCO – Action Research for CO-Development – and a post-doctoral researcher at the University of Florence. His research focuses on social inclusion, analysis of marginalisation processes and resilience. He has strong experience in the field of quantitative data analysis and econometric techniques.

Edmund Coleman-Fountain is a lecturer in Sociology at Northumbria University, UK. He was previously a research fellow in the Social Policy Research Unit at the University of York, UK. His interests are in narrative identities, disability and youth.

Timo Dins is a junior researcher at the Institute for Pedagogy and Rehabilitation for Persons with Intellectual and Severe Disabilities at the University of Cologne, Germany. His research interests include disability studies, disability ethics and capability theory.

Eilionóir Flynn is Deputy Director of the Centre for Disability Law and Policy and Senior Lecturer with the School of Law, National University of Ireland, Galway, Ireland. Her interests in disability law include assisted and supported decision-making, rights-enforcement mechanisms and access to justice.

G. Anthony Giannoumis is Assistant Professor of Universal Design at the Department of Computer Science at Oslo and Akershus University College, and an international research fellow at the Burton Blatt Institute at Syracuse University. His research interests include universal design, international governance, sustainable development, social regulation and standardisation.

Giampiero Griffo is Co-director of the Robert Castel Center for Governmentality and Disability Studies at the Naples University 'Suor Orsola Benincasa', Italian member of the European Academic Network on Disability, Disabled Peoples International world council member, European Disability Forum board member and chairperson of the Italian network on disability and development.

Rune Halvorsen is Associate Professor in Social Policy in the Department of Social Work, Child Welfare and Social Policy, Oslo and Akershus University College, Norway. His research focuses on comparative and international social policy, social movements and social citizenship.

Bjørn Hvinden is Professor in Sociology and Head of Research at Norwegian Social Research (NOVA), an institution in the Oslo and Akershus University College, Norway. His main research interests are comparative and European social policies, social citizenship, climate change and welfare, disability, poverty and youth job insecurity.

Šárka Káňová is a researcher in the Department of Special Education, Charles University in Prague and a senior lecturer at the Faculty of Education, University of West Bohemia in Pilsen, Czech Republic. Her research interests include the issue of the life course of people with disabilities and exploring the possibilities of fulfilling the roles associated with their Active Citizenship.

Anemari Karačić is a junior researcher at the International Research Unit in Disability Studies, University of Cologne, Germany. Her research interests include disability studies, the cultural and political sociologies of 'dis/ability' and biopolitics.

Sinéad Keogh is a post-doctoral researcher at the Centre for Disability Law and Policy at the National University of Ireland, Galway. She has previously worked as a lecturer in economics and researched time use patterns of farm household members in the West of Ireland.

Anna M. Kittelsaa is a senior researcher at NTNU Social Research and holds a part-time position as Professor at the Arctic University of Norway. Her main interests are the lives and living conditions of people with disabilities, especially the first person perspectives of individuals with intellectual disabilities on their own identities and life circumstances.

Jennifer Kline is a post-doctoral researcher at the Centre for Disability Law and Policy at the National University of Ireland, Galway. She has expertise in immigration, human rights and disability law.

Rafael Lindqvist is Senior Professor in the Department of Sociology, Uppsala University, Sweden. His main research interest is the emergence of the Nordic welfare states, with an emphasis on reforms and organisation in sickness insurance, vocational rehabilitation and disability policy.

Roy Sainsbury is Professor of Social Policy in the Department of Social Policy and Social Work at the University of York, UK. His main research interests are reforms in social security systems, administration and delivery of benefits and the relationship between social security, disability and the labour market.

Victoria Schuller is a PhD student in Health Sciences and Health Policy at the University of Lucerne, Switzerland. Her research interests include gender and disability, Active Citizenship and social inclusion of persons with disabilities.

Marie Sépulchre is a PhD candidate in the Department of Sociology, Uppsala University, Sweden. Her research interests centre on citizenship, disability, activism and digital media.

Jan Šiška is Associate Professor at the Faculty of Education, Charles University, Prague and West Bohemia University, Pilsen, Czech Republic. His main research interests include disability-related policies, special/inclusive education and development, de-institutionalisation and community living.

Andreas Sturm is a junior researcher at the International Research Unit in Disability Studies, University of Cologne, Germany. His research focuses on biopolitics, the cultural and political sociologies of 'dis/ability', the disability rights movement and interest representation of persons with disabilities.

Jan Tøssebro is Professor of Social Work and Director of NTNU Social Research, Trondheim, Norway. His primary research interest is disability policy, notably deinstitutionalisation, inclusive education, families with disabled children, standards of living and working life experience.

Bruno Trezzini is Group Leader in the Empowerment, Participation and Social Integration Unit, Swiss Paraplegic Research, Nottwil, Switzerland. His research interests include work and employment across the life course of persons with disabilities, vocational rehabilitation of persons with spinal cord injury, welfare regimes and social insurance reforms as well as disability studies.

Anne Waldschmidt is Professor of Sociology, Politics of Rehabilitation and Disability Studies and Director of the International Research Unit in Disability Studies at the University of Cologne, Germany. Her research focuses on the cultural and political sociologies of 'dis/ability', body sociology, contemporary disability history, the political participation of persons with disabilities and transnational disability policies.

Preface

This book is the second of two volumes on Active Citizenship and disability in Europe. The two volumes – *The Changing Disability System* and *Understanding the Lived Experiences of Persons with Disabilities in Nine European Countries* – are the results of the collective effort of a team of European researchers working together within a project co-funded by the European Union's Seventh Framework Programme for research, technological development and demonstration (FP7). The full title of the project is 'Making Persons with Disabilities Full Citizens – New Knowledge for an Inclusive and Sustainable European Social Model (DISCIT)' (grant agreement number 320079). Bruno Trezzini and Victoria Schuller gratefully acknowledge additional financial support from the Swiss National Science Foundation (grant agreement no. 150229). The project was coordinated by Bjørn Hvinden, Bettina Uhrig and Rune Halvorsen, Norwegian Social Research (NOVA), an institution in the Oslo and Akershus University College.

We would like to thank the contributors to this book for their enthusiasm in writing their chapters. During our work with the book, we have benefited from encouragement and support from a number of people. In particular, we would like to mention Carlotta Besozzi, Peter Blanck, Jerome Bickenbach, Mary Ann Kenny, Monica Menapace, Jan Monsbakken, Catherine Naughton, Inmaculada Placencia Porrero, Gerard Quinn, Robert Salais, Marta Szebehely, Lisa Waddington and Jenny Williams. In preparing this book, we have benefited enormously from the participation of the European Disability Forum and the Mental Disability Rights Initiative – Serbia as consortium members in the project. The European and national stakeholder committees in the DISCIT project have provided invaluable support and advice in all stages of the preparation of this book. We would also like to extend our thanks to all interviewees who have shared their views and experiences with the researchers in the Czech Republic, Germany, Ireland, Italy, Norway, Serbia, Sweden, Switzerland and the UK.

The information and views set out in this book are those of the authors and do not necessarily reflect the official opinion of the European Union. Neither the European Union and bodies nor any person acting in their behalf may be held responsible for the use which may be made of the information contained therein.

Rune Halvorsen, Bjørn Hvinden, Julie Beadle-Brown, Mario Biggeri, Jan Tøssebro and Anne Waldschmidt
Oslo/Kent/Florence/Trondheim/Cologne, August 2017

1 Changing opportunities for Active Citizenship

Understanding the lived experiences of persons with disabilities

Rune Halvorsen, Bjørn Hvinden, Julie Beadle-Brown, Mario Biggeri, Jan Tøssebro and Anne Waldschmidt

Since the 1990s, a number of reforms have taken place in European social policy that have impacted the opportunities for persons with disabilities to be full and active members of society. The policy reforms have aimed to change the balance between citizens' rights and duties, and their opportunities to enjoy choice and autonomy, to live in the community and to participate in political decision-making processes that impact their lives. At the centre of the policy reforms are notions of Active Citizenship. Citizens are encouraged, provided with resources and sometimes coerced into taking more responsibility for their own self-sustainability, the care of others, the well-being of the community and a more vibrant polity. Not only have European governments adopted policy reforms to stimulate more citizens to become active in the labour market – they have stimulated and provided opportunities for the more active involvement of citizens in welfare and health-care services, in informal care for family members, in civil society organisations and in community work.

This book centres on how persons with disabilities experience their opportunities to exercise Active Citizenship. Based on coordinated semi-structured and retrospective life-course interviews in nine European countries (the Czech Republic, Germany, Ireland, Italy, Norway, Serbia, Sweden, Switzerland and the United Kingdom (UK)), we examine the scope for agency on the part of persons with disabilities (i.e. the extent to which men and women with disabilities are able to make choices and pursue the lives they have reasons to value). We map the diversity in their experiences and identify factors and mechanisms that enhance or prevent the Active Citizenship of persons with disabilities. Furthermore, we compare the variations we find between persons with disabilities, analyse how public policies have shaped their lived experiences and discuss potential improvements in policies promoting Active Citizenship.

This book contains the findings from the first cross-national comparison of how Active Citizenship of persons with disabilities varies across Europe. The investigation builds on the collective efforts of researchers collaborating within the context of the project 'DISCIT – Making Persons with Disabilities Full Citizens – New Knowledge for an Inclusive and Sustainable European Social

Model'. The project received funding in 2013–2016 from the European Union's (EU's) Seventh Framework Programme for Research, Technological Development and Demonstration (grant agreement number 320079).

This chapter introduces the major issues discussed in the book and presents the key concepts adopted to produce new and relevant knowledge about these issues. At the centre of our research is the concept of Active Citizenship. As a backdrop for the empirical analyses that comprise most of the chapters of this book, this chapter outlines some of the main policy reforms passed in the last three decades aimed at persons with disabilities and the variations we have found in disability policy among the European countries (see also Chapter 2, Volume 1). We then identify some factors and mechanisms that may explain why we find variation in the Active Citizenship of persons with disabilities among countries, between women and men, and among different disabilities, age groups and birth cohorts.

Active Citizenship as a multidimensional concept

While existing scholarship provides a number of definitions of social citizenship in general, more precise conceptualisations of Active Citizenship are rare. To the extent that we find such conceptualisations, they tend to focus on one particular and rather narrow aspect, for instance linked to active labour market policy, the privatisation of social risk protection, citizens' education to promote socially responsible participation in the local community or political activism (Johansson & Hvinden, 2007; Halvorsen & Hvinden, 2013).

By contrast, the research project this book reports from has adopted a unified and multidimensional concept of Active Citizenship. Scholars have seldom discussed the Active Citizenship of persons with disabilities and, when they do, it is rarely in a systematic way, or they mention it only in passing or in dismissive ways (e.g. Barnes & Mercer, 2003, pp. 20–22; Priestley, 2003, pp. 116–142; Dwyer, 2004, pp. 116–117; Gilbert, Cochrane & Greenwell, 2005; Annetts, Law, McNeish & Mooney, 2009, pp. 12, 20–28; Hall, 2011; Pound, 2011; Roulstone & Prideaux, 2012, pp. 34–35). Important exceptions are publications by Power, Lord and de Franco (2013) and Christensen, Guldvik and Larssen (2014), who analyse disability measures such as personal assistance and personal budgets in terms of Active Citizenship; they emphasise the self-determination dimension of such citizenship. Similarly, Hästbacka and Nygård (2013) investigate the shifting rationale for Finnish disability policy, finding that Finnish members of parliament do frame such policy in terms of Active Citizenship to a limited extent; however, they do so with a focus on how services and support enhance the independence of disabled persons in their everyday lives.

Together with Volume 1 (Halvorsen, Hvinden, Bickenbach, Ferri & Guillén Rodriguez, 2017), this book constitutes the first extensive, systematic, theoretically informed and empirically based comparative analysis of the scope and prospects for the Active Citizenship of women and men with disabilities in Europe. Our conceptualisation of Active Citizenship focuses on three dimensions (while acknowledging that there may also be others):

- *security:* whether public policy, (largely) through redistributive measures, enables citizens to maintain a sense of security by effectively using the social rights meant to protect them against major life risks and contingencies such as illness, poverty and violence;
- *autonomy*: whether public policy, through a mix of redistributive and regulatory measures, allows citizens to decide for themselves what is valuable, living their lives in accordance with this decision (i.e. that they are capable of defining their needs, making their own choices and pursuing the life they have reasons to value);
- *influence*: whether public policy creates the conditions for citizens' participation in public deliberation and decision-making processes, creating the framework for their own lives as well as promoting common good and regulating social behaviour, given the interdependence of human action (such citizens' participation may take place at the individual level or collectively through citizens' groups and interest organisations, including organisations of persons with disabilities (DPOs)).

While treating these three dimensions (security, autonomy and influence) as analytically distinct, we expect them to be overlapping in practice, that is, in the lives and practices of people. Moreover, we assume that the three may interact and mutually support each other. For instance, we find it improbable that citizens would be able to enjoy real possibilities for exercising independence and influence on matters of importance for their lives, unless they can use their social rights to a predictable and adequate income and have access to necessary and high-quality services (e.g. education, social and health services). Conversely, we find it difficult to imagine that citizens will be able to claim social rights, unless they are capable of expressing and entitled to express their needs and wants. Altogether, the understanding of Active Citizenship presented here is very close to the 'full and effective participation in society on an equal basis with others' as laid out by the United Nations Convention on the Rights of Persons with Disabilities (CRPD) (United Nations, 2006, Preamble, Item E, see Articles 1 & 3). While the CPRD does not codify social citizenship as such, its overall vision is very much the same as the one reflected in our conceptualisation of Active Citizenship.

In practice, public policy designs have often been oriented towards securing or improving the situation of persons with disabilities along one or more of the three dimensions (security, autonomy, influence) without framing policies in terms of promoting 'Active Citizenship'. Yet, the common element of all three dimensions is whether public policy enhances or prevents citizens' sense of their own agency (i.e. their ability to act, participate in and be in charge of their own lives) (Lister, 2003, p. 39).

Following our definition of Active Citizenship, being an active citizen involves exercising social rights and duties, enjoying choice and autonomy and participating in political decision-making processes that are important for one's life and society as a whole. In other words, in this book, we focus on the social practices of persons with disabilities and the persons they interact with, not only the formal status bestowed upon them.

In his now classic essay 'Citizenship and Social Class', T. H. Marshall (1965) defines citizenship as 'a status bestowed on those who are full members of a community. All who possess the status are equal with respect to the rights and duties with which the status is endowed' (p. 92). From Marshall's perspective, citizenship can be regarded as an inclusionary social institution, codifying societal membership as well as a contractual relationship between the individual citizen and society at large. To the extent that previously excluded population groups are included by being accorded equal rights and duties combined with opportunities for participation, we regard this as a process of democratisation (i.e. more people are attributed the same level of autonomy and opportunities to choose the life they have reasons to cherish).

Citizenship, however, is not only about social status or the extent to which people are recognised as full and effective members of society, regardless of differences in social position or other characteristics. Citizenship is equally as much about the social and cultural practices that shape opportunities for participation. We follow the prevailing understanding of citizenship used in the social sciences today:

> But being a full and equal citizen is, basically, a question of *practices*: living a decent life in accordance with the prevailing standards in society, being able to act autonomously, being able to participate in social and political life in the broadest sense, and having 'civic' orientations to the political community and to one's fellow citizens.
>
> (Andersen & Halvorsen, 2002, pp. 12–13, our emphasis)

Often, the concept of *social* citizenship has been used to describe the relationship between the citizen and public institutions in terms of the provision of social security. As we have already explained, we have adopted a broader concept of Active Citizenship. Feminist scholars emphasise social citizenship as follows:

> social citizenship is not only a question of entitlement, it also involves participation in all realms of public and societal life: not only in political institutions or bodies but also in neighbourhoods, at workplaces, in charity work or voluntary organisations and social movements.
>
> (Lister et al., 2007, p. 37)

Many scholars construct the citizen as an agent with the capacity to make individual choices and take part in decision-making (e.g. Williams, Popay & Oakley, 1999; Hoggett, 2001; Le Grand, 2003; Deacon, 2004; Jensen & Pfau-Effinger, 2005). However, persons with disabilities have often been excluded from access to the resources and opportunities required to participate on a par with non-disabled persons. Some persons with disabilities have been deprived of the legal capacity and competence to make their own choices. Others have been excluded from access to education, employment, opportunities for community living and political activity. Yet, we find it reasonable to assume that there will be broad variations in lived experiences among persons with disabilities across Europe.

Policies fostering or hampering Active Citizenship

Here, we provide a brief background for understanding the variation we have found in experiences between the nine countries and some of the policy transformations that women and men with disabilities have experienced.

As mentioned, we have witnessed a number of reforms in public policy that could potentially enhance the Active Citizenship of persons with disabilities, particularly since the 1990s. How the EU, international organisations, European governments, DPOs and other stakeholders think about social policy for persons with disabilities has become broader in scope. Especially since the 1990s, more policy areas have come to be considered relevant for persons with disabilities. While 'disability policy' in the last century was largely confined to the provision of separate and segregated services in cash and in kind, the needs of persons with disabilities have been incorporated or mainstreamed in an increasing number of policy areas, including access to public transport, the built environment and information and communication technologies (Chapter 12, Volume 1). In this context, we see the growing importance of the EU and the United Nations (UN) in setting minimum standards for member states in their policies for persons with disabilities, as well as the emergence of new arenas for influence and co-decision from individuals and DPOs.

First, at the international level, the UN has played a key role in codifying legal and other requirements to enable persons with disabilities to exercise agency and also Active Citizenship. In 1975, the UN set forth the 'Declaration on the Rights of Disabled Persons' that called for the member states to promote the full integration of disabled persons into all aspects of economic and social life (United Nations, 1975). Later, it adopted the 'Standard Rules on the Equalization of Opportunities for Persons with Disabilities' (United Nations, 1993). While the 'Standard Rules' were not legally binding, they represented a clear commitment by the member governments to work towards equal opportunities for all, including persons with disabilities. With the adoption of the 'Convention on the Rights of Persons with Disabilities', the international community has taken a large step in the direction of defining legal obligations for the parties of the convention to ensure opportunities for 'full and effective participation' for persons with disabilities (United Nations, 2006).

Second, since the mid-1990s, the EU has been a driving force for more and stronger regulatory social policy measures for ensuring equal treatment for all, independent of disability or impairment. Social regulation policy is concerned with removing physical, organisational and attitudinal barriers that limit or preclude participation or hinder an assessment based on an individual's qualifications or achievements. The directives on equal treatment in employment, occupation and web accessibility are the main advances in the EU thus far regarding the rights of persons with disabilities (European Union, 2000, 2016). Additionally, separate disability-related provisions have been included in an increasing number of general directives and regulations to safeguard and advance accessibility to goods and services for persons with disabilities (Waddington, 2017). While the EU's power is limited when it comes to the coordination or even harmonisation of social security and services between the countries (Chapter 12, Volume 1), since 2014, it has promoted de-institutionalisation and community living through its structural funds (Chapter 13, Volume 1).

Third, at the national level, there are significant differences in disability policy, creating intended and unintended consequences for persons with disabilities. Most obviously, the nine DISCIT countries exhibit considerable differences in the levels and profiles of public expenditures on disability-related income maintenance programmes and social services (Table 2.1, Volume 1). While we found little evidence to support the assumption that the volatile international economy in the 2000s has forced governments to cut disability-related social protection, the share of means-tested disability benefits increased, particularly in Ireland, the UK, Germany and Switzerland (Table 2.3, Volume 1). Available data for 2003–2012 indicate that, among the DISCIT countries, only the UK has a clear trend towards a lower level of spending on disability benefits in terms of purchase power standards, whereas Ireland and Norway have a significant increase (Hvinden, 2016). Overall, there are remarkable path dependencies in the levels and profiles of disability-related public expenditures. Earlier analyses of the diverse institutional contexts demonstrate how these distinct policy profiles have been influenced by different national policy traditions, public–private divisions of labour and the roles of social partners and DPOs (Halvorsen & Hvinden, 2009; Waldschmidt, 2009; Halvorsen, 2010; Halvorsen & Hvinden, 2011).

A country's actual configuration of social provision and risk protection is always more complex than the pure and simplified picture drawn by a model. Nonetheless, it is fair to say that the disability policy systems of some countries (e.g. Norway and Sweden) have placed relatively greater emphasis on the public redistribution of resources and collective risk protection ('security') than others. Other countries have, in diverse ways, granted a greater role to individual or family responsibility and risk protection ('autonomy') than others, which has given occupation- or market-based insurance a more prominent role in overall disability-related provisions (e.g. Germany, Ireland, Italy and the UK).

The data presented in Volume 1 confirm that European countries not only use different policy instruments – their efforts to enhance the Active Citizenship of persons with disabilities also have distinct profiles. Volume 1 presents a tentative typology of six redistributive disability policy systems in Europe. The typology distinguishes between 'high spenders', 'mixed spenders' and 'low spenders' and whether the system gives means testing a strong or weak role (Table 2.6). The findings suggest that high spenders (Germany, Norway, Sweden and Switzerland) provide better conditions for the Active Citizenship of persons with disabilities than the mixed spenders (Italy and the UK), which in turn provide better conditions than the low spenders (the Czech Republic and Ireland). High spenders tend to have lower mean values on the share of persons with disabilities living in households with very low work intensity, which puts them at risk of material deprivation and relative poverty. We must be careful not to interpret these findings as causal relationships. Tøssebro and Hvinden (Chapter 4, Volume 1) discuss some of the reasons for why we should be cautious when making such inferences.

In addition to the path dependencies in the national disability policy systems, we also found some evidence of 'equifinality' (Gresov & Drazin, 1997): arriving from different initial conditions, many European countries (e.g. Norway, Sweden, the UK and Switzerland) have introduced reforms that have led to improvements in the conditions for exercising autonomy in everyday life (e.g. by closing down previous institutions and offering persons with disabilities the opportunity to live independently in the community; by providing personal assistance or budgets, care and support; by implementing the innovative use of new technologies; by introducing universally designed or appropriate accommodation for persons with disabilities and by facilitating accessible physical environments and transport systems). In other European countries (e.g. the Czech Republic and Serbia), the number of persons with disabilities living in large institutions is stagnating, while a few countries have seen the emergence of new forms of institutional living (e.g. Italy, Norway and the UK) (Chapter 4, Volume 1).

Fourth, a more dynamic relationship between welfare states and disabled citizens is evolving, since citizens themselves expect (or are expected) to play a more active role in handling a diverse set of risks and promoting their own welfare. At the individual level, European governments have introduced various forms of user involvement, consumer choice and control for persons with disabilities. The amount of autonomy and influence that persons with disabilities have achieved through such reforms depends on whether choice is built into the services in cash or in kind, whether conditionality and 'self-responsibility' have been attached to the receipt of the services and what kind, quality and level of services persons with disabilities have been entitled to. In particular, persons with intellectual and psychosocial disabilities have experienced constraints in their opportunities to choose and influence service provision (European Union, 2013; Priestley et al., 2016; Lindqvist & Sépulchre, 2016).

At the collective level, DPOs have achieved new opportunities to sidestep national authorities by directly contacting supranational authorities in the EU and UN systems. In efforts to achieve policy change in their home countries, DPOs may aim to influence the recommendations and requirements of EU and UN bodies. The relations between European governments and DPOs vary. Despite the adoption of the CRPD, the involvement and influence of DPOs are not necessarily increasing at the national level. In certain countries, there are trends towards less priority being given to communication with and involvement of DPOs, the closing down of consultation mechanisms with DPOs and less priority accorded to the national coordination of disability policy across government ministries (Chapters 10, 11, 13, Volume 1). Overall, the nine countries covered by the two books reveal broad variations in the conditions for the Active Citizenship of persons with disabilities.

What do we mean by a life-course approach to Active Citizenship?

The empirical chapters in this book examine in detail how the varying conditions for exercising Active Citizenship have been experienced by persons with disabilities. We do this by adopting a life-course approach, defined as 'a sequence of socially defined events and roles that the individual enacts over time' (Giele & Elder, 1998, p. 22). To others, the life course 'denotes a temporal order of life shaped by institutions and public policies and propelled by continual biographic decisions made by the individual' (Leisering & Walker, 1998, p. 9). The life-course approach differs from a focus on the 'life cycle', which usually refers to a biological or psychological approach to the various stages of the individual life from birth to death (Yerkes, Peper & Baxter, 2013, pp. 105–106). Sociologically speaking, the idea of the life course describes important events that people experience over time related to education, work and employment, establishing a separate household, marriage, parenthood, retirement, etc. The life course is constructed on the basis of dominant expectations about the normal timing of life events, and it defines the un-normal timing of events as 'too early', 'too late' (Hagestad & Neugarten, 1985) or being of un-normal duration (Merton, 1984). Persons with disabilities may experience that their timing of events is considered appropriate and in compliance with dominant expectations or that they are moving out of their parents' house 'too late', they achieve paid work 'too late' or they become dependent on health care services 'too early' according to dominant expectations (Thorsen & Jeppsson Grassman, 2012).

By adopting a life-course approach, we are interested in how the Active Citizenship of persons with disabilities evolves over time. We focus on how disability-related policies impinge on the timing of life events, what level and type of education disabled persons are able to achieve and whether they manage to achieve paid work, live in the community and participate in political decision-making processes. Lutz Leisering (2003, p. 2) argues the following:

> out of the major forces that shape the life course – family, work, social networks, state – the state is the only overarching agency that extends to the entire life-course, including periods of non-work and lack of a family. Still, only small groups like long-term welfare recipients or in sheltered workshops are set on a lasting and exclusive welfare state trajectory.

Persons with disabilities are more likely than others to be dependent on the welfare state over a long period of time. Yet, to examine the relationship between public disability policy and the life course is not a simple task. By adopting a life-course approach, we are by definition focusing on individual persons with disabilities as a unit of analysis. Our major focus is on individual agency and the conditions that can be conceptualised and measured at the individual level (Mayer & Schoepflin, 1989, p. 190). Almost no direct link exists between the official disability policies at the EU and national levels and the lives of individuals with disabilities. Rather, the policies are mediated through interaction processes between units at different levels: national governments, organisations, social groups and individual citizens. One important task for life-course studies on the Active Citizenship of persons with disabilities is to examine how such processes (sequences of actions) impinge on the opportunities for exercising Active Citizenship over time.

Hubbard (2000, para. 11.4) argued that 'life histories have the potential to reveal how people interpret and understand social structures and encourages an exploration of how social structures are perceived by individuals at key turning points in their lives'. Yet, life history and life-course studies more generally have the capacity to contribute beyond exploring the phenomenology of the individual citizens (Shah & Priestley, 2011, p. 19). While we take the individual subjectivities as a starting point for our analyses, we want to interpret the statements and stories of persons with disabilities in light of what we otherwise know about their biographies and social positions.

Objectives of the book

Existing research has rarely examined in a systematic and thorough way the conditions that hamper or enable persons with disabilities to exercise Active Citizenship. In most existing research, issues or challenges related to this topic are completely absent or invisible. While the opportunities for full and effective membership of society, living a decent life in accordance with the prevailing standards in society, being able to act autonomously and participate in social and political life in the broadest sense have become more salient on the national and international policy agenda, the research literature about the mechanisms and processes influencing the opportunities for Active Citizenship is still limited. Therefore, we have set ourselves the task of identifying the conditions that are required for Active Citizenship to become an experienced reality for persons with disabilities.

Adopting a life-course perspective, we examine the links between the *conditions* for being active citizens, the *interaction processes* between persons with disabilities, their significant others and achieved *outcomes*, and how the conditions develop over time both in individual life courses and between age cohorts. We ask how national- and EU-level disability policies have influenced the scope for agency and capability on the part of persons with disabilities (i.e. the extent to which women and men with disabilities have been able to make choices and pursue the life objectives they have reasons to cherish, or whether rules, resources and practices outside the control of the welfare states are of equal or more importance). By comparing the experiences of women and men with disabilities in three age cohorts and in four broad categories of disabilities across Europe, we analyse under which conditions European welfare states are most likely to contribute to the full and active participation of persons with disabilities. A basic goal is therefore to determine the extent to which persons with disabilities exercise Active Citizenship, and, if they do not, the factors or mechanisms behind this absence.

To provide the necessary information to achieve the objectives, the researchers behind this book have carried out coordinated life-course interviews with equal numbers of women and men with four types of disabilities belonging to three different birth cohorts in nine countries. In the context of DISCIT, we have collected life-course data from women and men born around 1950, 1970 and 1990 (i.e. the interviewees were 25, 45 and 65 years old +/– 5 years at the time of the interview). The nine DISCIT country teams interviewed women and men with visual, mobility, intellectual and psychosocial disabilities in each of the age groups.

The data have ensured sensitivity to the heterogeneity of the situation and circumstances of persons with disabilities. *First*, comparison of the life courses of three birth cohorts of persons with disabilities belonging to partially overlapping time spells has enabled us to create new and systematic knowledge of the impact of changes in policy and social environments within each country. *Second*, we examine the development and continuity in individual life courses in light of changes in public policy and opportunities for Active Citizenship. *Third*, based on comparisons across countries, we analyse the impacts of inter-country differences in overall disability policy design, implementation and enforcement. *Fourth*, we compare the experiences of four broad categories of disabilities. *Fifth*, we examine how gendered norms and expectations impinge on the Active Citizenship of women with disabilities.

In Volume 1, we examined disability policy, policy coordination and implementation, investigating whether and to what extent European and national policies included explicit goals, appropriate means and coordinated efforts to enhance the Active Citizenship of persons with disabilities. Additionally, we identified factors and mechanisms that influence the extent to which persons with disabilities are able to exercise Active Citizenship: competing policy paradigms, underlying ambivalence towards target groups, deficits in institutional and policy design and implementation deficits (Halvorsen et al., 2017).

By contrast, in Volume 2, we focus on the lived experiences of individuals with disabilities, their social practices, their coping and negotiation strategies and their interaction with significant others, including family and kin, employers, people in their local communities and organised civil society. This allows us to take the investigation of factors and mechanisms that enhance or undermine the Active Citizenship of persons with disabilities one step further than we accomplished in Volume 1.

Factors that may hamper or enhance the Active Citizenship of persons with disabilities

When analysing the data in this book and the accompanying Volume 1, we find it useful to distinguish three types of factors that may influence the Active Citizenship of persons with disabilities (Hvinden, Halvorsen, Bickenbach, Ferri & Guillén Rodriguez, 2017):

- meta-political factors
- factors related to policy design and institutions
- factors related to the take-up and use of disability-related cash benefits, services and regulations by disabled persons.

Meta-political factors

A fundamental set of factors is the processes that allow or prevent the interests and demands of persons with disabilities from entering the political agenda. Two rather different strands of literature have inspired us to think about such processes.

First, social philosopher Nancy Fraser (1995, 2000) has developed a normative theory of social justice, in which she initially distinguishes between the redistribution of resources and the socio-cultural recognition of status as two complementary ways of ensuring participatory parity. While redistribution refers to processes for achieving the fair allocation of resources, typically economic in nature, recognition refers to the processes whereby people achieve or are bestowed the requisite standing in society (Fraser, 2008, p. 16). She later revises her theoretical framework to include political representation as a third process, seeing it as equally important as redistribution and recognition (2008, pp. 17, 60). She refers here to political processes in a constitutive sense, as mechanisms and decision-making rules that structure whose claims for redistribution and recognition will be discussed and decided upon. In other words, she focuses on the factors that include some people's claims, as well as factors that exclude other claims from consideration and adjudication. Moreover, she distinguishes between two levels of political misrepresentation. 'Ordinary political misrepresentation' is when a particular decision-making rule makes it difficult for some people to participate fully in political decision-making. The other level of misrepresentation, which she calls 'misframing', refers to when some people are excluded completely from participation or consideration in decision-making forums (Fraser, 2008, pp. 19, 147).

Second, political scientists Anne Schneider and Helen Ingram (1993, 2005; see also Schneider & Sidney, 2009) have formulated a general framework for understanding how cultural characterisations or popular images of various categories of citizens and potential target groups of public policy affect the policy agenda and choice of policy instruments. They also examine how policy agenda and design influence the political orientations and participation patterns of target populations. One dimension is whether elected officials regard a certain category of citizens as 'strong' or 'weak' in terms of power and access to political resources. Another dimension is whether public officials tend to regard a category of citizens in positive or negative terms. The authors argue that various combinations of such constructions are important for what public officials will expect of members of a category in terms of capacity, participation and contribution to society, or conversely in terms of demands, lack of capacity and burdens on society (e.g. whether target populations are asked to find their own solutions to problems and are attributed the qualities of being responsible and capable of making good choices for themselves and society at large). To the extent that public officials build on such constructions in the direction of policy and the allocation of resources to categories of citizens, the constructions are to some extent self-confirming, reinforcing the relative and differentiated positions of persons belonging to these categories. Based on this conceptual framework, Schneider and Ingram suggest how one can imagine that some categories of persons with disabilities risk being seen as less able to exercise active agency, and consequently that political elites will be less concerned about creating conditions to help members of these categories exercise Active Citizenship.

Schneider and Ingram (1993) argued that target populations can use and manipulate social constructions to their advantage, depending on their positive or negative experiences with governments. Yet, one can object to Fraser's and Schneider and Ingram's frameworks by pointing out that they tend to be somewhat static and do not account for the possibility of transformational social change. For instance, members of marginalised and apparently politically weak groups may turn out to be able to exercise active agency, both at the collective and individual level. Through social mobilisation and organising, persons with disabilities have managed to achieve considerable political impact both at the national and supranational level (see Chapters 10, 11, 13, Volume 1). At the individual level, we argue that persons with disabilities control resources of value and interest to politicians and public officials by contributing information about their own needs and experiences, collaborating about practical solutions and accepting responsibilities. By criticising the policy and questioning the intentions of politicians and help providers, they may deprive them of a positive self-esteem or even undermine the legitimacy of disability-related policy measures. When such resources are available, women and men with disabilities are more likely to be able to exercise active agency.

Factors related to policy design and institutions

As lived experience, citizenship needs to be examined in its social and economic context. Indeed, to understand how disability-related policies affect the Active Citizenship of persons with disabilities requires an examination of national variations. Volume 1 documented systematic and lasting differences in disability policy profiles – or disability policy systems – between European countries

(Halvorsen et al., 2017). Additionally, the countries have developed institutional differences in terms of how public disability policy intersects with processes in the market, family and organised civil society. The empirical chapters in Volume 2 use findings from the policy analyses in Volume 1 to interpret some of the country differences in the interview data. They also examine the intersection between the national disability policy systems and processes in the market, family and organised civil society.

Factors related to the take-up and use of disability-related cash benefits, services and regulations by disabled persons

By including a focus on the relationships between citizens (the horizontal dimension of citizenship, to use Pfister's (2011) term), we allow for analyses of how informal norms and values (i.e. the attribution of meaning and perceptions of persons with disabilities) influence their opportunities for participation in the local community, labour market, civil society and political activism. While social policy measures are likely to influence the opportunities for Active Citizenship (the vertical dimension of citizenship) (Pfister, 2011), how they are implemented matters. A large body of research on policy implementation gives us reason to expect that what happens to the disability-related policy measures in the end is constructed through a social, rather than entirely policy-driven, process. Hence, the empirical chapters in this book examine factors and mechanisms that structure the interaction between persons with disabilities, help providers and their significant others such as family members and peers. In some cases, the informal relations and the resources to which they provide or prevent access may turn out to be of equal or more importance than public policy. Thus, the empirical chapters in this book examine both the vertical and horizontal dimensions of Active Citizenship for persons with disabilities (Pfister, 2011), the interaction between citizens themselves and the interaction between citizens and public institutions.

References

Andersen, J. G. & Halvorsen, K. (2002). Changing labour markets, unemployment and unemployment policies in a citizenship perspective. In J. G. Andersen, J. Clasen, W. van Oorschot & K. Halvorsen (Eds), *Europe's new state of welfare. Unemployment, employment policies and citizenship* (pp. 1–19). Bristol: Policy Press.

Annetts, J., Law, A., McNeish, W. & Mooney, G. (2009). *Understanding social welfare movements*. Bristol: Policy Press.

Barnes, C. & Mercer, G. (2003). *Disability*. Cambridge: Polity.

Christensen, K., Guldvik, I. & Larsson, M. (2014). Active social citizenship: The case of disabled people's rights to personal assistance. *Scandinavian Journal of Disability Research*, *16*(1), 19–33.

Deacon, A. (2004). Review article: Different interpretations of agency within welfare debates. *Social Policy & Society*, *3*(4), 447–455.

Dwyer, P. (2004). *Understanding social citizenship*. Bristol: Policy Press.

European Union. (2000). Council Directive 2000/78/EC of 27 November 2000 establishing a general framework for equal treatment in employment and occupation. *Official Journal of the European Communities*, *L 303*, 16–22.

European Union. (2013). *Legal capacity of persons with intellectual disabilities and persons with mental health problems*. FRA – European Union Agency for Fundamental Rights. Luxembourg: Publications Office of the European Union.

European Union. (2016). Directive 2016/2102 of the European Parliament and of the Council of 26 October 2016 on the accessibility of the websites and mobile applications of public sector bodies. *Official Journal of the European Communities*, *L 327*, 1–15.

Fraser, N. (1995). From redistribution to recognition? Dilemmas of justice in a 'post-socialist' age. *New Left Review*, *212*, 68–93.

Fraser, N. (2000). Rethinking recognition: Overcoming displacement and reification in cultural politics. *New Left Review*, *3*, 107–120.

Fraser, N. (2008). *Scales of justice: Reimagining political space in a globalizing world*. New York: Columbia University Press.

Giele, J. Z. & Elder, G. H. (1998). *Methods of lifecourse research: Qualitative and quantitative approaches*. Thousand Oaks, CA: Sage.

Gilbert, T., Cochrane, A. & Greenwell, S. (2005). Citizenship: Locating people with learning disabilities. *International Journal of Social Welfare*, *14*, 287–296.

Gresov, C. & Drazin, R. (1997). Equifinality: Functional equivalence in organization design. *The Academy of Management Review*, *22*(2), 403–428.

Hagestad, G. O. & Neugarten, B. L. (1985). Age and the life course. In B. Binstock & E. Shanas (Eds), *Handbook of aging and the social sciences* (pp. 35–61). New York: Van Nostrand Reinhold.

Hall, E. (2011). Shopping for support: Personalisation and the new spaces and relations of commodified care for people with learning disabilities. *Social & Cultural Geography*, *12*(6), 589–603.

Halvorsen, R. (2010). Digital freedom for persons with disabilities: Are policies to enhance e-accessibility and e-inclusion becoming more similar in the Nordic countries and the US? *European Yearbook of Disability Law*, *2*, 77–102.

Halvorsen, R. & Hvinden, B. (2009). Nordic disability protection meeting supranational equal treatment policy – A boost for the human rights of persons with disabilities? In H. Sinding Aasen, R. Halvorsen & A. Barbosa da Silva (Eds), *Human rights, dignity and autonomy in health care and social services* (pp. 177–202). Antwerp: Intersentia.

Halvorsen, R. & Hvinden, B. (2011). *Andre lands modeller for å fremme sysselsetting blant personer med nedsatt funksjonsevne [Models for promoting labour market participation of persons with disabilities in Europe and USA]* (NOVA Report 14/11). Oslo: NOVA Norwegian Social Research.

Halvorsen, R. & Hvinden, B. (Eds). (2013). Active citizenship for persons with disabilities – Current knowledge and analytic framework: A working paper (DISCIT Deliverable 2.1, 31 August 2013). Retrieved 2 May 2017 from https://blogg.hioa.no/discit. Oslo: Oslo and Akershus University College.

Halvorsen, R., Hvinden, B., Bickenbach, J., Ferri, D. & Guillén Rodriguez, A. M. (Eds). (2017). *The changing disability policy system. Active citizenship and disability in Europe Volume 1*. London & New York: Routledge.

Hoggett, P. (2001). Agency, rationality and social policy. *Journal of Social Policy*, *30*(1), 37–56.

Hubbard, G. (2000). The usefulness of in-depth life history interviews for exploring the role of social structure and human agency in youth transitions. *Sociological Research Online*, *4*(4). Retrieved from www.socresonline.org.uk/4/4/hubbard.html.

Hvinden, B., Halvorsen, R., Bickenbach, J., Ferri, D. & Guillén Rodriguez, A. M. (2017). Introduction: Is public policy in Europe promoting the Active Citizenship of persons with disabilities? In R. Halvorsen, B. Hvinden, J. Bickenbach, D. Ferri & A. M. Guillén Rodriguez (Eds), *The changing disability policy system. Active citizenship and disability in Europe volume 1*. London: Routledge.

Hästbacka, E. & Nygård, M. (2013). Disability and citizenship. Politicians' views on disabled persons' citizenship in Finland. *Scandinavian Journal of Disability Research*, *15*(2), 125–142.

Jensen, P. H. & Pfau-Effinger, B. (2005). 'Active' citizenship: The new face of welfare. In J. Goul Andersen, A.-M. Guillemard, P. H. Jensen & B. Pfau-Effinger (Eds), *The changing face of welfare* (pp. 1–14). Bristol: Policy Press.

Johansson, H. & Hvinden, B. (2007). What do we mean by active citizenship? In B. Hvinden & H. Johansson (Eds), *Citizenship in Nordic welfare states: Dynamics of choice, duties and participation in a changing Europe* (pp. 32–49). London: Routledge.

Le Grand, J. (2003). *Motivation, agency, and public policy*. Oxford: Oxford University Press.

Leisering, L. (2003). Government and the life course. In J. T. Mortimer & M. J. Shanahan (Eds), *Handbook of the life course* (pp. 205–225). New York: Springer.

Leisering, L. & Walker, R. (Eds). (1998). *The dynamics of modern society: Poverty, policy and welfare*. Bristol: Policy Press.

Lindqvist, R. & Sépulchre, M. (2016). Active citizenship for persons with psychosocial disabilities in Sweden. *Alter – European Journal of Disabilities*, *10*(2), 124–136.

Lister, R. (2003). *Citizenship. Feminist perspectives*. Basingstoke, UK: Palgrave Macmillan.

Lister, R., Williams, F., Anttonen, A., Bussemaker, J., Gerhard, U., Heinen, J., … Gavanas, A. (2007). *Gendering citizenship in Western Europe: New challenges for citizenship research in a cross-national context*. Bristol: Policy Press.

Marshall, T. H. (1965). Citizenship and social class (first published 1950). In *Class, citizenship, and social development* (pp. 71–134). New York: Anchor Books.

Mayer, K. U. & Schoepflin, U. (1989). The state and the life course. *Annual Review of Sociology*, *15*, 187–209.

Merton, R. K. (1984). Socially expected durations: A case study of concept formation in sociology. In W. W. Powell & R. Robbins (Eds), *Conflict and consensus: In honor of Lewis A. Coser* (pp. 262–283). New York: Free Press.

Pfister, T. (2011). *The activation of citizenship in Europe*. Manchester: Manchester University Press.

Pound, C. (2011). Reciprocity, resources, and relationships: New discourses in healthcare, personal, and social relationships. *International Journal of Speech-Language Pathology*, *13*(3), 197–206.

Power, A., Lord, J. L. & de Franco, A. S. (Eds). (2013). *Active citizenship and disability: implementing the personalisation of support*. Cambridge: Cambridge University Press.

Priestley, M. (2003). *Disability: A life course approach*. Cambridge: Polity.

Priestley, M., Stickings, M., Loja, E., Grammenos, S., Lawson, A., Waddington, L., & Fridriksdottir, B. (2016). The political participation of disabled people in Europe: Rights, accessibility and activism. *Electoral Studies*, *42*, 1–9.

Roulstone, A. & Prideaux, S. (2012). *Understanding disability policy*. Bristol: Policy Press.

Schneider, H. M. & Ingram, A. L. (1993). Social construction of target populations: Implications for politics and policy. *The American Political Science Review*, *87*(2), 334–347.

Schneider, H. M. & Ingram, A. L. (2005). *Deserving and entitled: Social constructions and public policy*. Albany, NY: State University of New York Press.

Schneider, A. & Sidney, M. (2009). What is next for policy design and social construction theory? *The Policy Studies Journal*, *37*(1), 103–119.

Shah, S. & Priestley, M. (2011). Disability and social change: Private lives and public policies. Bristol: Policy Press.

Thorsen, K. & Jeppsson Grassman, E. (2012). *Livsløp med funksjonshemming [Life courses with disabilities]*. Oslo: Cappelen Damm Akademisk.

United Nations. (1975). *Declaration on the Rights of Disabled Persons* (resolution adopted by the General Assembly, 9 December 1975, A/RES/30/3447).

United Nations. (1993). *Standard Rules on the Equalization of Opportunities for Persons with Disabilities* (resolution adopted by the General Assembly, 20 December 1993 (resolution 48/96 annex).

United Nations. (2006). *Convention on the Rights of Persons with Disabilities* (resolution adopted by the General Assembly, 24 January 2007, A/RES/61/106).

Waddington, L. (2017). The potential for, and barriers to, the exercise of active EU citizenship by persons with disabilities. The right to free movement. In R. Halvorsen, B. Hvinden, J. Bickenbach, D. Ferri & A. M. Guillén Rodriguez (Eds), *The changing disability policy system. Active citizenship and disability in Europe, volume 1*. London: Routledge.

Waldschmidt, A. (2009). Disability policy of the European Union: The supranational level. *ALTER: European Journal of Disability Research*, *3*(1), 8–23.

Williams, F., Popay, J. & Oakley, A. (Eds). (1999). *Welfare research: A critical review*. London: UCL Press.

Yerkes, M. A., Peper, B. & Baxter, J. (2013). Welfare states and the life course. In B. Greve (Ed.), *The Routledge handbook of the welfare state* (pp. 105–114). Milton Park: Routledge.

2 Connecting lived lives and disability policy

Active Citizenship from a life-course perspective

Rune Halvorsen, Bjørn Hvinden, Mario Biggeri and Anne Waldschmidt

In this chapter, we discuss scholarly perspectives on life courses, especially the life courses of persons with disabilities. We are particularly interested in what analyses of life courses tell us about changes over time in the scope of exercising Active Citizenship in the nine countries studied. In principle, we are also looking for possible links between developments in public policy, especially disability-related ones, and the changing and diverse life-course experiences of persons with different kinds of disabilities. At the same time, we acknowledge the possibility of many intervening and mediating factors between the two, not least those related to family relations, gender, class and local community life or culture. Furthermore, it would be unreasonable to expect our interviewees to have precise knowledge about the content of and developments in public policy. Realistically, we mainly gain insights into their experiences, life worlds and practices.

Trajectories, transitions and turning points during the life course

This volume primarily focuses on the *practices* (active agency) of persons with disabilities that are relevant for achieving Active Citizenship (as defined in Chapter 1) – both routine (habitual) everyday actions and reflexive purposive actions (O'Reilly, 2012; Stones, 2005). In this context, we are interested in our interviewees' experiences of – and ways of coping with – living with disabilities or the impacts of chronic health issues. To increase our understanding of how and to what extent the actions taken by persons with disabilities or other actors (and their interactions) at one point (Time 1) influence the same persons' opportunities for participation and inclusion subsequently (Time 2), it is important for the data to capture *trajectories, transitions* and *turning points*.

First, *trajectories* point to the organisation of particular experiences over the life course. For George (2009), a trajectory typically refers to stability and change in an individual life. Similarly, a "trajectory can be conceptualized as 'a pathway or a line of development over the life span' through time and space" (Sampson & Laub, 1993, p. 8, as cited in Carlsson, 2011, p. 3). For Elder (1985, p. 31), a trajectory is a "pathway defined by the ageing process or by movement across the age structure". The temporality of a life and the patterns of life experiences (e.g., in employment) that emerge over time are important in this case. Green (2010, p. 25) argues that trajectories are typically long term, covering "trajectories of schooling, work and parenthood". In this respect, a life course incorporates multiple trajectories that "interweave […] such as work careers and family pathways" and are "subject to changing conditions and future options" (Elder, 1994, p. 5). However, trajectories are "marked by transitions" (Carlsson, 2011, p. 3).

Second, *transitions* are "embedded in trajectories and evolve over shorter time spans. […] Some transitions are age-graded and some are not" (Sampson & Laub, 1993, p. 8). Trajectories are subject "to short-term transitions ranging from leaving school to retirement" (Elder, 1994, p. 5). These transitions comprise a larger trajectory, which evolves over the course of a life. Distinct events often mark transitions – for instance, moving from school to work or from one job to another – but do not necessarily alter the course of a life. Thus, they do not carry the significance of turning points. Transitions "refer to changes in status and role which are generally known about and prepared for – such as from being single to being married, or from student to full-time worker" (Green, 2010, p. 25). These lead to changes in the organisation "of the daily functions of life" (Russell & Lee, 2006, p. 3). Such transitions do not necessarily carry expectations for radical changes in a life trajectory.

In contrast, *turning points* lead to more fundamental changes in a person's life. Scholars have described them as "biographical bifurcation" (Supeno & Bourdon, 2013), "critical" (Holland & Thomson, 2009) or "fateful moments" (Merrill & West, 2009). A turning point signifies "a change in the direction of the life course, with respect to a previously established trajectory, that has the long-term impact of altering the probability of life destinations" (Gotlib & Wheaton, 1997, p. 5). It reflects "an alteration or deflection in a long-term pathway or trajectory that was initiated at an earlier point in time" (Sampson & Laub, 2005, p. 16).

In sum, these three concepts mean that we have to be attentive to both continuity and the more substantial changes in the life course of persons with disabilities. We want to find out about the circumstances in which the participants have lived and how they have responded accordingly. At all times, therefore, we want to know about the contexts of their lives, the opportunities and the barriers they have come across, the decisions they have made in those contexts and the significant interactions they have had with others.

A life-course perspective on citizenship and disability

A life-course perspective has allowed us to identify barriers to and facilitators of Active Citizenship as they evolve over the life course. The notion of the life course draws attention to the limited value of chronological age per se as a sociological explanation. Rather, the life-course perspective offers a framework for examining the following aspects:

- the specific expectations, rights and obligations to participate in different life-course stages;
- the kinds of mechanisms and social processes that shape the experiences of persons with disabilities in these life-course stages; and
- how persons with disabilities cope with the dominant expectations about participation over their life course.

Generally, a person's life course tends to be constructed on the basis of dominant expectations about the "normal" timing of life events, and such expectations define the abnormal timing of events as (too) "early" or "late" in relation to the social timetable for such events (Hagestad & Neugarten, 1985, p. 50). In DISCIT, we have examined how persons with disabilities cope with the dominant expectations about participation in society and how this has influenced the unfolding of an individual life experience over time.

Research into life-course issues intersects with disability issues in important ways. Persons with disabilities may experience that their timing of events is considered inappropriate and not compliant with dominant expectations, that they are moving out of their parents' houses "too late," land paid jobs "too late" or become dependent on healthcare services "too early," according to dominant expectations (Priestley, 2003, pp. 26–27; Thorsen & Jeppsson, 2012).

Priestley (2000, 2003, p. 118) has highlighted parallels between the experiences of members of marginalised life-course groups, such as senior citizens and persons with disabilities, emphasising the ways that modern welfare systems have constructed and marginalised these groups in Western industrialised societies. More recently, Shah and Priestley (2011, p. 2) have examined the "relationship between changes in public policies and people's private lives". They argue that "public policies and institutions have a powerful influence in shaping life choices and chances" (p. 2). Using the broad historical changes in disability policies as the background, they explore the variety of lived experiences among persons with disabilities who grew up in England in the 1940s, the 1960s and the 1980s.

Based on 70 life-course interviews with persons with disabilities born in the 1930s, the 1950s and the 1970s, Sandvin (2003) analyses how social change and the evolution of the welfare state have influenced life conditions and opportunities for participation in Norwegian society. Reporting on not only the diversity but also the commonality among people with disabilities in terms of how they have coped with barriers to participation in society, he argues that the self-identity and the collective identity of persons with disabilities have changed from one generation to another.

Irwin (2001, p. 19) contends that citizenship is an important yet under-theorised life-course dimension. The life course can be described as an age-structured process that reveals differential access to citizenship rights and to meaningful participation of children and young persons, adults and senior citizens. Different age groups are attributed "different rights, duties, status, roles, privileges, disenfranchisements" (Foner, 1988, p. 176). *Childhood* has commonly been regarded as the phase of socialisation and learning, as well as dependency. *Youth* has been characterised as the transition to adulthood and the stage of becoming independent. As young people gain rights and assume obligations at different ages in various areas of their lives, they will in certain respects be considered semi-citizens and semi-dependants. For *adults*, financial independence, paid employment, establishing a separate household and parenthood are fundamental to social identity and prestige. Men and women who are not engaged in such activities tend to be marginalised in a variety of ways. *Senior citizens* will sooner or later depend on assistance in cash and in kind (e.g., old-age pension to ensure income after retirement, healthcare and social care services). In their capacity as welfare beneficiaries, older people are to a larger extent dependent on biased social exchange relations. A large body of literature has demonstrated how societal expectations are gendered and thus differ between men and women in the four life stages.

By adopting a life-course approach, we are able to examine social inequalities across the life span, not only within a particular age group (Priestley, 2003, p. 22). In present-day Europe, young people and seniors are usually more dependent on help from others. However, a common expectation has been that, over their life course, people will contribute as much as they receive from others. According to Priestley (2003, p. 4), "disability carries a different significance for people of different ages and stages of life". Similarly, as persons with disabilities age, their opportunities to exercise citizenship are likely to change. In this respect, the literature has demonstrated a large diversity of life courses among persons with different types of disabilities (Buchner et al., 2015; Johnson & Traustadottir, 2005; Priestley, 2003). Nonetheless, earlier research has provided limited and fragmented insights into how persons with disabilities cope with the dominant expectations to reciprocate over the life course and to adjust to the expected timing of life events.

Focus on generative processes enabling and disabling Active Citizenship

When we took on the task of analysing the conditions for the Active Citizenship of persons with disabilities, we could have chosen a different explanatory framework. For instance, structural or materialist accounts of disability locate "past experiences of disability within the political, social and cultural organization of society" (Borsay, 2004, p. 12). Prominent academics in disability studies have held the view that the emergence of capitalism – the demand for productivity and the drive for profit in a capitalist society – further excluded and disenfranchised people with disabilities from society (Barnes, 1997; Oliver, 1990).

While materialist accounts may have provided insights about the *longue durée* in the history of disability, more finely tuned explanations are needed to have a better grasp of the complexity of social relations that influence the opportunities for Active Citizenship on the part of persons with disabilities. Structural explanations of the resources and the position of persons with disabilities have provided insights into how the productivity system may influence the opportunities for participation (Thomas, 2007, p. 59). Nonetheless, increased sensitivity to the interaction *between* agency and structure is necessary to build realistic models of how opportunity gaps between people with and without disabilities are produced, reproduced and transformed (Thomas, 2007, p. 181).

We aim to move beyond descriptive accounts of the experiences of persons with disabilities to explanations of how and under which conditions Active Citizenship is likely to emerge. It does not mean that we are aiming at uncovering universal laws that claim to operate similarly in all situations or under all conditions. Our ambition is more modest – to identify and build models of the processes (mechanisms) through which Active Citizenship is generated (see Merton, 1968). According to Hernes (1998, p. 95), "a social mechanism is a device for *combining* actors with a given set of characteristics (casting) with a particular social structure (staging) in order to infer what outcomes will result (plotting)" (our emphasis). While we focus on generative processes of this kind, we are not exclusively interested in disabling processes (Thomas, 2007) but equally in *enabling* processes that facilitate the opportunities for exercising Active Citizenship.

Connecting conditions, practices and outcomes – a process-oriented perspective on life courses

Based on the findings in DISCIT, in this volume, we examine the links between the *conditions* for exercising Active Citizenship, the *practices* of persons with disabilities and the *outcomes* achieved, as well as how such links develop over time. In doing so, we are wrestling with sociology's enduring challenge of capturing the dynamic agency/structure linkages in a convincing way. In DISCIT, we have explored whether the structuration theory (O'Reilly, 2012; Stones, 2005) may provide a fruitful perspective, especially when used critically and taking into account the body of criticism directed against it (Archer, 1995; Elder-Vass, 2010; Mouzelis, 1995; Sewell, 1992). Combining several threads in the structuration theory, we have sought to establish a set of useful concepts that can be applied in the empirical analysis of the processes affecting the opportunities for exercising Active Citizenship. Our proposed framework identifies broad social processes that are involved in (re-)producing, shaping and reshaping the conditions for exercising Active Citizenship.

The structuration theory is closely associated with Anthony Giddens' work, going back to the early 1970s and later developed in several publications, notably in his book *The Constitution of Society* (1984). The structuration theory presents a meta-theory and a social ontology about how we can understand the social world and its elements, rather than clear propositions about how this social world works (Giddens, 1984, pp. xvii, xx–xxi, xxx). Giddens highlights the role of social practices in the linking of agency and structures, perceiving social practices as both producing and being produced by structures (pp. 5, 29–30). However, Giddens rejects the idea that structures exist independently of social actors. Instead, he argues in favour of regarding structures as *rules* (norms and interpretive schemes) and *resources* (p. 17), which actors produce and reproduce through their semi-reflexive and habitual practices. Giddens captures this idea in his conception of the "duality of structure": structure is conceptualised as both the medium and the outcome of social practices (pp. 25–28). This conception of structure, as well as other features of the structuration theory, has meant that many people have viewed the theory as overly abstract, open-ended and indeterminate, making it difficult to adopt it as a source of guidance and a framework for empirical research (McLennan, 1984, as cited in Stones, 2005, p. 76; see also Sewell, 1992; Stones, 2005, pp. 13, 34–40).

Stones (2005) has codified a theoretical framework informed by Giddens' theory but has also de facto reinterpreted the conceptualisation of social structures and the intersection between agents and structures to make the framework useful for designing empirical investigations and analysing empirical materials. According to Stones, the conceptualisation of the "duality of structure" is the key to understanding how the structuration theory models social processes, practices and relations:

> Giddens argued that structures enter into the constitution of the agent, and from here into the practices that this agent produces. Structure is thus a significant *medium* of the practices of agents. There is a complex and mediated connection between what is out-there in the social world and what is in-here in the phenomenology of the mind and body of the agent. Structure is also, however, the outcome of these practices of agents.
>
> (2005, p. 5)

Building on the criticism of Giddens' early version of the structuration theory, Stones (2005, p. 9) introduces a model of a "quadripartite cycle of structuration [...] in order to elaborate upon and clarify the variety and nature of the elements involved in the 'duality of structure' ". This cycle of structuration has the following four elements (Stones, 2005, pp. 84–94):

1. *External structures* as the conditions for actions include both constraints on and opportunities for action. The agent experiences external structures directly in his or her local context or indirectly and mediated even if the agent does not acknowledge them as conditions for action.
2. *Internal structures* within the agent include his or her more lasting dispositions and world views, as well as his or her more situated and time-dependent interpretation, learning, ways of thinking and responding. Internal structures comprise both general-dispositional media used by the same agent across different situations (reminiscent of Bourdieu's (1977) conceptualisation of habitus) and an agent's conjuncturally specific knowledge of particular settings and contexts.
3. *Active agency* encompasses a range of aspects involved when an agent draws on internal structures to produce practical action. Active agency has

three elements – habitual or routine action, practical considerations and responses vis-à-vis events in the broader or immediate contexts, and projective action by imagining alternatives to the current situation, as well as creating and pursuing goals.

4 *Outcomes* can be the specific events taking place in a person's life. At the same time, such events can be conceptualised as part and parcel of the new or elaborated external and internal structures. In other words, the effects or consequences can be both external and internal, affecting the objective social conditions, as well as the subjectivity of the agent. Outcomes can take the form of the reproduction or the transformation of social life. Social change may manifest itself in reshaping or shaping (new) external and internal structures, that is, conditions for action. "The impact on internal structure can be thought of as part of the overall effect of external structure on agents" (Stones, 2005, p. 85). For example, this can come about through processes of primary and secondary socialisation, learning processes, adjustments and changes in what the agents believe is possible and their opportunities for participation.

This approach builds on two basic assumptions. First, structure necessarily predates the actions that reproduce or transform it; second, outcomes (i.e., structural elaborations) necessarily post-date those actions. At Time 1, the initial structural conditions (established rules and allocation of resources) are the consequence of prior interactions. This situation conditions the interactions among agents and their opportunities to change society at Time 2. In this conception of external structures, their "existence is autonomous from the agent-in-focus, which face that agent at time 1" (Stones, 2005, p. 109). External structures necessarily predate the internal structures of individual agents. While internal structures condition and enable the social practices of the agents, the latter produce the outcomes. In the next round or cycle of structuration, the outcomes constitute the new external and internal structures (Stones, 2005, pp. 85–86, 90, 110–111).

At this point, Stones' model incorporates a key argument in Archer's (1982, 1995, pp. 93ff.) criticism of Giddens for conflating agency and structure, with a bias towards agency. To be able to keep the structural and the agential effects analytically apart, a researcher needs data on how social conditions and events unfold over time. To avoid giving priority to either structure or agency, a researcher may want to examine "the interplay between them over time, and that without the proper incorporation of time the problem of structure and agency can never be satisfactorily resolved" (Archer, 1995, p. 65).

O'Reilly (2012, p. 149) summarises Stones' conceptualisation of structuration in a visual representation that brings out the dynamic linkages between the structures, on one hand, and the practices and active agency, on the other. Here, we have adjusted O'Reilly's visual representation to our research objective (see Figure 2.1).

In the context of DISCIT, the Structuration Approach allows us to examine different "degrees of freedom and restraint" (Craib, 1992, p. 151, as cited in

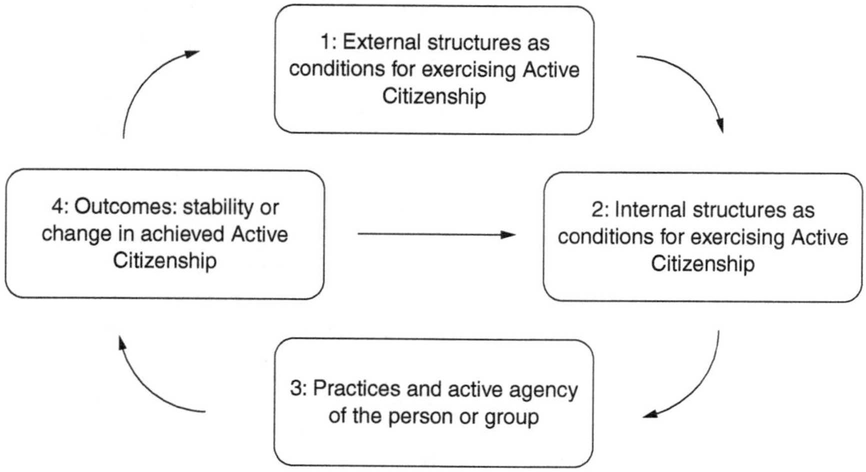

Figure 2.1 A simplified model of the dynamic relationships among structural conditions, agency and possible change, framed in terms of the Structuration Approach.

Source: adapted from O'Reilly, 2012, p. 149; see also Stones, 2005, p. 85.

Stones, 2005, p. 110) on the part of persons with disabilities. In this regard, the following aspects have evolved over the life course: opportunities for freedom of choice and influence, coping and resistance strategies among persons with disabilities, the extent to which persons with disabilities are limited or constrained by external social conditions or pressures, and the extent to which social structures impinge on the opportunities to live the life they have reasons to cherish and to realise their aspirations (Stones, 2005, pp. 77, 109–111). As suggested earlier, the life-course approach has allowed us to collect data on the interviewees' knowledge, aspirations and self-perceptions, along with their experiences of enabling and disabling social structures over the life course – as presented in retrospect by the interviewees. O'Reilly (2012, p. 5) argues that the individuals we interview and collect data from

> are usually unaware of the boundary between the circumstances that constrain their action, their knowledge of this [...] and their actions that take that knowledge into account, but that does not mean that a sociological researcher also needs to elide these movements: conditions are pre-dated, outcomes are post-dated.

Including a time perspective – how the Active Citizenship of persons with disabilities develops over the life course – enables us to keep structural and agential effects analytically apart.

We may state this view even more strongly; to qualify as structuration accounts, the interpretation of the data should not stop with the phenomenology of the subjective views and self-presentations of the interviewees (Stones, 2005, p. 81). The researcher should also aim to contextualise the interview data in view of the social position, the social network of the relevant others and other resources available to the interviewee. In the present volume, we identify trajectories, transformations and turning points and – when possible – relate the interview data to other information we have about local, national, regional and international policies of relevance to explain the lived experiences of the interviewees.

At the individual level, we have sought to examine how the interviewees' perceptions, values and aspirations for themselves were influenced by other people's reactions, support and criticism. We have also investigated how their own action choices (at Time 1) opened up new windows of opportunity for participation and closed down other alternative life choices (at Time 2), as well as how the opportunities for exercising Active Citizenship were influenced by external and internal structures.

The life-course data has allowed us to focus on "relations between specific events and agency, and relations between events themselves" (Stones, 2005, p. 82). The life-course interviews have provided data on trajectories, transformations and turning points over a period of 20–65 years, depending on the ages of the interviewees. To some extent, the data from three age cohorts (born around 1950, 1970 and 1990) has allowed us to examine how changes in external conditions have influenced the internal structures and the social practices of persons with disabilities in Europe between 1950 and 2014. The time perspective inherent in the life-course method has enabled us to identify specific mechanisms and processes "which can produce durable structures, regular patterns of interaction and developmental tendencies" (Parker, 2000, p. 107, as cited in Stones, 2005, p. 82) in the relationship between persons with disabilities and society at large.

Operationalisation of the structuration framework in DISCIT

The model of agency–structure dynamics reviewed here is at a relatively high level of abstraction and generality. The models outlined by Stones (2005) and O'Reilly (2012) primarily represent ways of thinking about such agency–structure dynamics. They do not spell out how we can expect the linkages between agency and structure to develop over time and the exact mechanisms and processes through which the linkages are likely to emerge, reproduce or change. For this purpose, we need more detailed and empirical examinations of the intermediary mechanisms. Taking as our point of departure the "cycle of structuration" and adapting it for our purpose, we suggest that the following elements are important to operationalise and use the framework in the data analysis:

External structures enabling or constraining persons with disabilities in achieving Active Citizenship

In Chapter 1, we outlined the main societal changes that have influenced the opportunities, rights and duties to exercise Active Citizenship in Europe. From policy analyses, available statistics and existing research, we have learned a great deal about the broader policy context for the lived experiences of individuals with disabilities.

At international and regional levels, we have observed several policy transformations of relevance for the lives of persons with disabilities, such as the emerging international human rights regime, in which the United Nations Convention on the Rights of Persons with Disabilities (UN, 2006) is now a key element. At national and local levels, we find country-specific disability policy measures that structure the opportunities for exercising Active Citizenship. Such measures include income maintenance systems, social service systems and regulatory systems that may facilitate or hamper the opportunities for security, autonomy and influence on the part of persons with disabilities (e.g., by providing more or less accessible built, transport and informational environments). We also find differences in the prevalence of discrimination, stereotypes and stigmatisation, as well as in the societal recognition and representation of persons with disabilities.

We follow O'Reilly's (2012, p. 24) work by conceiving these structural elements as "upper structural layers". When relevant, we situate the lived experiences of the interviewees in these broader contexts. In the life-course interviews, we asked the interviewees about their everyday life experiences, perceptions and practices as these had evolved over time, not their opinions about the disability policy as such. Nevertheless, some interviewees were explicit about their views on the disability policies and reforms in their respective countries of residence and related their personal experiences to the disability policies. This was the case with several interviewees who were active in politics and in organisations of people with disabilities. In most cases, however, this kind of contextualisation resulted from the researcher's interpretation of each interviewee's account. In this sense, references to the large-scale social forces that structure people's everyday lives have required a macro or a bird's-eye perspective on the experiences reported in the interviews. To achieve this, the authors of the empirical chapters of this volume have aimed at moving between investigating the phenomenology of the research subjects and contextualising the individual statements in their broader structural settings.

In the life-course interviews, our priority was to collect data about people's accounts of the main events and changes in their lives. This information included participation in education and training, employment, living arrangements, social activities, organisational and political activities, the use of technology, their experiences with claiming and receiving social services in cash and in kind, their financial situation, self-identity and views on disability, as well as biographical background data (including marital status and number of children).

To some extent, the data collection has allowed us to identify micro- and meso-level structures of direct and immediate relevance to the interviewees, such as stories about legislation and administrative rules, norms and values, representations of disability, housing arrangements, transport systems, the education system, the programmes and the organisation of the delivery of social services and the network of actors they identified as important and to whom they related (Stones, 2005, p. 83). Following O'Reilly's (2012, p. 24) study, we may conceptualise these features as "proximate structural layers", that is, factors of direct importance for "what is and is not (more or less) possible".

Internal structures enabling or constraining persons with disabilities in achieving Active Citizenship

Regarding the actors' enduring internal structures, we have collected data about their lengths of experience and ways of coping with restrictions in capacity or activity or with health issues, their habits, established ways of seeing and doing, perceptions and judgements of themselves and others. This information has included data on how the interviewees related to other persons with disabilities and whether they regarded themselves as disabled. As for temporary internal structures, we have collected data about the actors' reactions to existing patterns of norms, discourses and power relations and their critical awareness of the impacts of external and internal structures and of the possibility of change.

Social practices (active agency) of relevance for persons with disabilities in achieving Active Citizenship

Active agency takes place in reaction to specific circumstances but is always coloured by previous events and experiences. In the life-course interviews, we collected stories about events that involved direct interactions with other people and the relationships that the interviewees had developed with other people in their immediate proximity – including family members, fellow students and colleagues, staff in public agencies, friends and foes. In such cases, the interviewees often recounted how the interaction had evolved and what the outcome had been (e.g., how they dealt with that teacher, employer or social service office). Such interactions with others included both routine (habitual) and reflexive everyday actions or social engagement.

We invited the interviewees to describe both their practices and the links between events (what happened, when and how). By combining descriptive and evaluative questions, we collected data about their views on important life events: experiences of recognition and misrecognition, pride and self-blame, coping, resistance and negotiation strategies, and their possible visions of an alternative future.

The interview data has allowed us to examine how social practices unfolded on the ground in the so-called "communities of practice" (O'Reilly, 2012, pp. 9, 30). The communities of practice are the specific interrelationships of individuals who engage in social life and in negotiating or renegotiating social meaning. The active agency of persons with disabilities takes place in specific social spaces with other actors, such as family members, colleagues, health and social service providers, political parties or any other networks, organisations and groups they interact with. These other actors or agents – we use these terms interchangeably (see Giddens, 1984, p. xxii) – provide the contexts in which persons with disabilities are enabled or constrained in their efforts to negotiate opportunities for meaningful and equal participation in society. In this respect, communities of practice constitute "conjuncturally specific" external structures (O'Reilly, 2012, p. 31), constraining as well as enabling active agency.

Outcomes of relevance for persons with disabilities in achieving Active Citizenship

The life-course interviews sought to map whether key conditions (facilitators and barriers) for persons with disabilities in exercising Active Citizenship had changed during the life courses of the interviewees. Specifically, we collected data about the experiences of persons with disabilities, related to the following three dimensions of Active Citizenship (see Chapter 1, this volume):

- exercising rights and duties – the experience of reciprocity and complementarity of the individual's and the community's responsibilities;
- exercising freedom of choice – the experience of taking responsibility for one's own future and risk protection; and
- exercising co-determination – the experience of individually or collectively participating in self-organised, voluntary and political activities and in organised civil society.

The interviews have provided rich data on individual-level outcomes (e.g., improvements or deteriorations related to experiences of Active Citizenship). To some extent, the interviews have also provided data about group-level or collective outcomes, particularly from the interviewees who were active in organisations of people with disabilities. This information has included accounts of whether and how changes in public policies, available resources and cultural assumptions about disability have led to changes in the opportunities for full and effective participation in society on an equal basis with others, as perceived and experienced by the interviewees.

Conversion of resources into capabilities (and active agency) – a complementary perspective on generative processes

While the structuration theory provides a general framework for analysing how agency–structure dynamics influence the Active Citizenship of persons with disabilities, how you specifically model the linkages between external and internal structures and the agency of persons with disabilities remains an unanswered question. To enrich our conceptualisation of how agency–structure dynamics enable or prevent the Active Citizenship of persons with disabilities, we have found it helpful to refer to the Capability Approach's notion of "conversion processes". Broadly stated, the idea of conversion processes can sensitise our analysis to mechanisms and processes that can make it understandable why outcomes of relevance for achieving Active Citizenship do *not* take place in circumstances that seem promising for achieving change, as well as the opposite case – why change happens in circumstances that do *not* seem promising for achieving more Active Citizenship. The notion of conversion processes can be a tool for understanding the diversity among persons with disabilities and the conditions that need to be in place to enable them to exercise Active Citizenship.

In Amartya Sen's original version of the Capability Approach, the key issue is what ability a person possesses to act or reach states of being that the person has reason to value. Sen adopts *capability* as a term for "the *alternative combinations* of *things* a *person* is *able* to *do* or be – the *various 'functionings' he* or *she can achieve*" (1993, p. 30). He emphasises that the person's capability to achieve functionings constitutes his or her effective freedom – the freedom actually enjoyed by the person (Sen, 1992, pp. 40, 81). Sen has left open the question of exactly what functionings (combinations of doings and beings) one would generally expect a person to want to achieve. He argues that individuals are likely to give different weights to different functionings (perhaps beyond some basic capabilities, such as health and literacy) (Sen, 1992). Furthermore, Sen has repeatedly emphasised that, while the volume and nature of the various means (commodities, goods and resources, broadly defined) to which a person has access influence his or her capability set, these means do not determine this capability set in a uniform or definitive way.

Sen's Capability Approach sprang from a criticism of other scholars' reasoning about and evaluation of the relationship between the access to such means and the likely outcomes in terms of well-being, welfare, utility, and so on. In the 1979 Tanner lecture on "Equality of what?" Sen (1979) presented his original and then still tentative formulation of the Capability Approach, based on a critique of John Rawls' *A Theory of Justice* (1971), not least because Sen found that Rawls' theory of fairness dealt with persons with severe disabilities in an unacceptable way (Robeyns, 2009, p. 109).

Through several steps, Sen has developed the idea that the diverse characteristics of people and the particular circumstances in which they find themselves may affect their prospects of translating access to means into a capability set (and, as the next step, into achieved functionings). Since the experience of (or exposure to) such characteristics or circumstances will likely vary from person to person, their ability to convert means into a capability set (and then into achieved functionings) will also differ. For these reasons, Sen has argued that it is insufficient and misleading to evaluate the distribution of outcomes (however defined) solely based on the knowledge about a person's access to the means to attain such outcomes and, more generally, without taking into account human diversity and the heterogeneity of needs.

In more recent publications, Sen has identified five main sources of variations in the *conversion* of capability inputs into capability sets and functionings (1999, pp. 70–71, 2005, p. 154, 2009, pp. 254–255), as follows:

- *personal heterogeneities* (diversity in individual characteristics, physical and mental capacities, knowledge and skills);
- *distribution within the family* (intra-family distribution of paid and unpaid work, earnings and purchase power, gendered division of labour);
- *differences in relational positioning* (e.g., cultures, social norms and conventions negatively affecting the respect of others, as well as the person's dignity, self-respect and the "ability to appear in public without shame" (Adam Smith, as cited in Sen, 2000, p. 3);
- *varieties in social climate* (e.g., the quality of public services and community relations); and
- *environmental diversity* (e.g., climate, differential exposure and the risk of illnesses).

In Ingrid Robeyns' codification of the Capability Approach, she distinguishes among the following three main types of conversion factors, that is, the extent to which a person can transform a resource into a functioning (Robeyns, 2005, p. 99, 2010, p. 41, 2011, p. 7; see also Crockers & Robeyns, 2010, p. 68):

- *personal conversion factors* (e.g., metabolism, physical condition, sex, reading skills or intelligence);
- *social conversion factors* (e.g., redistributive and regulatory public policies, social norms, gendered division of labour, social practices that unfairly discriminate, societal hierarchies or power relations, including issues of the legitimacy and recognition of different impairments); and
- *environmental conversion factors* (e.g., physical or built environment where a person lives, climate, pollution, geographical location and topography).

An observation here could be that, not only are Sen's and Robeyns' examples for each type of conversion factor likely to interact with each other, but we also have good reason to expect interdependencies *among* the types. For instance, a person's reading skills will to a great extent depend on the existence of a system of universal education and the quality of the education the system provides. In this sense, the lists of types and examples are invitations to sociological theorisation about such interrelationships rather than a strict sorting of factors of relevance for conversion.

We incorporate these insights into our analytic framework for examining generative processes of significance for the opportunities to exercise Active Citizenship. We assume that broader societal, economic and political structures influence the nature of and interaction among what we (following Robeyns' classification) single out as conversion factors. We interpret conversion factors as consisting of a mix of external and internal structures, that is, patterns of some duration or stability, partly shaped by broader societal, economic and political structures and partly by an individual's background, circumstances and life course so far.

In the context of DISCIT, we have focused on factors and their interdependencies that facilitate and enable or constrain and prevent the conversion of resources into Active Citizenship. Perhaps most persons experience a combination of factors (conditions) constraining or enhancing their conversion processes. For instance, there may be not only discriminatory practices but also positive actions on the part of governments or employers (e.g., efforts to provide job openings for and accommodate the needs of persons with disabilities).

Conclusions

A main focus of this volume is what we call "social practices", to the extent that they include active agency directed towards exercising rights and duties, autonomy, choice and self-determination and/or influence through participation in decision-making or political processes. We also provide new knowledge about the consequences of the developments in external and internal structures for the social practices of persons with disabilities and their ability to use the opportunities created through changes and openings in external and internal structures. Likewise, we offer information about how new social practices – particularly the active agency of persons with disabilities – may in turn stimulate change (or contribute to it) in external and internal structures. This book identifies several cases of such dynamic relationships between structural conditions and the active agency of persons with disabilities and their organisations. We use the framework for the following aims:

- to identify the *difference* – even the *gap* – between *conditions* that ought to be favourable to Active Citizenship and the extent to which persons with disabilities are *actually becoming more active as citizens*; and
- to ask to what extent persons with disabilities believe they have *a real opportunity to* become more active citizens, whether they are *motivated* to do so or think that the prospect overall will likely mean *that their situation improves.*

Applying a generative–processual perspective, we aim to specify the relations between proximate structural features and other parts of the structuration cycle, the links between events and between events and agency that shape and reshape the opportunities for Active Citizenship (Stones, 2005, pp. 82–83). Admittedly, we have not been in a position to identify and examine all generative processes involved in the structuration of Active Citizenship. However, we hope that we have been able to identify key aspects in the structuration cycle (Stones, 2005, pp. 127, 142).

We have argued that a life-course perspective allows us to model the relationships among the practices of persons with disabilities, the external and the internal structures that influence the agency of these people and the achieved outcomes (more or less Active Citizenship). The process-oriented perspective inherent in the life-course data allows us to include time as an analytic dimension and thus examine the dynamics between external and internal structures, social practices and outcomes. Arguably, a process-oriented perspective may not only provide a better understanding of agency, but also allow us to distinguish analytically between the effects of agency and structure (and avoid the criticism about the agency/structure conflation that has been levelled against Giddens' early version of the structuration theory). At the same time, a process-oriented perspective may perhaps almost by definition provide a vaguer picture of social life – the relationship between social structures and their components – compared to studies that focus on the field situation at a given time.

One of the challenges is to recognise the connections between subjective considerations and objective structures while not conflating agency and structure. We have argued that pursuing a process-oriented perspective makes it possible to focus on the choices and considerations of persons with disabilities, their allies and adversaries, as well as to examine how the choices they make influence their future choice of actions. In this volume, we are interested not only in issues of subjectivity and identity but also in how the actors' former experiences, social positions and perceptions of their own opportunities for agency influence their actions and non-actions, as well as the relationships they develop with others in similar situations and with representatives of society at large.

This chapter has suggested several ways in which the analysis of life-course issues and processes can enhance our understanding of the nature and meaning of disability in contemporary European societies. Analyses of life-course data often involve a detailed inquiry into the dynamic interplay between structural conditions, on one hand, and people's individual considerations and action choices, on the other hand. The life histories of persons with disabilities not only provide information about the individual lives of the interviewees. Often, the life histories also teach us about how *other* people interact with and relate to persons with disabilities, about differences in opportunities for participation in society and cultural assumptions about disability and persons with disabilities.

References

Archer, M. S. (1982). Morphogenesis versus structuration: On combining structure and agency. *The British Journal of Sociology*, *33*(4), 455–483.

Archer, M. S. (1995). *Realist social theory: A morphogenetic approach*. Cambridge: Cambridge University Press.

Barnes, C. (1997). A legacy of oppression: A history of disability in western culture. In L. Barton & M. Oliver (Eds), *Disability studies: Past, present and future* (pp. 3–25). Leeds: The Disability Press.

Borsay, A. (2004). *Disability and social policy in Britain since 1750: A history of exclusion*. Basingstoke: Palgrave.

Bourdieu, P. (1977). *Outline of a theory of practice*. Cambridge: Cambridge University Press.

Buchner, T., Smyth, F., Biewer, G., Shevlin, M., Ferreira, M. A. V., Martin, M. T., … Káňová, Š. (2015). Paving the way through mainstream education: The interplay of families, school and disabled students. *Research Papers in Education, 30*(4), 411–426.

Carlsson, C. (2011). Using 'turning points' to understand processes of change in offending: Notes from a Swedish study on life courses and crime. *British Journal of Criminology, 52*, 1–16.

Crockers, D. A. & Robeyns, I. (2010). Capability and agency. In C. W. Morris (Ed.), *Amartya Sen* (pp. 60–90). Cambridge: Cambridge University Press.

Elder, G. H. (1985). Perspectives on the life course. In G. H. Elder (Ed.), *Life course dynamics: Trajectories and transitions, 1968–1980*. Ithaca, NY: Cornell University Press.

Elder, G. H. (1994). Time, human agency, and social change: Perspectives on the life course. *Social Psychology Quarterly, 57*, 4–15.

Elder-Vass, D. (2010). *The causal power of social structures. Emergence, structure and agency*. Cambridge: Cambridge University Press.

Foner, A. (1988). Age inequalities: Are they epiphenomena of the class system? In M. White Riley, B. J. Huber & B. B. Hess (Eds), *Social structures and human lives*. Newbury Park, CA: Sage.

George, L. K. (2009). Conceptualizing and measuring trajectories. In G. H. Elder (Ed.), *The craft of life course research*. New York: The Guildford Press.

Giddens, A. (1984). *The constitution of society*. Cambridge: Polity Press.

Gotlib, I. H. & Wheaton, B. (1997). *Stress and adversity over the life course: Trajectories and turning points*. Cambridge: Cambridge University Press.

Green, L. (2010). *Understanding the life course*. Cambridge: Polity Press.

Hagestad, G. & Neugarten, B. L. (1985). Age and the life course. In R. Binstock & E. Shanas (Eds), *Handbook of aging and the social sciences* (2nd ed.). New York: Van Nostrand Reinhold.

Hernes, G. (1998). Real virtuality. In P. Hedström & R. Swedberg (Eds), *Social mechanisms* (pp. 74–101). Cambridge: Cambridge University Press.

Holland, J. & Thomson, R. (2009). Gaining perspective on choice and fate: Revisiting critical moments. *European Societies, 11*(3), 451–469.

Irwin, S. (2001). Repositioning disability and the life course: A social claiming perspective. In M. Priestley (Ed.), *Disability and the life course* (pp. 15–25). Cambridge: Cambridge University Press.

Johnson, K. & Traustadottir, R. (2005). *Deinstitutionalization and people with intellectual disabilities: In and out of institutions*. London: Jessica Kingsley Publishers.

Merrill, B. & West, L. (2009). *Using biographical methods in social research*. London: Sage.

Merton, R. K. (1968). On sociological theories of the middle range. In R. Merton, *Social theory and social structure* (pp. 39–72). New York: The Free Press.

Mouzelis, N. (1995). *Sociological theory. What went wrong?* London: Routledge.

Oliver, M. (1990). *The politics of disablement*. London: Macmillan.

O'Reilly, K. (2012). *International migration and social theory*. Basingstoke: Palgrave Macmillan.

Priestley, M. (2000). Adults only: Disability, social policy and the life course. *Journal of Social Policy, 29*(3), 421–439.

Priestley, M. (2003). *Disability. A life course approach*. Cambridge: Polity.

Rawls, J. (1971). *A theory of justice*. Cambridge, MA: Harvard University Press.

Robeyns, I. (2005). The capability approach: A theoretical survey. *Journal of Human Development, 6*(1), 93–114.

Robeyns, I. (2009). Equality and justice. In A. Deneulin & L. Shahani (Eds), *An introduction to the human development and capability approach. Freedom and agency* (pp. 101–120). Ottawa: Earthscan & International Development Research Centre.

Robeyns, I. (2010). Capability approach. In J. Pell & I. van Staveren (Eds), *Handbook of economics and ethics* (pp. 39–46). Cheltenham: Edward Elgar Publishing.

Robeyns, I. (2011). Capability approach. In *Stanford encyclopaedia of philosophy.* Retrieved 5 April 2017 from http://standford.liberary.usyd.edu.eu/entries/capability-approach.

Russell, S. T. & Lee, F. (2006). Latina adolescent motherhood: A turning point? In J. Denner & B. L. Guzman (Eds), *Latina girls: Voices of adolescent strength in the U S* (pp. 39–46). New York: New York University Press.

Sampson, R. J. & Laub, J. H. (1993). *Crime in the making: Pathways and turning points through life.* Cambridge, MA: Harvard University Press.

Sampson, R. J. & Laub, J. H. (2005). A life-course view of the development of crime. *Annals of the American Academy of Political and Social Science, 602*, 12–45.

Sandvin, J. T. (2003). Loosening bonds and changing identities: Growing up with impairments in post-war Norway. *Disability Studies Quarterly, 23*(2), 5–19.

Sen, A. (1979). Equality of what? *The Tanner Lecture on Human Values, delivered at Stanford University, May 22, 1979.* The Tanner Lectures on Human Values, Lecture Library, University of Utah. Retrieved 11 September 2013 from http.//tannerlectures.utah.edu/_documents/a-to-z/s/sen80.pdf.

Sen, A. (1992). *Inequality reexamined.* Oxford: Clarendon Press.

Sen, A. (1993). Capability and well-being. In M. Nussbaum & A. Sen (Eds), *The quality of life* (pp. 30–53). Oxford: Clarendon Press.

Sen, A. (1999). *Development as freedom.* Oxford: Oxford University Press.

Sen, A. (2000). *Social exclusion: Concept, application, scrutiny.* Social Development Papers, No. 1, Office of Environment and Social Development, Asian Development Bank.

Sen, A. (2005). Human rights and capabilities. *Journal of Human Development, 68*(2), 151–166.

Sen, A. (2009). *The idea of justice.* London: Penguin.

Sewell, W. H., Jr. (1992). A theory of structure: Duality, agency, and transformation. *The American Journal of Sociology, 98*(1), 1–29.

Shah, S. & Priestley, M. (2011). *Disability and social change. Private lives and public policies.* Bristol: Policy Press.

Stones, R. (2005). *Structuration theory.* Basingstoke: Palgrave Macmillan.

Supeno, E. & Bourdon, S. (2013). Bifurcations, temporalités et contamination des sphères de vie. Parcours de jeunes adultes non diplômés et en situation de précarité au Québec. *Agora débats/jeunesses, 65*, 109–124.

Thomas, C. (2007). *Sociologies of disability and illness. Contested ideas in disability studies and medical sociology.* Houndmills Hants: Palgrave Macmillan.

Thorsen, K. & Jeppsson, E. G. (2012). *Livsløp med funksjonshemming.* Oslo: Cappelen Damm akademisk.

UN. (2006). *UN convention on the rights of persons with disabilities.* Resolution adopted by the General Assembly 13 December 2006. A/RES/61/106. New York: UN Documents. Retrieved 5 April 2017 from www.un-documents.net/a61r106.htm.

3 Life-course interviews on disability and Active Citizenship

Collecting and analysing big qualitative data

Rune Halvorsen, Kjetil Klette Bøhler and Jan Šiška

DISCIT's research design was developed in response to a call published in the European Commission's 7th Framework Programme under the general theme "Societal trends and lifestyles". The original call ("Understanding disabilities in evolving societies") reflected negotiations between actors with different interests and perspectives. Alluding to the UN Convention on the Rights of Persons with Disabilities (United Nations, 2006), the call text stressed the importance of examining how ongoing disability policy reforms affect opportunities for persons with disabilities to achieve "full and effective participation in society on an equal level with others". The call emphasised that "disability is an issue to be taken into account at every life-stage and for all age categories" (FP7-SSH-2012–2). This last sentence in the call text influenced the design of our data collection and methodology in the DISCIT project.

Given the attention paid to life-stages and age groups in the call text, life-course interviews with different age cohorts seemed to be an appropriate method for exploring the Active Citizenship of people with disabilities. In the literature, quite a few scholars have previously adopted life-course interviews as a method in disability policy research (Lillestø & Sandvin, 2012; Priestley, 2001, 2003; Sandvin, 2003; Shah & Priestley, 2011). Scholars have published results from life-course interviews amongst single-age cohorts, focussing on specific life-stages and impairment groups (e.g., Thorsen, 2000; Thorsen & Myrvang, 2008). Therefore, our method was not new in disability policy research. However, to our knowledge, no scholars had yet applied the method in cross-national and comparative research on the scale anticipated by DISCIT (see however Biewer et al., 2015; Buchner et al., 2015; Smyth et al., 2014).

The most common strategy in comparative social policy has been to rely on existing surveys and register data. For several reasons, this was not an option for DISCIT. Existing data on disability from Eurostat (the Labour Force Survey and EU-Statistics on Income and Living Conditions) has been limited – although progress is currently being made in this area. A national longitudinal register or national longitudinal survey data would have been useful but was, with a few exceptions, not available, and what was available was not easily comparable across countries (Tøssebro & Hvinden, 2017). Conducting a new longitudinal or cross-sectional survey would have required a substantial amount of resources.

Our time and financial resources required a more cost-effective strategy to collect new primary data.

This chapter reports our experience of collecting and analysing big qualitative data for cross-national and comparative purposes. First, we describe the selection of the sample. Second, we outline the recruitment strategies. Third, we describe the development and use of the interview guide. Fourth, we account for the data condensation process. Fifth, we identify ethical issues that arose in the project and explain how we dealt with them. Sixth, we then conclude by summarising the experience of collecting and analysing big qualitative data.

Selection of data sources

Our primary data source is a set of coordinated semi-structured life-course interviews with three birth cohorts of persons with disabilities (born around 1950, around 1970 and around 1990). We interviewed both males and females, and we gathered the same type of data in nine European countries (Sweden, Serbia, Switzerland, the United Kingdom (UK), Ireland, Italy, Germany, Norway and the Czech Republic). Table 3.1 summarises the composition of the data set.

During 2014, the team conducted 217 life-course interviews (25 in the Czech Republic, 24 in Germany, 24 in Ireland, 24 in Italy, 28 in Norway, 24 in Serbia, 24 in Sweden, 24 in Switzerland and 20 in the UK). In Norway, we received a positive response from more people than the 24 that we anticipated and we decided to interview all of them as they already had volunteered. The UK experienced greater difficulties in recruiting interviewees. The sample covers four broad categories of disability, two that have traditionally had high public awareness and interest-group support (mobility and visual) and two with less public recognition of their capabilities and contributions to society (psychosocial and intellectual). Due to limited resources, the team did not, for instance, include

Table 3.1 Life-course interviews with three cohorts of persons with disabilities

Disability/impairment	*Persons born around 1950*	*Persons born around 1970*	*Persons born around 1990*
Difficulties in seeing: blindness or limited eyesight	One female, one male in each country	One female, one male in each country	One female, one male in each country
Mild to moderate intellectual and developmental impairments	One female, one male in each country	One female, one male in each country	One female, one male in each country
Mild to moderate psychosocial difficulties	One female, one male in each country	One female, one male in each country	One female, one male in each country
Mobility difficulties: using a wheelchair, crutches or related devices	One female, one male in each country	One female, one male in each country	One female, one male in each country

persons with hearing difficulties in the sample. Increasing the sample would have made the task of collecting and analysing the data even more challenging. Also, hiring sign language interpreters was impossible within the budget available for the project.

When defining the disability categories, the important dimension was the extent to which people experienced disabling barriers to full and effective participation in society – not the medical diagnosis. Arguably, a narrower focus on specific diagnoses could have made the interviews more similar and easier to compare. However, even among persons with the same medical diagnosis, one is likely to find large variations in the severity of their impairments. Although we did not base our sampling on a specific diagnosis, all interviewees with an intellectual, visual or mobility impairment had a medical diagnosis, as did a majority of those with psychosocial disabilities (e.g., bipolar disorder, schizophrenia, depression or an eating disorder).

Because we primarily aimed to recruit interviewees through self-help groups, self-help activities and organisations of and for persons with disabilities, we largely relied on whether the person defined her- or himself as having a disability and/or was seen by others as having one. In relation to persons with mobility and visual disabilities, we recruited persons who used assistive technology (e.g., crutches, a wheel chair, Braille and/or text-to-voice software).

In comparison to other disability categories, the process of recruiting participants with "mild to moderate psychosocial disabilities" was more challenging and required more in-depth discussions amongst the research team. The category "mild to moderate psychosocial difficulties" covers a diverse set of individuals with various mental health-related issues (e.g., experiencing anxiety, depression, feelings of insufficiency, behavioural and personality issues and eating disorders). Even if we ideally wanted to focus on the same mental health-related issue across all countries, we had to remind ourselves that it was not the diagnosis per se but the restrictions and challenges that the person experienced in daily life that mattered for our research. Such restrictions and challenges, e.g., the risk of encountering prejudice or discrimination, do not follow directly from a single diagnosis.

From a medical model perspective, some persons are diagnosed based on the international psychiatric classification system. Yet, mental health issues also include forms of psychological distress that do not reach the threshold of a diagnosis (OECD, 2012, p. 19). For instance, the Swedish National Board of Health and Welfare has defined a person as having a psychosocial disability if he or she has fundamental difficulties in carrying out activities in important life areas and if these limitations have continued, or are expected to continue, over a longer period. Such difficulties must be a consequence of a psychiatric disturbance. The Swedish definition can be considered compatible with a relational model of disability (or a "gap model") (Shakespeare, 2006; Hvinden, 2012).

A pragmatic test to select persons with mild to moderate mental health issues was to ask what mental health issues were generally regarded as substantial in the country of concern. In cases where team members were in doubt, the coordinator encouraged them to consider which mental health-related issues were considered substantial in terms of being associated with difficulties of daily life in that country (e.g., regarding autonomy and freedom of movement, opportunities for independent living, entitlement to benefits, services and support, capacity to participate in working life) but not requiring long-term hospitalisation or institutionalisation.

This means that the sampling strategy adopted in DISCIT was not limited to specific medical diagnoses; instead, the selection criteria related to the experience of serious psychosocial difficulties in everyday life. Thus, "persons with psychosocial disabilities" include those who have long-term mental impairments which – in interaction with various social and cultural barriers – may hinder their full and effective participation in society on an equal basis with others. This term includes persons with very diverse psychosocial difficulties and mental health problems, including but not limited to depression, alcohol addiction, schizophrenia, bipolar disorder, an eating disorder, relational problems, intrusive thoughts, post-traumatic stress disorder, Asperger's syndrome and attention deficit hyperactivity disorder. Therefore, "persons with psychosocial disabilities" are not limited to those who fit the criteria of a medical diagnosis and can also include persons without a medical or psychiatric diagnosis (Lindqvist & Sépulchre, 2014; Lindqvist, Sépulchre & Thorén, 2014).

We limited our sample by excluding persons living in institutions at the time of the interview. Including this population group would have significantly increased variation in the data, would have made drawing comparisons more complicated and would have required more complex ethical reviews.

Given our focus on Active Citizenship it was more important to collect data from persons who had some experience of being active citizens. Because we wanted to identify favourable conditions for the Active Citizenship of persons with disabilities, we collected data on individual life trajectories from persons living in the community at the time of the data collection. Based on earlier research projects, we expected that we would collect data on many of the barriers the interviewees experienced in their efforts to participate as full and active members of society. However, there is no sharp division between the experiences of those with mild to moderate psychosocial difficulties and those with more severe and incapacitating problems. Even long-term, severe mental health issues may affect a person's life to a varying extent over time. Many of the interviewees had experienced difficulties that fluctuated or varied in severity. Several of them had stayed in psychiatric hospitals previously, either voluntarily or against their will.

We limited our sample to interviewees who had acquired a disability before the age of 20 and who had lived in the specified country for the majority of their lives. These criteria ensured that the interviewees had experienced the education system and the transition to the labour market as persons with disabilities in the same national contexts. It also meant that the interviewees had striking similarities because their experience of living with disabilities started early in life (in childhood or in youth) and had a long-term impact on their lives. A few interviewees turned out to have acquired their disabilities after the age of 20, but overall, we managed to collect rich data on the transition from education to employment. To examine the mechanisms and processes that promoted or hampered opportunities for labour market participation, the national teams recruited some persons who had achieved and sustained paid work over a longer period or who were currently participating in the ordinary labour market.

Recruitment strategies

We began recruiting interviewees through self-help groups, self-help activities and organisations of and for persons with disabilities. By recruiting interviewees through organisations of persons with disabilities, we ensured that the sample included persons who had been active in advocating for the rights and needs of persons with disabilities. Self-help activities included low-barrier meeting places, for instance for the psychiatric survivors movement, and social activities for and of persons with intellectual disabilities (sports activities, music or theatre groups). For persons with intellectual disabilities, such groups, activities and organisations sometimes also involved their parents or other relatives. Particularly for the two younger age cohorts (born around 1970 and 1990), a related strategy was to recruit through social media platforms established and operated by self-help organisations, networks and associations of and for persons with disabilities. The interviewees recruited through organisations of persons with disabilities or their social media platforms were not necessarily formal members of the organisations but also included individuals on their outskirts. A limitation of this approach was that some persons with disabilities find social media inaccessible or do not have the resources to benefit from it.

A second strategy was recruiting interviewees through our network, i.e., we adopted a snowball sampling strategy (Biernacki & Waldorf, 1981) by recruiting people we already knew or whom we met via others. To ensure that we covered all variations in the data matrix (Table 3.1), we sometimes asked key informants to help us recruit a person who fulfilled the desired criteria and whom they believed could be interesting to talk to.

In some cases, a last-resort strategy was to recruit interviewees through providers of services to people with disabilities. This turned out to be necessary, especially when recruiting interviewees with intellectual disabilities. One risk of this strategy was that the interviewee might feel he or she had to participate in the interview in order to continue receiving the service, which would, of course, not adhere to free and informed consent. When using this strategy, we were therefore careful to stress to potential participants that the service provider would not know whether they participated or not, that they were free to withdraw at any time and that the information they provided would not be shared with others in a non-anonymised format and would not affect their receipt of services in the future.

Overall, the country teams found that it was more difficult and time-consuming to recruit interviewees with psychosocial and intellectual disabilities, i.e., the two population groups with lower public recognition of their capabilities and contributions to society as a whole.

Designing and using the topic guide

The DISCIT project aimed to gather comparative data by using a common topic guide. However, at the same time, the team remained open to following up on individual accounts by the interviewees in order to achieve more elaborate responses and pursue issues that emerged in the interviews (e.g., Cohen, Manion & Morrison, 2007; Edwards & Holland, 2013; Kvale, 2006; Patton 2002).

When the consortium negotiated the content of the topic guide, the national teams wanted to ensure relevant data on the different topics we had committed ourselves to cover (organised in so-called "work packages"). The result was a quite detailed and complex interview guide. The topics included questions related to the experience of Active Citizenship under the following themes: (1) the life course in general, (2) education, (3) work, (4) living arrangements, (5) social participation, (6) participation in organisational and political activities, (7) use of technology, (8) self-identity and views on disability and (ix) concluding comments.

One reason the research teams wanted to include a number of more specific questions was to ensure that the interviewers in the nine countries covered more or less the same issues. In hindsight, we could perhaps have collected more narrative and in-depth data if we had simplified the topic guide and focussed on fewer main questions. In that case, however, we may have run the risk of more limited direct comparability between the interviews. Despite its breadth, there were limitations to how much could be anticipated and built into the topic guide. Conducting in-depth interviews is a craft that requires training in prompting – or following up on issues that emerge in the interviews and asking for more details. This skill requires, inter alia, that the interviewer has an understanding of the research objectives and analytic framework.

To this end, we organised a separate training session for the interviewers in Notwill, Switzerland, in April 2014. In the session, the interviewers tested parts of the interview guide on each other and discussed the DISCIT analytic framework. The final topic guide also included an introductory section that presented the project's key analytic concepts. The interviewers were encouraged to keep the key concepts and objectives in mind when conducting the interviews. Interviewers were thus encouraged to use the analytic framework to focus on the extent to which persons with disabilities experienced real opportunities to become active citizens, whether they were motivated to do so and whether they thought that becoming more active citizens would mean their situation would improve.

After the topic guide was finalised, the interviewers translated the questions into their respective national languages, either by improvising the exact wording during the interviews or by translating the topic guide before they carried out the interviews. In practice, the use of the guide varied. Not all team members had the same level of training in conducting in-depth interviews before the project, and the richness of the interviews varied considerably. This variation was reflected in the depth of accounts of different life events, trajectories, transitions and turning points. This partly resulted from some interviewees being more talkative than others. Also, some interviewers were more successful than others in establishing trust and a relaxed atmosphere. Some interviewers followed the guide literally and posed the questions in the way they had been formulated in writing. Others used the topic guide as a checklist to ensure that they had covered all the main topics. If questions did not seem relevant, some interviewers omitted them. Other interviewers felt they had to pose all the main questions. The length of the interviews ranged from 50 minutes to 3 hours. A few interviews were carried out over two sessions. Most of the interviews took place in the interviewees' homes. Some took place in an office of an organisation for persons with disabilities or at a university, especially those involving persons with psychosocial disabilities. For this population group, an office was a more "neutral" meeting place. This probably reflected the relatively larger vulnerability (more stigma) of this population group compared to many other groups of persons with disabilities.

Interviewing persons with intellectual disabilities

A specific challenge related to interviewing persons with intellectual disabilities, as their references to places, people and events were sometimes implicit. Both retrospection and abstraction were challenges for many within this group. To address this, when carrying out interviews at an interviewee's home, we sometimes pointed to pictures, memorabilia or furniture to illustrate our points or to ask for more information. Sometimes, we also asked the interviewee to bring photos from his or her life to the interview. In other cases, we tried to overcome these problems by asking relatives and social service staff for background information before we spoke with the interviewee. These strategies often improved the dialogue. Still, these challenges posed an ethical dilemma. On the one hand, we risked offending the interviewees if we were not able to ask relevant questions. On the other hand, we also risked insulting them if they perceived that we devalued their abilities to represent themselves.

Some team members had considerable experience of interviewing persons with intellectual disabilities. To avoid confusion, the teams generally tried to ensure the topic guide was written in plain language when translating it into the respective languages. We also developed general guidelines for the interviewers to facilitate dialogue, for instance by using examples that people know from their everyday lives, using the same word to describe the same thing throughout the interview and using layman's terms. The Irish team also developed an easy-to-read participant information leaflet with graphic illustrations and pictures.

Transcription and data condensation

When conducting the interviews, all team members used a digital voice recorder, provided that the interviewee agreed to this. While transcription of the recordings involved more work than only taking notes, it also allowed the interviewer to collect more detailed information and more precise (verbatim) quotes, as well as allowing for rechecking transcriptions or translations during the joint analysis with participating national teams.

Several of the country teams transcribed all their interviews into the national language. On average, it took six hours to transcribe one hour of a recorded interview. After the transcription was finished, the teams read it through several times to prepare an interview report, which portrayed an analytically focussed summary of the main features of the interview in the context of the research questions. However, as argued by Kvale (2007), it is important to stress that the transcriptions should not be considered objective descriptions of the real world, as several interpretive questions are linked to the processes of transcribing. The transcriptions prioritise the logic of the written word and do not always capture expression articulated orally (e.g., stress on certain words, repeating a word to emphasise its importance) or through body language (e.g., gestures). Still, we tried to incorporate these additional layers of meaning in the transcriptions through careful descriptions, e.g., by adding contextual information and early interpretations of the findings in brackets.

When conducting the interviews, some interviewers chose to use a timeline grid to systematise and chronologise life events (Parry, Thomson & Fowkes, 1999) (see Figure 3.1). They were able to use the grid to map and compare life events and to identify connections between different life events, e.g., changes in political participation and identification as "disabled". Other interviewers found it difficult to use the grid while they were interviewing people. Some found

Code: I__ __I - I__I I__ __I I__I

Country - Disability - Cohort - Gender

Year of birth: ______________

Timeline grid for persons born around <u>1950</u> (1945–1954)

Year	Education	Work (paid/unpaid)	Social, organisational and political participation	Living arrangement	Use of service	Use of technology	Health/ disability/ identity
1950							
1955							
1960							
1965							
1970							
1975							

Figure 3.1 DISCIT timeline grid for data condensation.

keeping track of the digital voice recorder, the topic guide and the grid to involve too much multitasking. In such cases, some interviewers completed the timeline grid after they had completed the interview.

To condense the interview data, the national teams filled in a report form (see Figure 3.2). Some did this after transcribing the interviews. Others filled in the reports directly from the audiotapes. The report form ensured that all researchers structured the findings from the interviews around the same topics. The interviewers completed one report for each individual interview, and each provided a detailed summary in English (5–15 pages).

The report form asked for key findings related to Active Citizenship (see Box 3.1). By using the sensitising concepts trajectories, transitions and turning points (see Chapter 2) the report form invited the researchers to summarise how opportunities for exercising Active Citizenship played out in each individual's life course. The report form also invited the researchers to provide an initial analysis of whether changes in the life course resulted from the interviewee's individual agency, external conditions (e.g., family, friends, organisations, new policies, etc.) or a mixture of both. In short, the report examined various facilitators and barriers that shaped the individual's access to Active Citizenship.

The strength of these interview reports was that they ensured the possibility of analysing all empirical data in the light of questions about Active Citizenship and also enabled various forms of comparison (see Box 3.1, Figure 3.2). A challenge was that the research teams interpreted the report guidelines differently. This resulted in descriptions that differed in length and depth. Some reports were only four to five pages long, provided little empirical information (e.g., quotes)

Code:
Country - Disability - Cohort - Gender

Report from DISCIT life course interview

Name of interviewer:	Date of interview:

Basic biographical data of interviewee			
Year of birth:	Disability/ impairment:	Employment status:	Other important information:

1. About the life situation and life course in general (Section 1)

Briefing note: About 0.5–1 page. Please summarise the main findings from the interview regarding main trajectories, transitions and turning points. What have been the big and important changes with lasting effects on the person's life? Changes caused by others or external factors? Changes through the person's choices and active agency? To what extent did gendered norms and expectations emerge as an issue in the interview?

Figure 3.2 DISCIT interview report form.

Box 3.1 Main topics in the DISCIT interview report

1. *The life situation and life course in general*: big and important changes with lasting effects on the person's life.
2. *Participation in education and training*: key features of the individual's participation in education, such as whether he or she had participated in mainstream or segregated education, the extent to which education had been completed and the individual's social relationship to his or her peers at school.
3. *Participation in employment*: findings relevant to the individual's participation in the ordinary and sheltered labour market. The section asked for information about work experience throughout the life course, duration of employment and relationships with colleagues at work.
4. *Living arrangements*: whether the individual had lived in institutions, residential care arrangements, segregated housing arrangements or had lived independently in the community, including whether the person had lived with his or her parents as an adult.
5. *Social participation*: data on social participation and activities such as involvement in sports, culture, the arts, leisure activities and travelling.
6. *Participation in organisational and political activities*: data on trajectories, transitions and turning points in relation to organisational and political activities, including participation in political parties, organisations of persons with disabilities and other non-governmental interest organisations.
7. *Use of technology*: interviewee's use of technology, and whether it was accessible, available, affordable and usable. The interviewers mapped how specific types of technologies, e.g., mobile phones, computers and assistive technology, enabled or limited the Active Citizenship of the interviewee.
8. *Experience with public services, private services and services provided by NGOs*: whether the services the person received were relevant to and supported the Active Citizenship of the interviewee.
9. *Self-identity and views on disability*: data on the individual's self-identity, especially whether the interviewee identified as a person with disabilities.
10. *Concluding comments – your summary of the interview*: any additional points of relevance raised by the interviewee and an assessment of the overall quality of the interview.

and consisted mostly of summaries. Others were up to 15 pages and included long quotes from the interviewees. This complicated the comparative analysis.

The reports represented the selections and interpretations of the interviewer. With the exception of the interviews by the Irish team, full transcripts in English were not available. This limited insights into how the data had been constructed (i.e., the flow of communication between the researcher and the interviewee) and into the interviewees' own accounts of their experiences.

In certain respects, the reports share similarities with secondary data (Temple, Edwards & Alexander, 2006). Team members largely relied on original material collected and presented by other researchers in the team. To allow cross-language comparisons, all interview summaries were written in English. With the exception of team members from England and Ireland, English was the second or third language of the researchers. This meant that language barriers represented a potential risk for misinterpretation and misrepresentation of the data (Santos, Black & Sandelowski, 2015). However, the national teams were able to contact each other to ask for clarification, as well as assistance in finding verbatim quotes.

Some ethical issues

Participation in the interviews was voluntary. All the interviewees received a detailed information letter about the DISCIT research project and formally agreed to participate by signing a consent form before starting the interview. All interviews also complied with the guidelines of the Norwegian Data Protection Official for Research, and the interviewees had the option to withdraw from the study at any point without further explanation. Sensitive information regarding location, colleagues, family relations and employers, inter alia, was removed from the transcriptions and interview reports to avoid indirect identification. When required by national legislation, the DISCIT researchers also obtained approval from their country's board of ethics before starting the recruitment process. All audio files were erased after the interviews were transcribed and anonymised.

Only the team members directly involved in the data collection had access to the tape recordings, consent forms and participant contact details. The recordings, consent forms, contact details and transcripts were stored separately and in locked file cabinets. All contact details were deleted at the end of the DISCIT project. Unless national legislation required otherwise, the team members sought permission from the relevant research ethics committees to store anonymised transcripts and the summary reports for later reanalysis.

Some interview subjects were in vulnerable positions and life situations. Interviews with these subjects required particular care and sensitivity to ensure that taking part in the research did not create an additional burden or worsen a bad situation for the person (add insult to injury). For some interviewees, the interview initiated a process of self-reflection. In one case, we received several emails from a person after the interview. This person had very few other people to ask for help and assistance, and among the team members we discussed how we could best provide advice.

However, it is important to note that the justification for approaching persons in such vulnerable situations was to learn about the accessibility, adequacy, quality and practical value of the disability policy system (cash benefits, social services and social regulation) in their respective country (see Chapter 2 in the accompanying Volume 1), as perceived by the persons whom the disability policy system is meant to support and protect. Although the focus of DISCIT was not the problems or difficulties that persons with disabilities had experienced per se, a majority of the persons we interviewed described problems and difficulties in exercising Active Citizenship.

Additionally, we found that we had to be sensitive to participants' self-conception and identity. While DISCIT by definition undertook research on "disability", not all interviewees regarded themselves as "disabled" or having a "disability", or they expressed ambivalence about the label. Researchers usually asked direct questions about self-identity towards the end of the interview when we had a better understanding of the person's views and experiences. When recruiting interviewees with psychosocial disabilities, we emphasised that we were aware that not everybody considered themselves to be "disabled" (many preferred to say they had a temporary mental health problem).

Concluding comments

The DISCIT research team set itself the objectives of exploring a new analytic framework to study the opportunities for exercising Active Citizenship among persons with disabilities. Furthermore, the team adopted a data collection strategy that had not been previously tested on such a large scale. While only a few of the researchers had worked together before, the DISCIT project has shown that working together to prepare joint publications is a productive way to focus and integrate the efforts of many researchers based at different institutions within a given timeframe.

Cross-language collaboration meant that translations occurred prior to data collection (in the translation of the topic guide), during interviews to ensure conversation flow (improvisation and adjustment of the exact wording), during data condensation (writing up of the reports) and during verification of data interpretations amongst the national teams. Altogether, the cross-language and cross-national research design of the DISCIT project required active coordination between the national teams to ensure coherence in data collection and analysis, and to avoid misinterpretations of the data.

DISCIT collected and analysed 217 semi-structured interviews. On the one hand, the relatively large and diverse dataset contributed to higher data validity than a smaller and narrower dataset would have. On the other hand, a smaller and more narrowly defined dataset, and a smaller team, would have allowed more time to train the interviewers and to transcribe and analyse each individual interview. Given its budget and time constraints, the DISCIT consortium has largely relied on summary reports of the interviews from the nine national research teams.

When interpreting the data, the researchers have kept in mind that the interviewees' accounts were descriptions of important life events as they recalled and remembered them in retrospect. As explained by Brannen and Nilsen (2011), "a biography can be defined as a story told in the *present* about a person's life in the *past* and his or her expectations for the *future*" (p. 609). While the factual events of an interviewee's life were important, we were also interested in the meaning the events had for the person and how they presented them.

The interview data has provided information about some of the main types of relations between persons with disabilities and society at large. The dataset has been useful for developing analytic generalisations (Yin, 2014) and theoretical inference (Lloyd-Jones, 2005), i.e., identifying conditions for exercising active citizenship and making projections about the likely transferability of the findings. The dataset cannot, however, be used for numerical or statistical generalisations. It also does not allow us to conclude how common these experiences are or what the most important single mechanism or factor is for promoting Active Citizenship.

The life-course interviews have provided insights into the policies, social institutions and cultural assumptions that shape the experiences of people with disabilities. The life-course interviews have also provided insights into the diverse experiences of disability, contributing to a better understanding of why and how these experiences take different forms in different contexts.

The interview data has not provided systematic information about national disability policy systems, as such. However, many of the experiences the interviewees report reflect the disability policy and practices at the time they occurred. The extent to which the interviewees themselves made such connections between their experiences and official policy varied considerably. To a large extent, the researchers have had to clarify connections between the micro data and the meso and macro context. We found that only some contextual information was provided in the individuals' accounts. Because the team collected data about public policy in other parts of the project, we were nevertheless able to bring this contextual information to bear when interpreting the interview data (see Chapter 1, this volume).

References

Biernacki, P. & Waldorf, D. (1981). Snowball sampling problems and techniques of chain referral sampling. *Sociological Methods & Research*, *10*(2), 141–163.

Biewer, G., Buchner, T., Shevlin, M., Smyth, F., Šiška, J., Káňová, S., … Rodríguez Díaz, S. (2015). Pathways to inclusion in European higher education systems. *ALTER, European Journal of Disability Research*, *9*(4), 278–289.

Brannen, J. & Nilsen, A. (2011). Comparative biographies in case-based cross-national research: Methodological considerations. *Sociology*, *45*(4), 603–618.

Buchner, T., Smyth, F., Biewer, G., Shevlin, M., Ferreira, M. A. V., Toboso Martín, M., … Káňová, Š. (2015). Paving the way through mainstream education: The interplay of families, schools and disabled students. *Research Papers in Education*, *30*(4), 411–426. doi: 10.1080/02671522.2014.989175.

Cohen, L., Manion, L. & Morrison, K. (2007). *Research methods in education*. London: RoutledgeFalmer.

Edwards, R. & Holland, J. (2013). *What is qualitative interviewing?* London: Bloomsbury Academic.

Hvinden, B. (2012). Disability. In B. Greve (Ed.), *The Routledge handbook of the welfare state* (pp. 371–380). London: Routledge.

Kvale, S. (2006). Dominance through interviews and dialogues. *Qualitative Inquiry*, *12*, 480–500

Kvale, S. (2007). *Doing interviews*. London: Sage.

Lillestø, B. & Sandvin, J. T. (2014). Limits to vocational inclusion? Disability and the social democratic conception of labour. *Scandinavian Journal of Disability Research, 16*(1), 45–58. doi: 10.1080/15017419.2012.735203.

Lindqvist, R. & Sépulchre, M. (2014). Change and current status in the life course of persons with psycho-social disabilities. DISCIT Deliverable 4.2 report. Retrieved 10 April 2017 from https://blogg.hioa.no/discit.

Lindqvist, R., Sépulchre, M. & Thorén, K. (2014). Diversity and change of the life courses of persons with psycho-social disabilities: The impact of services. DISCIT Deliverable 4.1 report. Retrieved 10 April 2017 from https://blogg.hioa.no/discit.

Lloyd-Jones, G. (2005). Theoretical inference and generalisation within the case study. In G. Troman, B. Jeffrey & G. Walford (Eds), *Methodological issues and practices in ethnography* (pp. 73–94). Bingley, UK: Emerald Group Publishing Ltd.

OECD. (2012). *Sick on the job: Myths and realities about mental health and work.* Paris: OECD. Retrieved 10 April 2017 from: www.oecd.org/els/emp/49227189.pdf.

Patton, M. Q. (2002). *Qualitative research and evaluation methods.* London: Sage Publications.

Parry, O., Thomson, C. & Fowkes, G. (1999) Life course data collection: Qualitative interviewing using the life grid. *Sociological Research Online, 4*(2), U152–U165.

Priestley, M. (2001). *Disability and the life course: Global perspectives.* Cambridge: Cambridge University Press.

Priestley, M. (2003). *Disability: A life course approach.* Oxford: Polity Press.

Sandvin, J. T. (2003). Loosening bonds and changing identities: Growing up with impairments in post-war Norway. *Disability Studies Quarterly, 23*(2), 5–19.

Santos, H. P. O., Black, A. M. & Sandelowski, M. (2015). Timing of translation in cross-language qualitative research. *Qualitative Health Research, 25*(1), 134–144.

Shah, S. & Priestley, M. (2011). *Disability and social change: Private lives and public policies.* Bristol: Policy Press.

Shakespeare, T. (2006). *Disability rights and wrongs.* Abingdon, Oxon: Routledge.

Smyth, F., Shevlin, M., Buchner, T., Biewer, G., Flynn, P., Latimier, C., … Ferreira, M. A. V. (2014). Inclusive education in progress: Policy evolution in four European countries. *European Journal of Special Needs Education, 29*(4), 433–445. doi: 10.1080/08856257.2014.922797.

Temple, B., Edwards, R. & Alexander, C. (2006). Grasping at context: Cross language qualitative research as secondary qualitative data analysis. *Forum Qualitative Sozialforschung/Forum: Qualitative Social Research, 7*(4), Art. 10.

Thorsen, K. (Ed.). (2000). *Et langt liv med en alvorlig funksjonshemming. Utfordringer i et livsløpsperspektiv [A long life with a severe disability. Challenges in a life-course perspective].* Oslo: Nasjonalt kompetansesenter for aldersdemens.

Thorsen, K. & Myrvang, V. H. (2008). *Livsløp og hverdagsliv med utviklingshemning. [Life course and everyday life with developmental disabilities].* Tønsberg: Forlaget Aldring og helse.

Tøssebro, J. & Hvinden, B. (2017). Operational definitions of disability: Usable in comparative research on Active Citizenship? In R. Halvorsen, B. Hvinden, J. Bickenbach, D. Ferri & A. M. Guillén Rodriguez (Eds), *The changing disability policy system: Active Citizenship and disability in Europe, volume 1*, 55–71. London: Routledge.

United Nations. (2006). *Convention on the Rights of Persons with Disabilities* (resolution adopted by the General Assembly, 24 January 2007, A/RES/61/106).

Yin, R. (2014). *Case study research: Design and methods* (5th ed.). Thousand Oaks, CA: Sage.

4 Changes and diversity in community living in Europe

The experiences of persons with disabilities

Jan Šiška, Julie Beadle-Brown, Šárka Káňová and Anna M. Kittelsaa

Deinstitutionalisation and community living have been receiving growing attention in all European and most other Western countries since the 1990s. However, how welfare services should be organised has been discussed for much longer. It should be remembered that supporting the independence of persons with disabilities was an initial purpose of the first institutions, set up in the late 1800s. However, with the advent of the eugenic period, this function of such services disappeared and people with disabilities, in particular those with intellectual disabilities, became institutionalised, isolated and controlled. Passive maintenance of services was often assumed to be sufficient, and over time the number of people in institutions grew, strengthening institutional regimes and worsening living conditions. It became the common view that people with disabilities needed to be institutionalised, thus removing their potential to participate in the community (Power, Lord & de Franco, 2013).

In the 1950s, these regimes began to attract criticism and the institutions began to be seen as a barrier in themselves. Dissatisfaction with the institutional practices and public criticism of welfare gradually gave rise to a debate about innovative models of support. Such debates were initiated by professionals, policy makers, organisations of persons with disabilities as well as persons with disabilities themselves and their families. The reform in social care began in the 1970s, initially in Sweden, the UK and the US, but gradually spread to other countries. However, progress was slow and the original institutional practices of rigidity of routine, social distance, depersonalisation and block treatment (King, Raynes & Tizard, 1971) began to be replicated in the new community settings (Emerson, Cullen, Hatton & Cross, 1996; Ericsson, 2002). Even though people lived in the community, they did not necessarily participate or feel included in the community.

Within intellectual disability and mental health fields in particular, the multidimensional concept of 'quality of life' emerged as the guiding principle for services supporting people with disabilities (e.g. Schalock, 1996; Felce, 1997; Schalock et al., 2002; Connell, Brazier, O'Cathain, Lloyd-Jones & Paisley, 2012; Connell, O'Cathain & Brazier, 2014). There has also been some research exploring both objective and subjective elements of the quality of life for those with physical and sensory disabilities, but this is much less developed conceptually than for those with intellectual disabilities and mental health issues.

Research began to show that living in an ordinary home dispersed in the community (adequate, appropriate and adapted to people's needs) was a necessary but not sufficient condition to improve quality of life (Emerson & Hatton, 1994; Felce, 1996). At the same time, people with disabilities themselves began to agitate for better experiences for people with disabilities, and a greater focus on participation and self-determination began to emerge. In 2006, the UN Convention on the Rights of Persons with disabilities (CRPD) declared that people with disabilities have a right to live in the community, as independently as possible, with support to enable them to participate in the community as full and equal citizens, with freedom to make their own choices and have their voices heard (notably Article 19) (United Nations, 2006).

However, despite significant progress in some countries, the current picture is not encouraging. Even just looking at the number of people in institutions, never mind living and participating in their community, over one million people still live in institutions (in more than 30 places) in Europe (Mansell, Knapp, Beadle-Brown & Beecham, 2007). Research also suggests that persons with intellectual disabilities form over a quarter of this population and persons with mental health problems are the next largest group (Mansell, Beadle-Brown & Clegg, 2004; European Commission, 2009; Townsley, Ward, Abbott & Williams, 2010).

Looking at the countries involved in the DISCIT project, Šiška, Beadle-Brown, Káňová and Tøssebro (2017) concluded that there was still some way to go in many countries before the CRPD was fully implemented. However, as in previous research (e.g. Mansell et al., 2007), drawing any conclusions was hindered by a lack of complete and useful data, and the data that existed was often very general data around the number of places in particular institutions. Very little research or focus was found in any of the literature reviewed on the direct experiences of people with disabilities – for example, the nature of the support people received and the quality of their lives more generally as well as whether they were experiencing Active Citizenship in particular.

In this chapter, we focus on such experiences, i.e. the experiences of people with disabilities in terms of their living situation now, the path they followed to get there and the barriers they met along the way. We are interested in what their experiences can tell us about the achievements, shortcomings and possible gaps in existing arrangements and the potential for improvement in supporting Active Citizenship for all people with disabilities through community living and community-based support. We will focus primarily on their living situation and support. However, we will also give an overview of other areas associated with community living to set the scene for subsequent chapters which will explore specific elements in more detail. These include employment and political participation as well as issues for specific groups such as those with psychosocial disabilities and women with disabilities.

Living in the community (as opposed to an institution) is a central part of being an active citizen and is necessary for quality of life more generally – being a part of society physically as well as conceptually is crucial to being able to participate in society and to being seen by others as part of that society.

Participants and approach to analysis

Following the methodology described in Chapter 3, life-course interviews with 200 people were analsyed. Gender, age cohort and disability group were evenly distributed. Just under one third of the sample was, or had in the past been, actively involved in the work of organisations of persons with disabilities (DPOs). Involvement in DPOs varied by disability group (those with sensory (visual) and mobility disabilities were more likely to report being involved in the work of DPOs) and country (e.g. involvement in DPOs was very low overall in Germany and Ireland but very high in Sweden).

The first stage of analysis involved developing a framework for analysis by exploring emerging themes across different countries and different disability groups for a small sample of interviews. This framework was then used to analyse the full sample. Figure 4.1 summarises the thematic area extracted. Data related to living situation and life trajectories was then coded numerically for all 200 interviews to allow easier identification of patterns in the data.

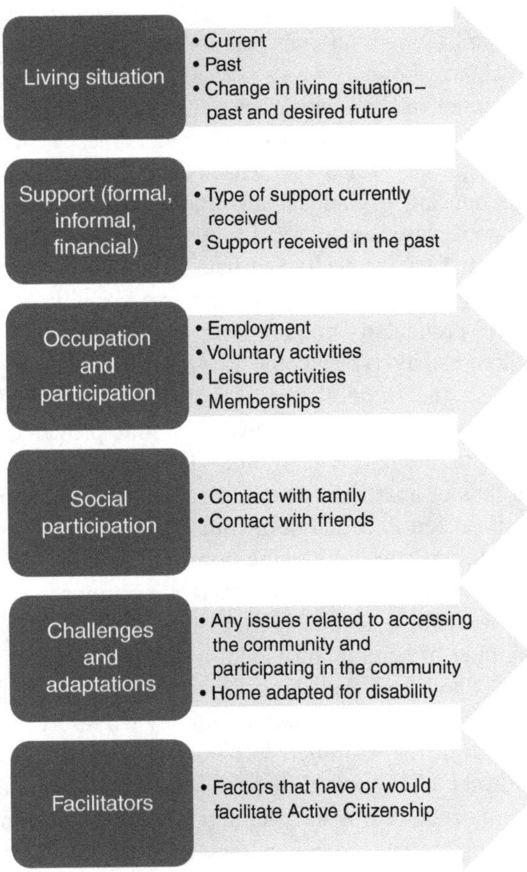
Living situation
• Current
• Past
• Change in living situation – past and desired future
Support (formal, informal, financial)
• Type of support currently received
• Support received in the past
Occupation and participation
• Employment
• Voluntary activities
• Leisure activities
• Memberships
Social participation
• Contact with family
• Contact with friends
Challenges and adaptations
• Any issues related to accessing the community and participating in the community
• Home adapted for disability
Facilitators
• Factors that have or would facilitate Active Citizenship

Figure 4.1 Thematic areas extracted for detailed analysis.

Finally, all interview reports ($n=86$) from four countries were coded across all thematic areas identified in Figure 4.1: the UK, Norway, Germany and the Czech Republic. These countries are all at different stages, and have followed different paths, in the process towards community living. They also have different welfare state systems, different systems for providing community living and have different relationships with the EU and UN. For the most part, findings are presented qualitatively and focus on living situation, support and community participation.

Findings

Living situation and support

For those with visual impairments, mobility difficulties and psychosocial disabilities, the most common type of current living arrangement was in their own house or flat (owned or rented), either on their own or with their partner and in some cases with their own children. Not surprisingly, those in the younger (1990s) cohort were more likely to be still living with their parents or grandparents or in their own place. For the most part, those living in normal flats (in some cases adapted to be accessible) dispersed in the community, reported having a good choice over where they lived, especially if they owned their own home. The exception to this were people who, for primarily financial reasons (e.g. lack of employment), were reliant on social housing from local government where rent was cheaper but choice limited. In most cases, people had to just 'take what they had been given'. Some people reported having to live in flats that were completely inadequate and in some cases dangerous and having had to move many times over the course of their lives. This was particularly true for those with psychosocial disabilities, a small number of whom had also spent some time homeless.

More of those who were older (nearly a quarter of those in the 1950 cohort and over a fifth of the 1970 cohort) were living in NGO- or state-provided settings with support available on site in one way or another. For the most part, this was in the form of individual flats or apartments clustered together – sometimes in smaller blocks of around six to ten flats and sometimes in larger clusters or attached to more institutional settings such as nursing homes or hospitals. For a smaller number of people, accommodation was in shared/group settings, some of which were quite large (over 10 people in one home). Some people reported having been able to visit a number of settings provided by the organisation and having had some choice as to which one they lived in as well as having had some choice as to which people from their previous setting they would live with. However, this choice was sometimes still limited in nature. For example, one man with visual impairments in the UK reported that the large institutional care home he was living in was being replaced by smaller supported living arrangements and residents were shown around the bungalows and invited to select where and with whom they wanted to live. He selected one house with four others and has lived there ever since.

For some people, support was available 24 hours a day within these settings, but for most people support was provided on an emergency basis or for particular activities. It was primarily people with intellectual disabilities, a few people with psychosocial disabilities and a few people with visual impairment in the UK who lived in shared, clustered or larger settings or who still lived with their families.

In terms of the nature and quality of support, a substantial minority of people were not receiving any formal support other than financial benefits or in some cases specific one-off help, e.g. with assistive technology, home adaptations, assistance dog, wheelchair, white cane etc.). For some people, especially those with mobility disabilities and some of those with sensory impairments, this was out of choice and a desire to be as independent as possible. Others were working and thus had to pay for their own support.

Choice of the type of support was less common than of the living situation, although most people reported being satisfied with the type of support – in particular if they had personal assistance. However, it appeared that this was limited in terms of having a choice about who supported them and when that support was available. Often people had to arrange their time and activities around when the support was available rather than the support being available to fit in with what people wanted and needed to do and when they wanted to do it. In addition a few people talked about having to take the type of support that was available rather than what they really wanted. A small number of people commented on the inefficiency of support or support that did not promote independence for people – for example, not providing the adaptations needed to someone's home but providing assistance instead. One issue that was repeatedly raised by people with psychosocial disabilities was that support was not flexible enough to meet their needs. The all-or-nothing approach did not match the fluctuating nature of most people's mental health conditions. Those with psychosocial disabilities needed support to be available during a crisis and in the background at other times but this rarely happened. They also often needed help to access more alternative types of support – self-help groups, support for exercise or support for maintaining their employment when they got into crisis. In some countries, for example the Czech Republic, some of the support they needed did not qualify as funded services – in particular services such as self-help groups.

Very few people mentioned anything about the quality of the support they received from assistants, although a few people commented on having to train their own staff so that they supported them in the way they wanted to be supported. This is likely to reflect the more able nature of this group of people, who in general were able to speak and tell staff what they wanted. For those with more severe and complex disabilities, the skills of staff become increasingly important (Mansell & Beadle-Brown, 2012).

Active Citizenship as participation in the community

This section explores whether people reported participation and inclusion in their local community – for example, whether they had a job, participated in voluntary activities and belonged to organisations as well as whether they engaged in community activities, hobbies, and social contact.

Interviewees identified substantial issues around getting and keeping jobs, partly through a lack of support to do so and partly through a lack of reasonable adjustments within the jobs. In some cases, bullying and discrimination were part of the reason people had to leave their jobs and why they had difficulty finding other jobs. Some people reported not having revealed their disability status until after their interview due to lots of experience of not getting invited for interview. Others reported a difficulty in finding employment that could be flexible enough during times of ill health – this was particularly so for those with psychosocial disabilities.

Whether people had jobs varied by country – with those in the UK least likely to report having a job. This is possibly due to what is referred to as the 'benefit trap' in the UK – in general, people lose at least some of their benefits if they earn too much money from work or have savings. Getting the benefits reinstated is very difficult and takes time. As such, working can be risky for people, especially if their condition means that they are more likely to be at risk of losing their job. Those with intellectual disabilities were more likely to be employed in sheltered workshops with only minimal pay, although many people expressed satisfaction with their work in sheltered workshops as it gave them something to do and a small amount of income.

Most people had contact with family and most people reported contact with at least one good friend. Just over half of the sample had at some point been married or in a relationship and one quarter had children. However, just over 15 per cent of people were currently married or in a relationship.

Most of those who were interviewed did take part in activities in the community such as shopping, leisure activities etc. and the majority reported hobbies including sport, music or the theatre. Many were involved in volunteering or unpaid work (although fewer of those with intellectual disabilities reported this type of activity).

However, the nature of all of these activities differed by country and disability group. Once again, those with intellectual disabilities were less likely to report hobbies, take part in volunteering and have contact with friends – contact with friends was more commonly with other people with disabilities and through organised activities. For those with psychosocial disabilities, participation varied according to how they were feeling at the time.

Self-determination was raised as an issue more generally, in particular for people with intellectual disabilities, especially in relation to how they spend their time and money, and there was variability even within countries and age cohorts. For example, one young woman with intellectual disabilities from the Czech Republic reported that she was afraid that her parents would not allow her to live independently and felt that she did not have a choice about who to have a relationship with. In contrast, a young Czech man with psychosocial disabilities reported that having moved from an institution to a community programme had meant more choice about how he spends his time:

> I mainly can go out whenever I want to. There is nobody who checked whether I returned until 7 p.m. I can go to the local pub if I want to. I only drink coffee or tea, of course as I said no drinking anymore. Less I drink alcoholic drinks, the more I drink coffee … so to sum it up basically I can do whatever I want to.

Barriers to Active Citizenship as community living

Barriers to Active Citizenship were identified by 45 interviewees, spread almost equally across the four countries. The majority of those with intellectual disabilities, mobility disabilities and sensory disabilities reported issues in accessing or participating in their community. This contrasted with people with psychosocial disabilities, where around 40 per cent reported such issues. What people described was analysed thematically and the themes are described below. However, it is also important to note that not everyone reported difficulties in accessing the environment and, even if they did experience barriers of any type, that did not necessarily mean they felt excluded from Active Citizenship. One man with a visual impairment from Norway reported that he had encountered barriers in terms of accessibility but yet in his neighbourhood he feels respected and not just the 'the blind man'. He regarded himself as a very active citizen.

There were five themes in terms of barriers identified. First, people identified issues with physical accessibility, in particular in Norway and the UK – access to shops, services and offices, wedding venues and holiday resorts were identified by some as problematic.

Second, people talked about barriers related to negative attitudes, low awareness and low expectations. Sometimes this related to the general public and local services such as insurance companies, shops and restaurants. For example, one woman reported that she was not allowed into many places because of her assistance dog, the reason given being that people might be allergic to dogs.

At other times, the issue was the attitudes of professionals. For people with psychosocial disabilities, the attitudinal barriers and low expectations sometimes came from professionals in the medical field. For others, in particular those with intellectual disabilities, the issue was the attitudes and low expectations of those providing support: for example, one man with intellectual disabilities from the 1970s cohort in the Czech Republic talked about freedom in how to spend his money:

> If I spend more, he scolds me, that I spend money on things that are not worth it … I have tried to argue that it was my money, but he was too squeamish. I thought it was not worth it to quarrel with him, he is strict.

For yet others, the low expectations came from family members and in particular affected those with an intellectual disability and their scope for choice and control.

Although some people had experienced a lack of awareness and low expectations, there was awareness from some of those interviewed that other people have much worse experiences. One man with visual impairments from Norway reported that he sometimes gets asked questions like, 'Can blind people have sex?' But he goes on to say that other people with greater visual impairments are met with far more prejudice than he is.

The third theme was around discrimination and bullying. For some people, this happened at school and, for others, when out and about in their community. One woman with intellectual disabilities from Germany (born around 1950) reported that people made fun of her and her brother when they went out in the community: 'when I and my brother … go for a walk … the, the people say: "Here come the disabled ones".'

However, for the majority who raised bullying as an issue, it happened in the workplace. For example, one woman with mobility difficulties from the UK reported that in the early days (in the 1970s) she was told that she was not wanted as a 'one-armed typist'. Later on she also experienced issues as she looked for work, saying: 'as soon as you said you had a disability they hadn't got vacancies'. In her most recent post, she experienced discrimination and negative attitudes towards her disability (which was surprising as it was a disability charity she was working for). But in this case she brought her manager to a tribunal and took action against her. She reported that having the equality legislation has helped, but that nevertheless there are still plenty of areas where discrimination exists.

The fourth theme related to barriers that emerged was a lack of financial resources or of [good] support to be active in the local community. Although for the most part having a personal budget was a facilitator for community living and Active Citizenship, for a small number of people this did not work out quite so well, partly because of a lack of funding for things not considered essential. For example, one woman with visual impairments from the UK reported how she would like to go out on a weekend but that there was never the staff available to support her. In other cases, the level of knowledge in local government and receiving poor advice had made things difficult for the individual and ultimately resulted in an inefficient use of resources. This was illustrated by one man with mobility issues from Norway, who had received advice from the municipality with regard to adaptations to his house. However, the advice was not good advice and he was now in the position of having to renovate the house again. He also reported that he was receiving support for personal assistance but that, if the house had been adapted properly, the authorities would have saved money because he would have needed less support.

For others, the experience was effectively a lack of useful support altogether and the difficulty of getting help, sometimes associated with institutional care for those with psychosocial disabilities. One young woman from the Czech Republic reported how she felt abandoned by the system – she needed help to manage her life again, but depression prevented her from taking the necessary steps in order to receive support. She also mentions a psychiatric clinic as an institution she never wants to return to, as according to her, 'nobody helps you there'.

Fifth and finally, there were a number of other barriers identified by a few individuals – in particular barriers associated with people's conditions such as for the woman in the paragraph above. This was particularly true for those with psychosocial disabilities, but also related to the emergence of physical or other medical issues in addition to psychosocial disabilities. For example, one man (born around 1970) from the UK reported that he started to experience changes in his disability – in particular problems with his stability – and was unable to walk very far without falling over. This, combined with the side-effects of his medication, which left him very fatigued and tired, had made getting back to work almost impossible, as well as sapping his motivation. He said that he feels that more recently he has started to let himself go and cannot motivate himself to do anything.

> As much as I can be enthusiastic one minute, I can be really down the next minute and out of it and not be bothered … and give up. It's very hard to be motivated on medication that really doesn't pick me up at all.

The other subtheme identified by a small number of people was the lack of staff knowledge and training and the fact that people had to train their assistants themselves. One woman with physical disabilities from the Czech Republic reported that whenever she gets a new personal assistant she teaches them to support her to be independent and not to work as a professional housekeeper or cook but rather to support her doing things for herself.

Facilitators of community living and examples of good practice

What had interviewees experienced as facilitative? The final example in the previous section along with a number of the other examples highlight some of the key themes that emerged around what facilitated community living. The first of these was the fact that direct support was critical for many of the interviewees but in particular for those with mobility disabilities and for some of those with intellectual disabilities. The availability of personal assistance had made a notable difference to the lives of many people with mobility issues (as well as to some people with sensory disabilities). Interestingly, very few of the interviewees with intellectual disabilities reported having personal assistants. They were more likely to be living with their families with very little formal support, living on their own with no support other than a family member or a guardian to help with financial issues, or living in supported accommodation with staff around to help. Another apparently important factor was the ability of staff and organisations providing support to involve and empower the individual in decisions around their own life, for example in a person-centred plan.

The second theme that emerged very strongly was that the individual's own resources – in some cases financial but primarily their personal resources, for example their ability to manage their own affairs, their tenacity, their ability to argue their case and to 'fight' for their rights and support – were critical. People developed strategies themselves to make things accessible. However, in particular for people with psychosocial disabilities, this was often very difficult. Many interviewees with psychosocial disabilities reported that getting treatment and in particular having access to self-help groups was very important to helping them move forward or to return to playing an active part in their local community.

Families were important facilitators for some people in terms of transitions in their living situations such as getting support or simply becoming more independent. This was true primarily for people with intellectual disabilities. It was not always the parents, but sometimes the grandparents or other relatives who provided support. As noted earlier, a change in government policy and the availability of funding streams in the UK was associated with a change in the nature of the living situation from larger residential care to small group homes and supported living for those with intellectual disabilities and some of the older people with visual impairments. This change was led by organisations providing services.

For other groups and in other countries the strength and support to fight for their rights often came from DPOs and sometimes from staff in NGOs.

Overall, those able to speak for themselves tended to, in the end, get what they needed. For those who found it more difficult to communicate or who, because of their disabilities, did not have the resources, strength or energy to fight, sometimes over many years, the experiences were less positive, in particular in terms of choice and control over their lives.

What did people say was needed to help people with disabilities experience Active Citizenship? As might be expected, the themes that arose in the area of facilitators of Active Citizenship related closely to the barriers identified above. Although many people noted that society had become more accessible to some extent, many people highlighted that improvements were still needed. Some people commented on things they thought were necessary to help themselves, such as creating accessible information and processes. For example, one man with intellectual disabilities from the 1970 German cohort said, 'To translate questions, er, well, I'd say, into easy language … so one can understand better'.

Others were also aware of issues encountered by other people and felt that society needed to be more accessible and more aware of disability issues. One man from the UK with mobility issues indicated that many things had changed since his youth and that in general buildings had become more accessible. He felt that the Disability Discrimination Act had played an important role in these changes.

More investment from governments, in particular in relation to supporting people into employment, was raised as important. One man with intellectual disabilities from Germany said that he wished that politics would 'engage more, care more and do more' and, in particular, he felt that government should do more to combat unemployment for people with disabilities.

As well as considering what governments and others could do to improve life in the community for people with disabilities, many of the interviewees were involved in making change happen for people with disabilities more generally. For example, one man with mobility issues from Norway uses photographs of the barriers he meets to show politicians and professionals what needs to be done – he said that he wanted anti-discrimination to be taken seriously in Norway.

Conclusion

In this chapter, we have focused on the experiences of people with disabilities, not just in relation to where they live now, where they have lived in the past and whether they have any choice in where they live, but also in how they participate in the community and the support they receive. In doing this, we have considered the barriers and facilitators people have encountered and have explored similarities and differences between those in different disability groups, in different countries and from different age cohorts.

While some people interviewed in this study regarded themselves as active citizens, others, in particular those with intellectual disabilities, were not yet experiencing community living in its fullest sense, as they were still living in congregated (or at least clustered) settings, with limited social networks and with limited support to access employment or individualised leisure activities. Their income was restricted and they were highly dependent on families in many cases to provide them with support and opportunities. They experienced limited choice and autonomy over some aspects of their day-to-day lives and often encountered barriers to their involvement in the community, in particular attitudinal barriers. Although, as acknowledged in Chapter 3, people with severe intellectual disabilities and complex needs were not included in the current study, on the basis of previous research it can generally be assumed that those with more severe disabilities are experiencing similar or even greater limitations on their quality of life more generally when compared to those who have less severe disabilities. This is partly because they are more highly dependent on staff to support them (Mansell & Beadle-Brown, 2012).

The other important issue to recognise was the fact that a substantial proportion of people who took part in the study, in some countries at least, were actively involved in DPOs – in particular, those with physical and sensory disabilities. Although no research exists to which we could compare level of DPO membership, it is possible that the people included in this sample might have more personal resources and support with which to fight for their rights than those who were not involved in DPOs.

However, as noted in Chapter 3, the intention behind the study was not to recruit a representative sample of people with disabilities but rather the findings are intended to be indicative of the situation and experiences of people with disabilities in Europe, who, for the most part, are already living in the community.

As had been noted in other research such as Mansell et al. (2007), there was substantial variation in the nature of services that were referred to as community living. This was particularly true for those with intellectual disabilities, with many people living in a group home or clustered apartment settings, which afforded them more choice and autonomy than in larger settings but at the same time may not have promoted their social inclusion as much as dispersed housing in the community might have done (Mansell and Beadle-Brown, 2009).

Comparisons, in particular across country and age cohorts, are also only indicative, as no account was taken of the severity of disability, which we know, at least for those with intellectual disabilities, accounts for a substantial amount of the variation in all aspects of quality of life including community participation and self-determination (e.g. Jones et al., 1999; Mansell, Beadle-Brown, MacDonald & Ashman, 2003).

Despite these limitations, the findings reported here give us substantial insights into the experiences of people with disabilities in terms of Active Citizenship through community living. They have allowed us to draw out similarities and differences across countries, across disability groups and across age cohorts. The validity of the findings is strengthened by the fact that the findings map very closely onto those from the review of previous research and official statistics, as well as the interviews with expert informants in each country (as reported in Šiška et al., 2017). This is particularly true with regard to the differences between disability groups. In addition, the facilitators for community living identified by interviewees also map closely on to those identified by the expert informants.

There were a number of factors that were identified as being important in determining how much people experienced Active Citizenship and which have implications for policy and service-funding decisions in EU member states (and beyond).

The first factor was that an individual's own capacity, in terms of awareness, knowledge, sense of control, strength and tenacity, was important in helping him/her fight for their rights and be an active member of society. Some groups were more vulnerable than others in this sense, in particular those with psychosocial disabilities and those with intellectual disabilities. This finding relates closely to Sen's (1999) Capability Approach (see Chapter 2, this volume). Sen argued that when evaluating well-being or quality of life it is essential to consider what a person can actually be and do. The extent to which people are capable of having a better quality of life is influenced by a wide range of factors, with the first being the individual physiology of the individual (Sen, 1999, pp. 70–71) – i.e. illnesses, disability and age, where some adaptations may be needed in order to allow people to be capable of taking the opportunities for quality of life (but acknowledging that this factor cannot always be completely eliminated – e.g. for many people, blindness cannot be remediated by operations, assistive devices or support. How much access people get to the adaptive solutions also depends both directly and indirectly on other factors. Resources such as wealth, and characteristics such as tenacity can play an important role in capability. Other determinants of capability include the services and support available as a result of social conditions, as well as cultural perspectives and attitudes and environmental issues such as climate, epidemiology and pollution. So, for example, if you live in a country with a cold climate where financial and social resources are limited, reducing how well the streets are cleared with snow and then having the money available to buy a wheelchair is unlikely to improve your capability to get to work during a spell of snowy weather. In a culture where people with disabilities are not seen as a valued part of the community, then it is less likely that people in your neighbourhood will come out to clear the footpaths and help you get to work. Many of the factors seen by Sen as influencing capability are reflected in other findings discussed below.

One of the factors identified as important for supporting people to have more awareness, capacity and confidence to fight for their rights was being part of self-help groups and self-advocacy groups. However, in some countries, this type of service was not funded by the local or national government but relied on charitable funding to exist, which in times of economic crisis sometimes meant that the service could not be sustained. These groups were also important because they allowed people with disabilities to help others experiencing similar difficulties, which in turn gave them more confidence and a reason for living.

The second factor that was particularly important was providing support that was flexible enough to respond to individuals' changing needs across time and which was not constrained by traditional ideas of what support should be but which allowed room for creative solutions. Both interviewees with disabilities and expert informants noted that often people had to take what support was available rather than getting the support they really needed or wanted. The failure to provide such support has potential cost implications, in particular through wasted or an inefficient use of funds. The right support provided at an early stage could potentially save money and allow more people to be supported in the long term. For example, this might take the form of:

- equipment or adaptations to the home that help people to remain as independent as possible for as long as possible;
- funding mentors or drop-in support volunteers to keep contact with individuals and help them access self-help groups etc;
- offering support to people who need medical treatment or who are looking for accessibility solutions or helping with decision-making before their condition worsens to the point where they lose their job, their home or their family;
- funding/providing advocacy and self-help services to help people exercise control over their lives;
- providing skilled support (if necessary 24-hour support) for those with more complex needs living in the community that focuses on helping people to develop self-help skills and have a good quality of life – this in turn will reduce the need for people to have to access intensive in-patient treatment for challenging behaviour or psychosocial disabilities;

- continuing to support people with benefits even when they are working, at least initially – in some countries this did happen but not in all;
- making it easy for people to regain benefits and support should their condition worsen and in particular if they are unable to work for some time;
- supporting people in whatever way necessary to access exercise or leisure activities and to maintain the social networks that help them to manage their physical or psychosocial state, thereby keeping them healthy and requiring less intensive support over time.

The third important factor that emerged was the role families continue to play in people's lives, especially the lives of those with an intellectual disability, even after they had left school. For many people, the family continues to provide day-to-day support and accommodation; for others, families help them to find accommodation in the community, facilitate applications for financial and other forms of support and manage their finances. This is not necessarily always the biological parents – for some of the people interviewed, it was grandparents or siblings. While in Norway there was an expectation that anyone who wanted to move into their own home as an adult should be supported to do so, this was not the case in the other countries included here. As such, families continue to be important sources of support and therefore need to be provided with support themselves. Good support for families when children are young can help prevent institutionalisation and support the development of the child so that, as they grow older, they have more skills and can become more active in their local community. This support includes respite or short-break stays for the person with the disability, regular in-home support to give the family a break and time with other family members etc. every week, training in how to support their son or daughter better, or even 24-hour in-home support for people who have complex disabilities.

The role and support provided by DPOs was highlighted as an important factor for a significant number of interviewees. DPOs had supported people in numerous different ways – helping to gain access to accommodation and to support, providing leisure activities and a chance to meet other people with disabilities, providing advocacy, information and advice, to name just a few. It is important that DPOs continue to be funded to provide social and practical support both to people with disabilities and their families. Such support includes having a place for people to meet, funding to produce accessible information about local services (how to apply for benefits or support, how to manage personal budgets where available), funding to offer training for families and support workers and support for self-advocacy.

Finally, the need for greater awareness of disability issues across public services and the community more generally was highlighted by some of the problems people had faced in terms of accessibility and the attitudes and awareness of others. Negative attitudes, often combined with an underestimation of the abilities of persons with disabilities, hamper people's opportunities for community participation and for control over their lives. This is particularly true for those with an intellectual disability. For some people, these negative attitudes and a lack of awareness went further than low expectations and lack of opportunities – a number of interviewees across different countries reported having experienced (and in many cases, continuing to experience) bullying and discrimination. For some, this took the form of being stared at and teased. For others, it was more serious physical harassment. Mostly commonly it happened in the workplace. The issue of disability-related victimisation has been the topic of substantial research in the UK in recent years (Beadle-Brown et al., 2014) and is currently attracting research interest in other countries including Norway and Sweden. One of the key recommendations from that research is the need for greater inclusion of disability issues in diversity and equality training in all public services as well as a much greater emphasis on educating children and young people in human rights and disability issues.

Creating greater public awareness of disability issues from the government down is an essential part of supporting greater Active Citizenship. However, the best way to do this is to help others to see the abilities – and not just the disabilities – of persons with disabilities; and to see people taking part in society and, more importantly, contributing to society. This is likely to be especially true for people with more severe intellectual disabilities, who will need support to take part and contribute. In addition, society is likely to be less positive towards these people as, until relatively recently, they had remained in institutional provision, segregated from societies that had started to become more accustomed to seeing people with physical disabilities and people with visual impairments in employment, on TV, in politics, competing in sport, etc. Some of the interviewees commented that the situation is changing, but that much more change is needed before everyone can experience Active Citizenship.

Some of the findings imply that a broad conceptualisation of how Security, Autonomy and Influence might look in the lives of people with all types of disabilities was needed. In order to be a useful framework for those working in the fields of intellectual disability and mental health in particular, the Active Citizenship framework should include participation in all aspects of life (at home as well as in the community). Even those with the most severe disabilities can be involved in political participation at a local level and beyond, influencing policy and practice development more generally. They can be employed and can also contribute to society in caring and volunteering roles. However, any conceptualisation also needs to consider and value participation in looking after their home and family as well as participation in neighbourly activities, leisure activities and relationships. These are also important for real social inclusion and acceptance.

Choice and control/autonomy/self-determination are just as important for those with more severe disabilities as for those who are better able to communicate their views, needs and desires verbally – but many people will need skilled support to get the experience necessary to be able to make choices and will need control to be made available to them in very different ways. Once our service systems and society more generally can support and accommodate this group of people as active citizens, then it is much more likely that all people with disabilities will be able to experience Active Citizenship.

As previously suggested in Mansell et al. (2007), the types of strategies discussed above require national and local government and those who are funding and/or commissioning services to take a long-term view. There are no one-off, 'quick fix' solutions to the issues raised by participants. Investment in preventative and ongoing (usually less intensive) services makes logical sense in terms of outcomes for people as well as potentially in terms of future costs. However, this is difficult to bring about in a climate of financial crisis and cuts, where the focus is usually on the current budget with little regard for the future implications of such cuts. Regular changes in government mean that both stability over time and sometimes even the memory of what has gone before is often compromised.

However, while financial crises might slow the process of deinstitutionalisation and the development of a wide range of living and support options available in the community, it is important not to take decisions that go in the wrong direction and make it difficult to move forward in the future. Some compromise might be necessary in order to make overall progress, but the ultimate goal of Active Citizenship in the form of community/independent living for all should be kept in focus.

References

Beadle-Brown, J., Richardson, L., Guest, C., Malovic, A., Bradshaw, J. & Himmerich, J. (2014). *Living in fear: Better outcomes for people with learning disabilities and autism.* Main research report. Canterbury: Tizard Centre, University of Kent.

Connell, J., Brazier, J., O'Cathain, A., Lloyd-Jones, M. & Paisley, S. (2012). Quality of life of people with mental health problems: A synthesis of qualitative research. *Health and Quality of Life Outcomes, 10*(1), 1–16.

Connell, J., O'Cathain, A. & Brazier, J. (2014). Measuring quality of life in mental health: Are we asking the right questions? *Social Science & Medicine, 120*, 12–20.

Emerson, E. & Hatton, C. (1994). *Moving out: Relocation from hospital to community.* London: Her Majesty's Stationery Office.

Emerson, E., Cullen, C., Hatton, C. & Cross, B. (1996). *Residential provision for people with learning disabilities: Summary report.* Keele University and the University of Manchester.

Ericsson, K. (2002). *From institutional to community participation: Ideas and realities concerning support to persons with intellectual disability.* Uppsala, Sweden: Uppsala Universitet.

European Commission, Directorate General for Employment, Social Affairs and Equal Opportunities. (2009). *Report of the ad hoc expert group on the transition from institutional to community-based care.* Retrieved on 22 April 2016 from http://docplayer.net/65632-Report-of-the-ad-hoc-expert-group-on-the-transition-from-institutional-to-community-based-care-european-commission.html. Brussels: European Commission.

Felce, D. (1996). Quality of support for ordinary living. In J. Mansell & K. Ericsson (Eds), *Deinstitutionalization and community living: Intellectual disability services in Britain, Scandinavia and the USA* (pp. 117–133). London: Chapman and Hall.

Felce, D. (1997). Defining and applying the concept of quality of life. *Journal of Intellectual Disability Research, 41*, 126–143.

Jones, E., Perry, J., Lowe, K., Felce, D., Toogood, S., Dunstan, F., Allen, D. & Pagler, J. (1999). Opportunity and the promotion of activity among adults with severe intellectual disability living in community residences: The impact of training staff in active support. *Journal of Intellectual Disability Research*, *43*(3), 164–178.

King, R. D., Raynes, N. V. & Tizard, J. (1971). *Patterns of residential care: Sociological studies in institutions for handicapped children*. London: Routledge and Kegan Paul.

Mansell, J. & Beadle-Brown, J. (2009). Dispersed or clustered housing for adults with intellectual disabilities: A systematic review. *Journal of Intellectual and Developmental Disability*, *34*(4), 313–323.

Mansell, J. & Beadle-Brown, J. (2012). *Active support: Enabling and empowering people with intellectual disabilities*. London: Jessica Kingsley Publishers.

Mansell, J., Beadle-Brown, J. & Clegg, S. (2004). The situation of large residential institutions in Europe. In G. Freyhoff, C. Parker, M. Coué & N. Greig (Eds), *Included in society: Results and recommendations of the European research initiative on community-based residential alternatives for disabled people* (pp. 28–56). Brussels: Inclusion Europe.

Mansell, J., Beadle-Brown, J., Macdonald, S. & Ashman, B. (2003). Resident involvement in activity in small community homes for people with learning disabilities. *Journal of Applied Research in Intellectual Disabilities*, *16*(1), 63–74.

Mansell, J., Knapp, M. R. J., Beadle-Brown, J. & Beecham, J. (2007). *Deinstitutionalisation and community living – Outcomes and costs: A report of a European Study: Volume 2 main report.* Canterbury: Tizard Centre, University of Kent.

Power, A., Lord, J. E. & de Franco A. S. (2013). *Active citizenship and disability: Implementing the personalisation of support*. New York: Cambridge University Press.

Schalock, R. L. (Ed.). (1996). *Quality of life: Conceptualization and measurement* (Vol. 1). Washington DC: AMMR.

Schalock, R. L., Brown, I., Brown, R., Cummins, R. A., Felce, D., Matikka, L., Keith, K. D. & Parmenter, T. (2002). Conceptualization, measurement, and application of quality of life for persons with intellectual disabilities: Report of an international panel of experts. *Mental Retardation*, *40*(6), 457–470.

Sen, A. (1999). *Development as freedom*. Oxford: Oxford University Press.

Šiška, J., Beadle-Brown, J., Káňová, Š. & Tøssebro, J. (2017) Active citizenship and community living in Europe – current policy, practice and research. In R. Halvorsen, B. Hvinden, J. Bickenbach, D. Ferri & A. M. Guillén Rodriguez (Eds), *Active citizenship and persons with disabilities in Europe: Volume 1* (pp. 72–89). London: Routledge.

Townsley, R., Ward, L., Abbott, D. & Williams, V. (2010). *The implementation of policies supporting independent living for disabled people in Europe: Synthesis report.* Retrieved on 22 April 2016 from www.disability-europe.net/content/aned/media/ANED-Task%205%20Independent%20Living%20Synthesis%20Report%2014.01.10.pdf. Leeds: University of Leeds, Centre for Disability Studies, Academic Network of European Disability Experts.

United Nations. (2006). *The United Nations convention on the rights of persons with disabilities. A/61/611.* Retrieved on 7 April 2016 from www.un.org/disabilities/convention/conventionfull.shtml. New York: United Nations General Assembly.

5 Diversity and change in the labour market careers of persons with disabilities

Edmund Coleman-Fountain, Roy Sainsbury, Bruno Trezzini and Šárka Káňová

The concept of Active Citizenship presumes that for 'full and effective' participation in society to be achieved, three principles must be observed. These are the principles of *security*, *autonomy*, and *influence* (see Chapter 1). Autonomy is of particular relevance for labour market participation. Active Citizenship is promoted when persons with disabilities make choices about work without the impediment of socially imposed barriers and sources of control not experienced by persons without disabilities. As employment is accorded the status of a right by the UN Convention on the Rights of Persons with Disabilities, and improved access to work is an established goal of the OECD, the EU and its member states, this chapter examines how persons with disabilities experience employment and the degree to which they make choices about employment.

To explore these questions, this chapter analyses life-course data from 217 interviews with persons with disabilities born around 1950, 1970 and 1990 in nine European countries (see Chapter 3). It asks how choice shaped people's employment trajectories 'within the opportunities and constraints of history and social circumstance' (Elder, Johnson & Crosnoe, 2003, p. 11). The chapter is divided into six parts. The first sets out how the data is used. Three further sections offer accounts of the diverse labour market experiences of individuals in the three age cohorts. The final part reframes the discussion about choice in terms of risk in order to make connections between the life courses of disabled persons and wider socio-economic structures. The chapter ends by drawing broad lessons for the future.

Interpreting the data on labour market careers

Methodological considerations

The data analysed in this chapter derives from questions asked about employment as one of several themes explored in the life-course interviews. Research participants were asked to provide biographical information on work they had done, choices they had made and about the ease or difficulty in accessing the labour market over their lifetime. Not all interviews were transcribed, nor were translations available to the study consortium. Instead, data from the interviews was summarised using a template in which researchers recorded the main trajectories, transitions and turning points from each interview (see Chapter 3). These offer rich data on labour market careers, but do not have the detail of full transcripts. Another challenge has been how to present findings from a large number of interviews. In this chapter, the summaries are used to identify broad trajectories, transitions and turning points – what Biewer et al. (2015) refer to as 'pathways' – and major sources of opportunity and constraint. In this chapter, individual accounts are aggregated to offer a thematic overview organised by age cohort rather than by country, gender or disability. Where relevant, however, these other dimensions are highlighted.

Structure, agency and narratives of disability

The structuration theory that guides the DISCIT study informs this chapter (Stones, 2005). Following Heinz (2003, p. 185), labour market careers are seen as shaped by a 'reciprocal relationship' between individual agency and structure. Accordingly the chapter highlights structures, conceived of as the enabling and constraining practices of powerful agents (e.g. employers, service providers and policy makers – at international, national, regional and local level) as well as the agency of disabled persons (Fraccaroli & Depolo, 2008; Heinz, 2003). Conceptually, the practices of state actors, employers and disabled persons are seen as guided by existing narratives of disability (alongside those of age and gender (Mik-Meyer, 2015; Vick & Lightman, 2010)). For instance, the labour market careers of persons with disabilities are often characterised by labour market exclusion, rationalised by a narrative of deficit (Barnes & Mercer, 2005). Such narratives have legitimised practices of exclusion and preference for income replacement. Challenging such narratives, social and relational models of disability argue that the 'limitations' of disability result from oppressive structures and practices (Traustadóttir, 2009). They tell a counter-narrative of inaccessible workplaces, discrimination and limited support.

By analysing the employment experiences of persons with disabilities, the chapter offers evidence of how choice has been promoted or constrained for this group. Also, by reframing some issues in terms of risk in the final section, it also highlights some concerns raised by the research participants about potential labour market outcomes.

Trajectories, transitions and turning points

Labour market careers are described in this chapter using the concepts of *trajectories, transitions*, and *turning points. Trajectories* are long-term patterns of stability and change, usually involving multiple transitions (Hutchison, 2010; Priestley, 2003). They represent progressions through the labour market over the life course. *Transitions* and *turning points* indicate progression and changes of direction within trajectories. Choice features as people make decisions about what they do, who with, and where (Elder, Johnson & Crosnoe, 2003). Importantly, in the case of persons with disabilities' labour market careers, choices are not always made by disabled persons themselves. The following sections explore the labour market careers of the three age cohorts. Each section provides an overview of trajectories, transitions and turning points and the factors that provided opportunities for or constraints on active agency in employment. A broader discussion of choice and risk is presented later in the chapter.

The 1950s cohort

Trajectories

Even more so than the other two cohorts, interviewees born around 1950 afford a long-term perspective on disabled persons' labour market careers. In the present context of employment histories, entering the labour market after school graduation and eventually retiring from working life represent two major life course transitions. Together, they set the perimeters of the 1950s cohort's career progression, which is interspersed with a variety of transitions and phases, including job changes and spells of unemployment. With the exception of persons with intellectual impairments, numerous participants had 'mainstream' employment biographies, although it became clear that they often had to overcome particular challenges and expend great effort to achieve these. While the available data (across all three cohorts) did not allow for a 'typology' of employment trajectories like, for example, that presented by Latcheva and Herzog-Punzenberger (2011) for migrant workers in Austria, factors such as gender, national disability policy frameworks and, in particular, impairment type seem to have had a certain structuring impact.

Transitions and turning points

One quarter of the cohort with early onset of their impairment had undergone vocational training and, partly overlapping with this group, one in three had pursued tertiary education. After completing secondary or tertiary education, most started out with a job in the open labour market with a range of employers from the private, public and the third sectors (e.g. organisations of persons with disabilities). There were, however, marked differences based on impairment group. While all persons with psychosocial impairments and most persons with visual or mobility impairments found employment in the open labour market, the majority of persons with intellectual impairments started work in sheltered settings, often continuing their previous segregated educational pathways. There was, however, some variation. At least six persons with intellectual difficulties from five of the DISCIT countries took up their first job in the open labour market, while two persons with mobility impairments (an Irish woman and a German man) started off in a sheltered workshop. A very small number of participants, for example one British man in the visual impairment category, and a Serbian man and a British man in the intellectual impairment group, reported no work throughout their entire adult life.

Securing a first job in the mainstream labour market was a relatively smooth transition for some, such as in cases where a person stayed on with an employer after an apprenticeship or where there were reserved occupations (e.g. telephone operators and masseurs) and quotas, as was the case in Italy and Sweden for persons with visual impairments. But work could also be a daunting experience. As in the other cohorts, participants with visual impairments spoke about applying for jobs but not receiving any response; for instance, a male Irish interviewee with a visual impairment had applied for over 70 jobs but got called for only 4 interviews. A female Irish interviewee got her first job after one attempt but reported being subjected to verbal abuse in the process due to her disability. People in other impairment categories spoke of long periods of unemployment, and feeling they were unable to get a job due to their disability (e.g. a male Czech interviewee in the mobility impairment category).

Employment patterns among the interviewees were varied. While part-time and temporary work was common, a number of participants had also worked full-time in permanent jobs and for an extended part of their careers. Most showed patterns of lateral career mobility, i.e. moving from one job to another at an equivalent skill and remuneration level. Vertical career advancement, either within the same organisation or by moving to better-paid and more prestigious jobs, was less prevalent. However, most people experienced lateral movements positively if they led to more suitable employment. In addition, unemployment and parenthood represented major changes. While only four persons were unemployed at the time of the interviews, many more instances of unemployment were mentioned. Periods of redundancy were generally difficult, but occasionally offered a time of personal reorientation, leading to new employment opportunities more attuned to people's interests and capabilities. Similarly, and notably for women, marriage and parenthood constituted significant turning points in their employment trajectories. These often led to temporary or extended withdrawals from the labour market, but could also open up new employment paths when they later returned to the labour force after, for example, having undergone occupational retraining or taking up further education.

Not surprisingly for this cohort, most participants' present status was (early) retirement, although a few continued to work beyond the official retirement age, were self-employed or pursued voluntary work. Early retirement was not always voluntary. Often people's pathways seem to have involved the gradual and sometimes early withdrawal from the labour market before reaching the official retirement age, due to a growing mismatch between increasing work demands on the one hand and limited work ability on the other. These trajectories also often involved a gradual shift from permanent full-time employment to a reliance on disability benefits, with temporary part-time jobs and unemployment benefits forming intermediate steps. This tendency might have been exacerbated by a perceived unwillingness of employers to hire persons who have a disability and/or are already past the age of 50. Disability benefits could then be seen as becoming a substitute for expiring unemployment benefits and a means of tiding recipients over until the official retirement age is reached.

Barriers and facilitators

The major personal and structural factors and dynamics influencing the careers of the 1950s cohort were similar to those found in other studies (e.g. Lindstrom, Hirano, McCarthy & Alverson, 2014; Vick & Lightman, 2010). In the interviewees' narratives, family members (e.g. parents, spouses or siblings) played either a constructive and supportive or, in contrast, a restrictive and constraining role. Similarly, there were stories about employers and co-workers who had been helpful and others who had not, depending on their attitudes towards persons with disabilities. In the case of persons with psychosocial difficulties, there was no discernible trend with regard to the (non)disclosure of their condition. In some cases, the interviewee preferred not to disclose their difficulties (e.g. the female Czech participant) and in others they found it helpful to let the employers and work colleagues know about their psychosocial issues (e.g. the Swiss male participant). Interactions with representatives of the various disability services were also often described as difficult and unsatisfactory, such as those featuring disagreements about retraining needs. The availability of appropriate state support and services was an explanatory factor for the participation in the mainstream labour market as well. The female Italian interviewee with psychosocial difficulties, for instance, was very dissatisfied that after her mental health problems had stabilised she was only offered a place in a co-operative and that no additional efforts were made to move her closer to the mainstream labour market over time.

The 1970s cohort

Trajectories

Individuals in the 1970s cohort entered the labour market at a time when a perception of persons with disabilities as rights-bearing subjects was developing (Waddington & Hendriks, 2002). Improvements in workplace accessibility, new technologies and anti-discrimination policies shaped the prospects of a group who, until the mid-1990s, had been marginal in employment policy (Hohnen, 2004). Whilst these developments were gradual and uneven (for example countries such as Serbia developed policies only relatively recently), they nonetheless shaped opportunities for people entering the labour market from the mid-1980s onwards. Most found regular work, securing a diversity of part- and full-time jobs, and some had opportunities for advancement. This cohort also had opportunities for education; over a third entered higher education and several studied to Masters or PhD level. Most in the mobility impairment and several from the visual and psychosocial impairment categories attended university.

Some took alternative pathways. In the UK, four participants were wholly supported by the social care and benefits systems. In Ireland, Norway and Sweden, men and women in the intellectual impairment category entered day services or activities. In Germany, Norway, Sweden and Switzerland, individuals from the same group spent large parts of their careers in sheltered contexts. One German woman spoke of the assumption that she was not 'fit' to work in the open labour market. In Serbia, participants in the intellectual and psychosocial impairment categories started in institutional settings, followed by un-contracted casual labour. Across several countries, women and some men in the intellectual and psychosocial impairment categories took low-paid jobs, as kitchen workers or cleaners for instance, either casually, in sheltered settings, or under integration schemes. A small number felt that long periods on training contracts had reduced their active agency.

Over time many participants reduced their work activities or left the labour market due to changes in health or impairment. Despite histories of work, some felt they got little support to stay on from the social security systems and employment services. Redundancy and non-renewal of contracts were also an issue, notably for women raising children. Dismissal protection kept people in work for only a short time. Others spoke of difficulties finding jobs relevant to their qualifications and skills, of the impacts of demanding and challenging roles, and of the effects of limited accessibility and discrimination on employment.

Transitions and turning points

In most cases participants started jobs after leaving education. Some were out of work initially, but these periods were not usually extensive. Many worked in part-time, temporary posts before moving on to longer-term roles. As is also the case for the 1990s cohort, work entry was usually facilitated by the *social service subsystem*. Vocational and skills-based training, employment subsidies and quota jobs were all identified. Many maintained their careers over time. The majority of the 1970s cohort was in work in 2014, either in a regular contract, subsidised or supported employment or a sheltered job. Few had had only one job, although some stayed on in sheltered, subsidised or quota jobs, only moving into new roles in the same company. Many spoke of leaving jobs and finding other work, and of undertaking retraining, particularly people in the visual and mobility impairment categories. One woman from Sweden retrained in computer science after a number of administrative roles. She went on to teach and become an author. Lateral career mobility allowed many to find work better suited to them. Several in the visual, psychosocial and mobility impairment categories also talked of vertical mobility, of promotion and career advancement, describing trajectories that led to a high level of satisfaction. This was often enabled by accessible working environments and support from colleagues and superiors.

There were differences between those in the open labour market and those in segregated employment. While a few had moved from sheltered work to regular or supported work, several had wholly segregated careers or moved into sheltered work soon after entering the open labour market. As in other cohorts, most movement into segregated work was among those in the intellectual impairment group. These respondents, many of whom had segregated school backgrounds, reported fewer opportunities to choose work in the open labour market, reflecting the influence of family and support workers. For instance, one Irish man in the intellectual impairment group held two non-contract jobs. These were identified by a support worker at the day centre he attended. While he was content with his situation, others felt more could be done to extend their range of options.

Employment downturns were also reported. By 2014, nearly half of the individuals in the psychosocial impairment group had retired as a result of ill health and time in treatment. This included one British man who, after a period of mental illness that led to reduced physical health, spent much of his time in a day centre. More broadly, a large portion of the cohort saw their health deteriorate. At times this preceded retirement from work or led to people re-entering work in a different way (e.g. part-time and with income maintenance). Changing family circumstances also influenced employment trajectories. Several women with visual, psychosocial and mobility impairments described leaving or taking time off to raise children. Some returned to jobs they were doing before they stopped work, some got different jobs, often in different conditions, and others stayed out of the labour market. Some made use of dismissal protection; a couple, however, had their contracts terminated after that protection ran out. One German woman in the psychosocial impairment group found that accessing employment services was made more difficult by being a mother. The view was that she should not seek work while her children were young.

Barriers and facilitators

A range of factors facilitated and restricted people's labour market careers. One major factor was health, which many saw as restricting their options (and thus as a barrier in itself). In some cases people spoke about the mismatch between their work capacity and the jobs available and about lack of support and inappropriate working expectations. Some entered the labour market with an ongoing mental or physical condition, while others faced new issues over time. Taking time out or changing working patterns (e.g. going part-time) were often mentioned as ways to adjust to changes in health and impairment that were not necessarily matched to existing work arrangements. Many decided to seek alternative employment, a decision that could be positive as people sought better roles.

Others talked about inadequate support. While some benefited from adaptations, in-work support and assistive technologies, others described the unavailability of these or difficulties accessing them. Others complained about restrictive assessments of work capacity and of a lack of opportunities to retrain (again including many in the psychosocial impairment group). One Norwegian man, who had previously been a successful businessman, felt that after changes in his physical health it was seen as easier to grant him a full disability pension than to help him find appropriate work. In such cases, barriers were the result of the attitudes of employment service staff and health professionals and the lack of or inefficiency of structures designed to promote labour market integration. Likewise, the attitudes of employers could be a barrier. Some people experienced difficulties getting work, while others described how they lost work due to assumptions about their ability. Some spoke of difficult relationships with supervisors and co-workers. Difficulties entering and staying on were further compounded by environmental factors, such as transport problems.

While barriers were numerous, there were also facilitators. Several people in the visual and mobility impairment groups noted how the workplace had improved as attitudes to inclusion changed and adaptations, technologies and personal support became more available. Others mentioned employers, service provider staff and other people who actively provided support or an accessible environment, and encouraged them to seek out what satisfied them. For instance, a German woman in the mobility impairment group, after completing a PhD, held a range of jobs, each of which was adapted to her needs. In addition people talked about training schemes as a way into work. Employment programmes, wage subsidies, quotas, rehabilitation services and support through the income maintenance subsystem structured the employment trajectories of the cohort. Finally, while there were accounts of discrimination, many also had support from employers. Family also provided support (frequently as sources of work) and disability organisations employed several participants.

The 1990s cohort

Trajectories

The employment trajectories of the 1990s cohort reflected young people's aspirations and efforts to 'get in' and 'stay on' at work. Trajectories were characterised by movements through training, education and early work experience as individuals hoped to find jobs they liked to do. In most cases their trajectories and concerns resembled those of young people in Europe generally (Mascherini, Ludwinek, Vacas, Meierkord & Gebel, 2014). Many described their hopes for work and their worries about navigating a competitive and demanding labour market. Experiences of work were also, for many, transitory, part-time, and punctuated by periods of unemployment. Across the countries, many had held non-standard jobs, including temporary, casual, freelance and voluntary roles.

There were differences from this picture, however. While most took 'mainstream' routes into work direct from school or following vocational training or higher or further education, a small number entered sheltered work or day services. Such pathways were structured by national policy systems. For instance, day services in the UK, Ireland and Sweden provided out-of-work activities, while sheltered work was still available to people in the Czech Republic, Germany and Switzerland (although with a greater range of options of employment and training, such as new social enterprises and government training schemes). Mostly these were provided to young people in the intellectual impairment category after segregated education, and to some in the psychosocial impairment category. In Serbia, one young woman described visiting an organisation where she made clothes and jewellery. This unpaid role provided her with activities through the day.

Those entering the open labour market also spoke of barriers such as a lack of accessible jobs, limited skills and qualifications, and discrimination from employers. Some remained unemployed or moved out of the labour market in the absence of effective early support (Greve, 2009). Formal assessments by state agencies determined access to benefits on the basis of work capacity. These incorporated different assumptions, ranging from medical models of functional deficit in countries such as Serbia and the Czech Republic to work capability models in the UK and Norway, to assess people as able to work or entitled to out-of-work support.

Transitions and turning points

Trajectories were typically characterised by engagement in employability schemes (run by public services, or alternatively NGOs as in the Czech Republic), which individuals from each country made decisions to enter. Participation in these schemes gave access to job placements, job search support, and job coaching. Such activities could enhance employment prospects where individuals experienced difficulty in finding work after education or vocational training, or, in a few cases, after a period of illness. One young Swedish man with a visual impairment had applied for multiple jobs over the course of seven months. He eventually got a permanent job contract after a short subsidised placement supported by the public employment service. In a small number of cases, participants had no access to such support. One young woman in the psychosocial impairment group in Serbia returned to the family home after school and carried out domestic work. In other countries, people entered a scheme but had not found work. Some made use of the available services but for others services were limited or unavailable and expectations that work could be found were reduced.

One feature of the employment trajectories of the 1990s cohort was the time spent in casual, short-term or temporary roles (such as seasonal work). Many labour market careers started in non-contract or seasonal jobs. For a small number still in education (including postgraduate education) this represented most or all of the work they had done. In addition, several people spent time doing freelance work. One young Czech woman in the psychosocial impairment category (the only woman in the cohort to have had children) had done home tuition while her children were young. Such work was often done without a regular contract, and provided income and experience in the absence of an employment contract. It was also common for participants to enter voluntary work to gain experience in the hope that such work would lead to a contracted and paid role. For example, this was reported by one young British man who was managing projects for a visual impairment charity – a common practice as young people approached organisations of persons with disabilities to strengthen their CVs.

Time in employability schemes and casual roles meant most young people had some experience of work. Most eventually entered periods of relative work stability (an artefact of the study sampling criteria which sought people with work experience, although not all people worked extensively). For some this happened soon after entering the labour market or after a period of skills development. It was common for people to highlight when they 'got in'. Many spoke of the importance of finding a first job, especially if they found they were not getting called for interviews, as many young people with visual impairments reported. Others also spoke about finding better work after doing jobs they felt were unsatisfactory. One young Czech woman in the intellectual impairment category decided to go back to school because her job in a sheltered workshop (which her mother had secured) was 'boring'. Two interviewees from the 1990s cohort in Ireland similarly attended a course designed to expand the options of people with intellectual impairments.

As a result there was movement for many into work, and some found work satisfaction after a while. There were multiple cases where people lost or left a job. People spoke of unrewarding or demanding jobs, or jobs in which they had been in conflict with colleagues or supervisors or had been labelled as 'underachieving'. Bad relations with supervisors featured in several of the summaries in the psychosocial impairment category. For instance, a young Italian woman was compelled to leave one job after complaints about her behaviour. After hearing about a job in another co-operative from her mother, she found work with a supportive supervisor. Having been employed since 2011, she was considering other ways in which she could be more independent. Leaving a job was not always a negative transition. In some cases it led to periods of unemployment, but often it eventually led to alternative opportunities in employment, education or training.

Barriers and facilitators

Some barriers related to personal circumstance. Across all nine countries, people said that lack of experience, qualifications or skills presented barriers to work. Many also felt that impairment made job entry harder. In contrast, there was less attention (even among young women) to unpaid domestic work as an employment barrier (Henriksson, Liedberg & Gerdle, 2005). These factors were seen as a barrier in relation to a job market that many said was competitive, demanding, and provided few job opportunities. One young Norwegian man spoke of a loss of practical jobs that visually impaired people could do, while a young Swedish woman said there were no longer any established career paths for visually impaired people. One common experience reported by young people with visual impairments was of applying for jobs but of hearing no response. Prejudice was also often cited as a barrier. Many said employer assumptions about their ability limited their prospects.

Combined barriers of personal circumstance, labour market and employer prejudice meant many young people in the 1990s cohort experienced difficulty finding work. These factors also shaped experiences in work. Some said they were working in jobs that paid low wages and gave few progression opportunities. Some also made conscious decisions around work, such as only to work part-time or to leave jobs in which they faced difficulties with supervisors or colleagues or with the allocation of tasks, and to enter employability schemes to boost their skills and experience. In this context, some spoke of efforts to minimise or conceal impairment (notably a psychosocial impairment) in order to prove their ability as reliable and productive employees (often, however, this led to periods of stress-related illness).

In some cases, barriers to work were not reduced by the disability policy system. For example, while services could positively influence employment trajectories, they were not always available or sufficient. In several countries, people described unhelpful employment service staff. One young Swedish woman felt she was not listened to by one employment agency. With the support of a new employment counsellor and an EU initiative, she eventually started her own business. Others highlighted the difficulty of getting technologies or support because of delay or lack of employer support. In addition, some spoke of the inadequacy of anti-discrimination laws and quota systems. One young German man said that quota systems set an informal upper employment limit for persons with disabilities. A young British woman in the visual impairment category said anti-discrimination laws failed to prevent discrimination. For those who relied on sheltered work programmes, some complained about a lack of range in their jobs, low pay and low prospects, and of difficult relationships with managers.

Not all relationships with colleagues and supervisors were problematic. For some, a good manager who showed confidence in them could be influential. It was also common for participants to identify the importance of support from family and friends. Several were employed by a family member. Relationships with staff from employment services were less often seen as influential, although the *social service subsystem* also featured prominently. Workplace adaptations, employability schemes and structured employment opportunities offered choices to disabled young people who found ‘getting in’ difficult. Jobs were also made sustainable by sheltered, subsidised or supported work programmes, or by technologies, adaptations or support. A few people who entered sheltered workplaces chose to change jobs without leaving the organisation. Finally, the *income maintenance subsystem* enabled some people classed as having a partial disability to work part-time. The presence or absence of appropriate services and support was crucial in determining if a person worked or not (Halvorsen & Hvinden, 2015; Mascherini, Salvatore, Meierkord & Jungblut, 2012).

Discussion: choice and risk

The previous sections have provided an overview of the labour market careers described by persons with disabilities in three age cohorts. Reflecting on the factors that enhanced or constrained labour market participation, it becomes possible to make some sense of the ways people seemed to have limited choice at times or no power to make a difference, and how governments can aim to influence choice. In this way, we can explore further the key Active Citizenship principle of *autonomy* and the extent to which persons with disabilities are able to exercise it. In addition, this section explores the issue of risk, and asks to what extent risk is a feature of life courses for persons with disabilities that might modify choice.

Exercising choice

Some participants in the DISCIT study described high levels of choice and control in their labour market careers. For instance, several in the 1950s and 1970s cohorts felt they had been able to decide which jobs they had done and where they had worked. Often they felt they had little use for employment services and had achieved things through their own efforts. Such narratives came mainly from people in the mobility impairment group whose careers unfolded in the open labour market in the context of support and modifications. Other people's trajectories were more marked by constrained choices. In the psychosocial and visual impairment groups, people talked about choice and lateral mobility. Having choice was realised in being able to take new jobs, although choices may have been made in consideration of things such as impairment and available support. In each case, choice was linked to expressed satisfaction.

Choices were not only experienced in open labour market trajectories. Different opportunities were available to people in segregated employment. For instance, people in sheltered employment, predominantly in the intellectual impairment group, felt they had chosen where they wished to work and what they had wanted to do. Typically this meant that they had been given a *limited range* of options by social workers and family. As in other cases, satisfaction was at times reported by individuals in the intellectual impairment group. Some, however, reported *very* limited choices in where they worked and what they did. This suggests that choices have historically been distributed differently to disabled persons. People with intellectual impairments have long been seen as having limited capacity to make choices, and other actors have stepped in to make decisions in their place. Indeed, across the older cohorts were people (notably in the intellectual impairment group, but in other categories as well) who had little employment history. In such cases, it seemed that a choice to work was not offered and that people were instead directed towards social care systems or had been in institutions.

Choices could also be restricted in other ways. For instance, many participants who made use of employment services spoke about having choices made for them, or having being offered a narrow set of choices. Women in particular talked about being denied opportunities to pursue work after having children. In these cases, people felt their choices were restricted, sometimes from vocational education onwards. These included people with visual and intellectual impairments. Another restriction, reported by persons in the psychosocial impairment group, was of people having failed to give them choice. For some the only option seemed to have been to exit the labour market and to move onto benefits.

In the 1990s cohort, choice was more often linked to the directions people hoped to take in life. Choices were available in education and in the kinds of jobs people hoped to get. More often, however, people in the 1990s cohort felt that labour market conditions restricted their choices. Just as young people felt empowered to make choices about their lives, they also felt that the structures were not favourable enough for the realisation of their aspirations.

Experiencing risk

The data not only showed the extent to which participants made choices but also provided evidence of the enduring degree of risk experienced by persons with disabilities, which influenced their labour market careers. These risks, for instance the sense that prejudice, ill health and lack of support might lead to unemployment and exclusion, were not necessarily 'new' although the experience of them could take on new forms as people felt compelled to see finding work as their responsibility (Taylor-Gooby, 2004). From the analysis of the life-course interview data, the *role of employers, public employment services* and the *state of the labour market* emerge as key determinants of people's labour market trajectories. This is not surprising – in difficult labour market conditions persons with disabilities are vulnerable to losing their jobs if companies reduce their workforces, and are disadvantaged in the open labour market as larger numbers of non-disabled people begin competing for fewer job vacancies. Here it is possible to identify the limitations of countries' disability policy systems that have no direct influence over labour market factors, particularly the demand for labour. There were examples of changes in the labour market that reduced opportunities for persons with disabilities. Lower numbers of secure low-skilled jobs and the difficulty of entering higher skilled occupations made finding work harder for persons with disabilities. These barriers could also be exacerbated by employment services not offering appropriate support, either due to lack of funds or due to the assumptions of service provider staff about the capacity and willingness of individuals to work.

For younger individuals, emerging labour market conditions, underfunding of services and the apparent weakness of anti-discrimination legislation forged *new experiences of risk*. For example, across all age cohorts, people with visual impairments felt that employers were less willing to take them on in jobs generally advertised. This barrier was heightened for younger people by the loss of established career paths for visually impaired people, in part due to technological changes making roles such as telephone operator less necessary, but also due to an emphasis on individual aspiration. Prejudice was not necessarily reduced by new assistive devices and in-work supports. While many in the 1970s and 1990s cohorts felt these could be effective, too often they were hard to access due to slow administrative processes, tough entitlement criteria and under-resourced employment services. Some thus felt that an emphasis on open labour market entry and individual choice increased risk, as routes to work were largely on the same terms as non-disabled people. As one young participant said:

> In reality I think people would rather employ somebody with no disabilities whatsoever because it's less hassle. You know, what's easier? Getting an ergonomically adapted chair for someone with a spinal injury or saying here's a normal chair, crack on?
>
> (UK, Female, 1990s cohort, visually impaired group)

For many of the younger participants, the emphasis seemed to be on creating their own paths in the absence of large structures designed to guide the labour market careers of disabled persons. Risk appeared to have been individualised for these participants (O'Rand, 2003). Conversely, across all the countries in the DISCIT study some people referred to improved *attitudes towards persons with disabilities* and a greater recognition of persons with disabilities as valuable employees. In other cases people spoke of good services, of securing technologies, adaptations and support, and of the positive effects of a general 'consciousness' about disabled persons' rights. This mirrored suggestions that people had benefited from changes in anti-discrimination law and policy, and indicated the positive influence of government policy on the life course (Leisering, 2003). However, it must be added that for some the benefits of improved attitudes were reduced by other shifts in the economy (such as the introduction of austerity measures) and the labour market (such as the loss of jobs particularly suited to persons with disabilities). In the accounts of their employment trajectories, many people also described *changes in their health* as influencing their work and work prospects. For some, health improvements enabled them to think about work if they were unemployed and make progress towards the labour market, but declining health meant reducing their labour market participation or leaving the labour market completely. These experiences point to *risk as an enduring feature* of the life course of persons with disabilities.

Conclusion

This chapter has presented findings from the DISCIT study about the labour market careers of persons with disabilities in three age cohorts. It has reflected on the diverse trajectories *across* and *within* the three age cohorts and also for men and women in different impairment groups. It has shown the different routes by which people entered the labour market and the different forms of employment they took up. It has also shown the divergent paths people embarked on as a product of changes in family life, the labour market, policy, health and impairment, and public provisions. Importantly it has shown some of the continuing and common difficulties persons with disabilities face, such as the challenge of discrimination, and of fluctuations in people's capacity to enter work over time. As should be expected from such a diverse sample, careers varied in a large number of ways. This was because of (1) varying labour market conditions and levels of labour market integration, (2) key stakeholders' perceptions of employability and work capacity (e.g. family, employers, health professionals and service providers), (3) the availability of services, regulations and social protection, and (4) individual and collective decisions around education, training, work, family life, health and welfare. These factors represent a range of opportunities and constraints.

In general, it has been possible to identify factors that have shaped the employment trajectories of the persons with disabilities participating in the DISCIT project and to identify transitions and turning points that have been associated with employment progression. The life-course approach also provides some detail on how changing labour market conditions and developments in countries' disability policy systems were experienced across the different age cohorts, although the degree to which these can be reviewed systematically or in detail is restricted by the limitations of the DISCIT data. It must be remembered that this chapter is based on an innovative qualitative design with a large sample spread across multiple countries. It is currently not methodologically appropriate to try to derive any generalised conclusions from such data about the employment trajectories experienced by the three age cohorts. What has been possible, however, is to demonstrate the diversity in people's experiences and trajectories over time, and from these to raise some issues that may be considered in further research.

For instance, one enduring issue across the three cohorts is employers' attitudes and behaviour towards persons with disabilities, often experienced as prejudice and discrimination, and thus as a source of risk in that labour market exclusion entails a range of other problems for persons with disabilities. This presents a persistent challenge for policy makers, NGOs and others seeking to promote employment opportunities. A focus on potential risks created by the practices of external agents, including employers, but also state actors, is as important as any emphasis on the degree to which persons with disabilities feel empowered to make choices.

One policy lesson emerges from the finding that *all* forms of policy and programme initiatives have produced some beneficiaries, i.e. persons with disabilities who have found meaningful and satisfying work, including policies such as quota systems and sheltered employment that have fallen out of favour or been rejected in some countries. This is not to suggest a return to large, segregated institutions as the settings for providing employment opportunities for persons with disabilities. Rather the findings suggest that some useful lessons could be learned about what was valued by the people working within those structures and about how that might inform practices in other, less stigmatising environments. More widely, in thinking about the future there is arguably merit in reconsidering the full range of policy mechanisms used over the past 50–60 years and reassessing them in the light of current economic and social conditions.

At a theoretical level, the life-course data collected in the DISCIT study provides further evidence of how the interaction between structure and agency shape labour market trajectories of persons with disabilities. We can also see how structures, in the form of components of countries' disability policy systems, can increase or restrict agency. The 1950s cohort arguably had fewer opportunities to benefit from social services provision compared to the two later cohorts for the simple reason that fewer services existed. However, the data also suggests that they had more chances to enter the open labour market in the mid- to late 1960s when the economies of Europe provided more employment opportunities compared with those open to the 1990s cohort. The 'labour market exclusion' narrative of Barnes and Mercer (2005) certainly finds support in the accounts of people in the interview sample from all three cohorts, while a narrative of oppressive structures and practices argued by Traustadóttir (2009) is also identifiable in accounts that describe restricted choice and the experience of discrimination.

To conclude, this chapter shows the need to recognise the continuing challenges faced by persons with disabilities in the labour market and the need for increased efforts to design appropriate support and help that gives persons with disabilities real choice and autonomy in pursuing their individual labour market goals and aspirations. Until that has been accomplished, the prospects for persons with disabilities achieving full and active participation in society will continue to be severely limited.

References

Barnes, C. & Mercer, G. (2005). Disability, work, and welfare: Challenging the social exclusion of disabled people. *Work, Employment & Society: A Journal of the British Sociological Association*, *19*(3), 527–545.

Biewer, G., Buchner, T., Shevlin, M., Smyth, F., Šiška, J., Káňová, Š., … Rodríguez Díaz, S. (2015). Pathways to inclusion in European higher education systems. *ALTER – European Journal of Disability Research*, *9*(4), 278–289.

Elder, G. H., Jr, Johnson, M. K. & Crosnoe, R. (2003). The emergence and development of life course theory. In J. T. Mortimer & M. J. Shanahan (Eds), *Handbook of the life course* (pp. 3–19). New York: Springer.

Fraccaroli, F. & Depolo, M. (2008). Careers and aging at work. In N. Chmiel (Ed.), *Introduction to work and organizational psychology: A European perspective* (pp. 97–118). Oxford: Blackwell.

Greve, B. (2009). *The labour market situation of disabled people in European countries and implementation of employment policies: A summary of evidence from country reports and research studies*. ANED. Retrieved from: www.disability-europe.net/content/aned/media/ANED%20Task%206%20final%20report%20-%20final%20version%2017-04-09.pdf.

Halvorsen, R. & Hvinden, B. (2015). *New policies to promote youth inclusion: Accommodation of diversity in the Nordic welfare states*. Copenhagen: Nordic Council of Ministers.

Heinz, W. R. (2003). From work trajectories to negotiated careers. In J. T. Mortimer & M. J. Shanahan (Eds), *Handbook of the life course* (pp. 185–204). New York: Springer.

Henriksson, C. M., Liedberg, G. M. & Gerdle, B. (2005). Women with fibromyalgia: Work and rehabilitation. *Disability and Rehabilitation*, *27*(12), 685–694.

Hohnen, P. (2004). Experiences of participation citizenship: A bottom-up analysis of the social rights and obligations of work-disabled employees in Denmark and the Netherlands. *European Spine Journal: Official Publication of the European Spine Society, the European Spinal Deformity Society, and the European Section of the Cervical Spine Research Society*, *6*, 205.

Hutchison, E. D. (2010). A life course perspective. In E. D. Hutchison (Ed.), *Dimensions of human behavior: The changing life course* (pp. 1–38). Thousand Oaks, CA: Sage.

Latcheva, R. & Herzog-Punzenberger, B. (2011). Integration trajectories: A mixed method approach. In M. Wingens, H. de V. M. Windzio & C. Aybek (Eds), *A life course perspective on migration and integration* (pp. 121–142). Berlin: Springer.

Leisering, L. (2003). Government and the life course. In J. T. Mortimer & M. J. Shanahan (Eds), *Handbook of the life course* (pp. 205–225). New York: Springer.

Lindstrom, L., Hirano, K. A., McCarthy, C. & Alverson, C. Y. (2014). 'Just having a job': Career advancement for low-wage workers with intellectual and developmental disabilities. *Career Development and Transition for Exceptional Individuals*, *37*(1), 40–49.

Mascherini, M., Ludwinek, A., Vacas, C., Meierkord, A. & Gebel, M. (2014). *Mapping youth transitions in Europe*. Luxembourg: Publications Office of the European Union.

Mascherini, M., Salvatore, L., Meierkord, A. & Jungblut, J.-M. (2012). *NEETs: Young people not in employment, education or training: Characteristics, costs and policy responses in Europe*. Luxembourg: Publications Office of the European Union.

Mik-Meyer, N. (2015). Gender and disability: Feminizing male employees with visible impairments in Danish work organizations. *Gender, Work, and Organization*, *22*(6), 579–595.

O'Rand, A. M. (2003). The future of the life course. In J. T. Mortimer & M. J. Shanahan (Eds), *Handbook of the life course* (pp. 693–701). New York: Springer.

Priestley, M. (2003). *Disability: A life course approach*. Cambridge: Polity.

Stones, R. (2005). *Structuration theory*. Basingstoke: Palgrave Macmillan.

Taylor-Gooby, P. (2004). *New risk, new welfare: The transformation of the European welfare state*. Oxford: Oxford University Press.

Traustadóttir, R. (2009). Disability studies, the social model and legal developments. In O. M. Arnardóttir & G. Quinn (Eds), *The UN convention on the rights of persons with disabilities* (pp. 1–16). Leiden: Martinus Nijhoff.

Vick, A. & Lightman, E. (2010). Barriers to employment among women with complex episodic disabilities. *Journal of Disability Policy Studies*, *21*(2), 70–80.

Waddington, L. & Hendriks, A. (2002). The expanding concept of employment discrimination in Europe: From direct and indirect discrimination to reasonable accommodation discrimination. *International Journal of Comparative Labour Law and Industrial Relations*, *18*(4), 403–428.

6 Identity and political participation throughout the life course

The experience of persons with disabilities in European countries

Anemari Karačić, Andreas Sturm, Anne Waldschmidt and Timo Dins

For a long time, persons with disabilities have been regarded merely as recipients of welfare without any possibility of exercising influence in political life and public affairs. This situation has gradually changed, mostly as a result of the international disability rights movements that emerged in the 1970s. Largely as a response to disability rights activism, Article 29 of the United Nations Convention on the Rights of Persons with Disabilities has established the right of disabled persons to full and effective 'participation in political and public life' on an equal basis with others. Accordingly, DISCIT's concept of Active Citizenship focuses not only on the dimensions of social security and personal autonomy, but also on political influence. These three dimensions are interrelated, i.e. security and autonomy are substantial preconditions for influence in political matters. For pragmatic reasons, however, we only consider the latter in the following.

The life course greatly determines whether a person remains a passive political citizen or becomes actively involved in politics and public affairs, be it individually, e.g. as a voter, or collectively, as a member of civil society organisations (Acheson & Williamson, 2001; Sandvin, 2003; Schur, Kruse & Blanck, 2013; Schur, Shields & Schriner, 2005; Shah & Priestley, 2011). Earlier research has also indicated that there are close links between political engagement and individual self-concepts (Anspach, 1979; Crenshaw, 1991; Miller, Gurin, Gurin & Malanchuk, 1981; Putnam, 2005; Sandvin, 2003; Scotch, 1988; Shakespeare, 1996). Within the field of disability studies, different self-concepts are discussed with reference to different models of disability (Oliver, 2013). In this contribution, we are interested in the question of how the life courses of persons with disabilities, their individual identities and their forms of political (non-)engagement are interrelated.

In the beginning of this chapter, we discuss possible connections between the life course, identity and political participation of disabled persons from a conceptual point of view. By reviewing existing studies, we aim to develop a heuristic approach for our empirical analysis. Based on guided interviews with men and women with different disabilities from four European countries, belonging to three age groups (see Chapter 3), we first present a system of categorisation and then offer an overview of the data; second, we focus on the (inter-)relations between the life course, identity and political participation; and third, we offer an empirically grounded typology of (non-)engagement in organisations representing persons with disabilities. We conclude this chapter by discussing the results of our analysis.

Linking life course, political participation and identity – a relational concept

Following DISCIT's approach of structuration theory (see Chapter 2), this contribution explores the complex relationships between external and internal structures as well as individual practices, with special regard to the life courses of persons with disabilities. When analysing the interdependencies between life courses, forms of political engagement and individual identities we intend to think in circles and processes instead of assuming fixed structures resulting in pre-determined actions. To apply this complex approach, we first need to consider each of the relevant three notions – the life course, political participation and identity – in relation to one another. We start with defining our basic concepts.

First, when using the life course approach we follow Priestley (2003: 4), who understands life courses as 'the ways in which disabled lives are understood, organized and governed within societies', thus focusing not only on individual biographies, but also on the wider social context, and exploring the relationships between structures and practices. Second, for practical reasons our understanding of political participation is based on the aforementioned Article 29 of CRPD and its section (b), thus restricting our analytical perspective to individual engagement in collective forms of political action such as organisations representing disabled persons. Third, concerning our notion of identity, we draw upon Siebers (2013: 278), who outlines the social embeddedness of identity formation as follows:

> [I]dentity is not the structure that creates a person's pristine individuality or inner essence but the structure by which that person identifies and becomes identified with a set of social narratives, ideas, myths, values, and types of knowledge of varying reliability, usefulness, and verifiability. It represents the means by which the person, qua individual, comes to join a particular social body.

Before we present our own empirical data, we review earlier research on these three concepts. What do we already know about the interconnections and links between the life course, identity formation and political participation?

The relations between the *life course* and *identity formation* have already been discussed widely in sociological research, since identity formation is essentially a social process. Mead (1969 [1934]) highlights the relevance of society and the environment for individual identities. Similarly, Goffman (1986 [1963]) distinguishes three components of a person's identity (personal, social and ego identity), each of them contributing to the individual self-concept. Drawing on Goffman, Anspach argues that the role-taking process has cognitive and normative constituents, which must be differentiated (Anspach, 1979: 768). While the former refers to the person's awareness of how he or she is perceived by others, the latter stands for the integration of this perspective into one's own self-concept (ibid.). This aspect is of importance for our analysis, as persons who are aware of a certain disability image do not necessarily incorporate this perspective into their self-concept. They have the option of either accepting or distancing themselves from this image or role.

Further, existing studies highlight the relationship between the *life course* and *political engagement*. As regards persons with disabilities, contacts with social services and incidents of discrimination are common, and these life course experiences are linked with political participation (Acheson & Williamson, 2001; Beckman, 2007; Schur, 1998; Scotch, 1988; Shah & Priestley, 2011). For example, rehabilitation services are considered to foster an image of disabled persons as 'dependent and in need of professional help' (Scotch, 1988: 162). This image contrasts with the model of the democratic citizen acting rationally and independently (Beckman, 2007), which is often denied to disabled persons, in particular to persons with psychosocial or learning difficulties. Following Hahn (1988), who argues that traditional rehabilitation programmes foster depoliticisation processes, not only because of their patronising imagery of disabled persons, but also because they imply that the problem lies within the disabled person and not within society, Schur (1998) contends that tracing disability-related problems back to the environment is a necessary prerequisite, among others, for the political activism of disabled persons.

In addition, the literature regards the impact of institutional settings as either enabling social contacts among peers or preventing social contacts with the outside world. While some works highlight the positive effects of special institutions as places where disabled persons can meet, interact and possibly develop shared identities (Acheson & Williamson, 2001; Shah & Priestley, 2011; Shakespeare, 1996), others focus on the negative effects of institutions and point out that they prevent the accumulation of social capital (Schur, 1998; Schur, Shields, Kruse & Schriner, 2002; Schur, Shields & Schriner, 2003).

Other research addresses the links between the life course and political participation by investigating discriminatory events and interactions in the social environment. Inaccessibility as a form of discriminatory experience is regarded as producing depoliticising effects, since environmental barriers prevent people from attending official meetings or entering polling stations (Guldvik, Askheim & Johansen, 2013). Interestingly, the literature discusses experience with discrimination not only as an inhibiting factor, but also as possibly fostering political engagement (Schur et al., 2003).

Further, the relationship between *political participation* and *identity* needs consideration as well. As mentioned above, several works (Anspach, 1979;

Crenshaw, 1991; Miller et al., 1981; Putnam, 2005; Sandvin, 2003; Scotch, 1988; Shakespeare, 1996) show that identities have an impact on whether persons become politically active or not. On the one hand, connecting with other disadvantaged persons can stimulate collective political action; on the other hand, a person's self-concept and its impact on political engagement are relevant. Concerning the former point, Crenshaw describes identity as 'a site of resistance for members of different subordinated groups' (1991: 1297). As regards the latter aspect, Schur (1998: 7) mentions four preconditions for disability rights engagement by an individual. First, the disabled person has to realise that there are disability-related problems. Second, he or she should perceive these problems to be resolvable. Third, the person has to consider the problems and their solution as a shared issue. Fourth, he or she should be of the opinion that politics is responsible for the problem solving. This catalogue is helpful for our study in order to better understand the relevance of identity for political participation.

This approach leads us to the consideration of a further important factor. Schur's third dimension, whereby a problem is regarded as a shared one, implies that the person identifies with other persons who are in a similar situation, thus forming a reference group. At this point, the notion of 'group identity' comes into play. Acheson and Williamson (2001: 89f.) define group identity as a precondition for political activism in the interests of a minority group. However, minority group identification does not necessarily lead to political activism. Miller et al. (1981) differentiate between group identity and 'group consciousness'. The former means 'a psychological feeling of belonging to a particular social stratum' (ibid.: 496) and is only one, albeit important, component of group consciousness. The latter 'involves identification with a group and a political awareness or ideology regarding the group's relative position in society along with a commitment to collective action aimed at realizing the group's interests' (ibid.: 495). While group consciousness implies 'a perception of deprivation' (ibid.: 495), group identity does not. This differentiation is helpful in explaining why an individual's understanding of being disabled as a result of environmental and societal barriers may lead to group consciousness, thus constituting a stimulus for political engagement. In other words, whereas identifying as a disabled person is important, but does not sufficiently motivate a person to join in collective political action, group consciousness is a necessary prerequisite for political engagement. Likewise, Putnam emphasises that having a positive self-identity as a disabled person does not necessarily lead to a 'political identity based on disability status' (Putnam, 2005: 189).

In order to trace back the political engagement of disabled persons to their self-concepts, Anspach (1979: 769) has adapted Goffman's stigma theory to develop 'a typology of four modal responses to stigma'. Although we consider her approach as somewhat problematic, as it tends to reduce engagement in disability rights organisations to 'stigma management' and ignores the role of culture and society in processes of stigmatisation, it introduces important aspects which are of relevance in understanding disabled persons' political activism.

Anspach regards this engagement as being influenced by, first, a person's self-concept, which is either positive or negative, and second, a person's attitude to societal values, be it rejection or acceptance (ibid.). According to this author, political activism only happens when both a positive self-concept *and* the rejection of existing societal values come together. The latter point is linked to the aforementioned concept of group consciousness which also implies that the perception of deprivation needs to be accompanied by a critical stance to societal values. Anspach's differentiation of a positive or negative self-concept and a person's rejection or acceptance of societal values is taken up by Schur, Kruse and Blanck, who distinguish three 'response[s] to disability' (2013: 96) which involve different forms of political engagement. *Fatalists* tend to practise role distance and not identify with other persons with disabilities; they are characterised by a 'lack of personal efficacy' (ibid.: 94) which leads to non-engagement. *Normalisers* stress their commonalities with non-disabled persons and their political activism does not revolve around disability-related topics. In contrast, *disability activists* identify with other disabled persons and also consider disability-related problems as societal rather than individual problems (ibid.: 95f.).

Following these findings, we can draft a heuristic approach by operationalising our three relevant concepts as follows. First, we differentiate the life course from the concept of biography (Voges, 1987) and consider the category of the *life course* as an element of external structures, which are characterised by

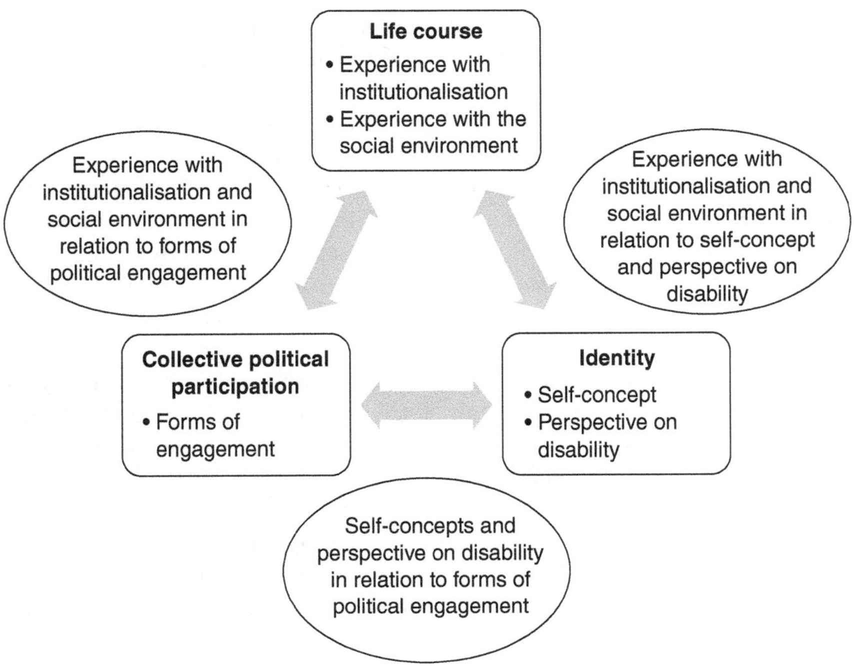

Figure 6.1 Heuristic approach: (inter-)relations between main categories and codes.

'objective existence' (Stones, 2005: 59), influencing personal agency and embracing a whole range of aspects in society and the environment. As regards disabled persons, external structures such as institutions and societal reactions greatly influence and regulate their life courses (Shah & Priestley, 2011). For reasons of feasibility, we focus on 'experience with institutionalisation' and 'experience with the social environment' as two relevant aspects in disabled persons' life courses. Second, we understand the category of *identity* as one dimension of internal structures, i.e. 'internal perceptions of external conditions' (Stones, 2005: 56). Here, we concentrate on the two aspects 'perspective on disability (models)' and 'self-concept', with the former's subcodes (see below) reflecting the differentiation of group identity and group consciousness. As outlined above, these factors are of importance when it comes to political participation on one's own behalf. Lastly, by employing the category of collective *political participation* we intend to explore practices. For this purpose we distinguish different 'forms of engagement'. Figure 6.1 depicts this system of categorisation in visual form.

Data, methods and description of sample

Our empirical analysis is based on life course interviews generated within the DISCIT research project. Because of the recruitment strategy, the results of our study are not representative for persons with disabilities in general, since a higher rate of political engagement than usual among our interview partners is likely. Besides, the experiences with institutionalisation are probably not typical either, as the sampling left long-term hospitalisation or institutionalisation out of consideration. Aiming for an in-depth approach, we focus on four countries: the Czech Republic, Germany, Ireland and Sweden. In other words, we examine a subsample of 96 interviews from the DISCIT data set (see Chapter 3). This selection is primarily guided by the number of relevant thematic sections in the interview reports, since a substantial empirical basis for our analysis is needed. In our analysis, we focus on categories which are consistent across the whole sample, such as gender, age and kind of disabilities. Further, we neglect country differences, as the material does not allow for a meaningful differentiation of nationalities.

The interviews which form the basis of our empirical data were conducted in national languages and structured by a joint topic guide. In particular, we examine data generated from these five questions that explore interviewees' experience with political participation:

1 Are you generally interested in politics and political activities?
2 Over the years, have you been a member of or participated in any self-help group, citizens' initiative or organisation that advocates the rights of persons with disabilities or any other organisation?
3 If you think back on your life so far, would you say that you yourself have decided how much you have participated in organisations and politics?

4 Over the years, have you experienced any barriers to participating in groups or activities?
5 Today, do you regard yourself as disabled (a person with a disability)?

Our analysis is based on summarised interview reports in English. From a methodological point of view, it needs to be mentioned that the summaries are likely to include interpretations by the persons writing the reports. Wherever possible, we use direct quotes to provide for original insights into the interviewees' perspectives.

Life course, identity and political participation as analytical categories

This chapter employs multifaceted concepts that we need to simplify before we can apply them in empirical analysis. In the following, we describe our three main categories (life course, identity and political participation) with their five codes and 16 subcodes by offering empirical material for illustration.

First, the analytical category of the *life course* includes the two codes 'experience with institutionalisation' and 'experience with the social environment', which are of special relevance for disabled persons and their life courses. The code 'experience with institutionalisation' refers to special institutions or community living, and it comprises the three subcodes 'less', 'mixed' and 'more'. Predominant experience with special institutions corresponds with the subcode 'more', while predominant experience with community living falls under the subcode 'less'. Personal experience with both situations is coded as 'mixed'. Similarly, the code 'experience with the social environment' includes the two subcodes 'experience with discrimination', understood here as personal disadvantages, and 'positive experience'.

Within our sample, more than half of the interviewees have less experience with institutionalisation, followed by those who have mixed experience and some with more experience. Persons with learning difficulties are dominant in the latter two categories. Further, men are slightly underrepresented among those with less experience and more frequent among those with mixed experience. As regards age, the oldest group is underrepresented among those with mixed experience and slightly more numerous in the group with less institutionalised life courses. Concerning the code 'experience with the social environment', the material includes considerably more narratives on discriminatory experience than on positive experience. Women are dominant in both subcodes, but report on experience with discrimination in particular. Persons with psychosocial difficulties are less frequent among those who report positive experience.

Next, the category *identity* includes the two codes 'self-concept' and 'perspective on disability (models)'. The former has the following subcode: narratives alluding to abilities, activity, self-confidence etc. are coded as 'positive' self-concept. A 'negative' self-concept is assumed when stories refer to helplessness, passivity, low self-esteem, etc.

In the data, positive self-concepts appear twice as often as negative self-concepts. Again women are represented slightly more often in both subcodes. As regards age, the oldest group mentions a negative self-concept less often, whereas the youngest interviewees do so most frequently. At the same time the youngest age group is the least numerous among those with positive self-concepts. Persons with psychosocial difficulties indicate negative self-concepts most often and positive ones less often, whereas persons with mobility disabilities show little evidence of negative self-concepts.

Concerning the code 'perspective on disability (models)', we differentiate the three subcodes 'social model', 'individual model' of disability and 'role distance'. First, the 'social model' of disability refers to statements featuring disability as grounded in the environment and society rather than in impairments. Second, the subcode 'individual model' implies that the person considers disability as rooted in his or her own shortcomings or identifies it with impairment; this subcode is also applied when statements on the term disability or the role of the environment are not specified. Third, the subcode 'role distance' includes statements in which interviewees explicitly distance themselves from their impairments or their role as disabled persons.

In our sample, the middle-aged group refers to the social model of disability most frequently, whereas the majority of the youngest interviewees indicate distance from being regarded as disabled. The individual model is mentioned equally often among the 1950s and the 1990s cohort and less often among interviewees in the 1970s cohort. As regards different kinds of disabilities, persons with psychosocial difficulties show role distance slightly more often and, together with persons with learning difficulties, indicate an individual model of disability most frequently and a social model less often.

Last, the category *political participation* has the code 'forms of engagement', which we differentiate into six subcodes. First, 'active member' implies that the interviewee is a member of a disability (rights) organisation, which involves attending meetings, taking part in organisational activities or holding an official function within the organisation. Second, the subcode 'staff or official in organisation' covers those who engage in an organisation as (part of) their job, either on an honorary or paid basis. Third, the subcode 'active, but not a member' covers a person's involvement in organisational activities without being a member of this association. Fourth, 'inactive member' comprises official members who do not take part in the organisational life, but are content to be kept informed. Fifth, 'not a member yet, but interested' is used when interviewees indicate that they may become a member in the future. Sixth, the subcode 'non-member' relates to persons stating explicitly that they are not members of a disability (rights) organisation.

As regards our data, about half of the interviewees are active members, and about a quarter have a job or position in an organisation. Another quarter are not members, some are inactive members and very few are either not members yet or are active without being members.

(Inter-)relations between life course, identity and political participation

As outlined above, identity formation is a dynamic process and is shaped by experience within a person's life course. In this section we examine how the life courses of persons with disabilities, their individual identities and their forms of political (non-)engagement are interrelated. We present our findings in three steps.

Experience with institutionalisation and social environment in relation to self-concepts and perspectives on disability

A defining feature of many life courses of disabled persons is *experience with institutionalisation*. What impact does this have on self-concepts? In our sample, the experience with special institutions is frequently accompanied by negative self-concepts, whereas persons who have experienced community living tend to have positive self-concepts. Many interviewees relate their self-confidence to supportive families. The experience of a German woman with mobility disabilities from the 1970s cohort illustrates this point: She has 'the luck to be very self-confident and ascribes that to her family and the way she was brought up'. Similarly, other interviewees, e.g. in Ireland and Sweden, link their self-confidence to experience with integrated/inclusive education, work and other relevant life situations.

As regards the (inter-)relations between institutionalisation and a person's perspective on disability (models), the data indicates that those interviewees who have had more experience with institutions are more likely to follow the individual model of disability as well as to adopt a role distance approach rather than adhering to a social model perspective. The following statement of a Swedish man with visual disabilities in the 1950s cohort highlights the influence of special institutions: 'It was when I came to special education [...] that I started to perceive myself as disabled – it was difficult to stand'. The same can be observed in the case of those persons who have experienced both special institutions and community living. The experience of a visually impaired man from Ireland in the 1970s cohort is described as follows: 'He said that for a long time he didn't identify as a person with a disability in part to get away from the institutionalisation of his youth'. A Czech man with mobility disabilities in the 1970s cohort highlights as a turning point when he started 'attending hospital institutional school. At that time, he first noticed his differences to other people. He was not able to understand why he did not go to the same school as his parents did. In contrast, persons who adopt a social model perspective tend to have less experience with special institutions. These findings emphasise the impact of special institutions on personal perspectives on disability.

Next, we look at how *experience with the social environment* is linked to self-concepts and perspectives on disability. Strikingly, experience with discrimination is mentioned more often by persons with a negative self-concept. Further, those who report positive experience with their social environment tend to display a positive self-concept more often than a negative one. A Swedish man in the 1950s cohort with mobility disabilities is reported to partly owe his self-confidence to 'the education he got in school and to his parents who believed in him'. Considering the relationship between discriminatory experience and a person's perspective on disability, we find that persons with an individual model or a role distance approach mention far more negative experience with the social environment than positive ones. Although we cannot determine which of the three factors – environmental experience, self-concepts or perspectives on disability – are causes and which are effects, we can conclude that persons with different environmental experience also show differences as regards their self-concepts and perspectives on disability.

With regard to the intersections between personal *self-concepts* and *perspectives on disability*, our analysis indicates that interviewees who follow a social model perspective tend to have positive self-concepts. The life course of an Irish woman with visual disabilities in the 1970s cohort illustrates this:

> In the last 15 years she has begun to see herself as a person with a disability and sees the barriers and obstacles she encounters as not her problem but a result of how society is constructed. She now says she sees her disability in a positive light. She said she is no longer ashamed to tell people that she has a disability and if they have a negative reaction that's on them: it reflects nothing on her. She said this shift occurred as she became more confident in her abilities, which led to her becoming more comfortable requesting supports or talking about her disability.

This description exemplifies how the development of a positive self-concept is linked with different perspectives on disability. As a result, the interviewee does not equate disability with impairment, but rather emphasises the responsibility of society.

To sum up, although the findings cannot be interpreted in a causal sense, we find interesting (inter-)relations between experience with institutionalisation and social environment on the one hand, and personal self-concepts and perspectives on disability on the other.

Experience with institutionalisation and social environment in relation to forms of political engagement

Our analysis shows that the life course of a disabled person is an important factor when it comes to identity formation. In this section we are interested in the impact of institutionalisation and social environment on political participation.

First, we look at *experience with institutionalisation* and how it relates to different forms of engagement. It appears that active forms of engagement – i.e. active membership, being a staff member or an official in an organisation as well as being active, but not a member – appear with less institutionalisation experience. Among those who hold positions in an organisation or are active, but not members, nearly all interviewees have more experience with community living. This is also the case for the majority of active members. In contrast, interviewees who are neither members nor active show a different picture. The majority of this group can be divided into two subgroups, one experiencing both institutionalised settings and community living, the other predominantly experiencing institutionalised settings. Those interviewees who are either inactive members or interested, but not yet members, have an ambivalent position. Their life courses are characterised by both mixed experience and experience with community living. Among those persons whose life courses mostly include experience with special institutions, none holds a position in an organisation or reports activism apart from organisations representing the interests of persons with disabilities. Interestingly, the group of non-members is largely formed of those who have mixed experience with institutionalisation.

As regards the relationship between *experience with the social environment* and forms of engagement, positive experience is mentioned more frequently among those who are inactive members. For example, a German woman with mobility disabilities in the 1970s cohort 'never protested by addressing official positions as she never experienced bad treatment as a structural discrimination'. Active forms of engagement are present with discriminatory experience, which are mentioned frequently, but positive experience is reported as well.

To sum up, our data reveals that there are specific relations between the life course and political participation, in particular with regard to experience with special institutions. Persons who have more experience with institutionalised settings tend to be less engaged than those with more experience with community living. Further, the prevalence of positive experience with the social environment is linked to a tendency to non-engagement or non-affiliation.

Self-concepts and perspectives on disability (models) in relation to forms of political engagement

As a next step, we consider the links between identity (formation) and political participation. First, we look at *self-concepts* and their (inter-)relations with forms of political engagement. Interviewees who indicate a positive self-concept tend to be politically active. However, we cannot verify whether the positive self-concept influences political engagement or vice versa, as effects obviously operate both ways. The report on a visually impaired woman of the 1970s cohort from Germany illustrates the latter aspect: 'she got more self-confident. She is not as intimidated at the age of 40 as she was at the age of 20.' The increased self-confidence is also related to her work in an organisation for blind and visually impaired persons: 'if you know your rights better, you also can appear more self-confident compared to when you are not that confident'.

An Irish man of the 1950s cohort with mobility disabilities points out the other side of the coin, namely 'that self-belief has enabled him to participate to the degree that he does'. Some interviewees refer to this aspect as a crucial precondition for future engagement. The position of an Irish middle-aged woman with visual disabilities in the 1970s cohort is described as follows: 'She might get more involved in the future as she gets more confident and comfortable and is better prepared to be involved in issues that concern her'.

Among the interviewees with negative self-concepts, those who are active members and those who are non-members are equally represented, complemented by some who are not members yet, but interested. Remarkably, inactive members predominantly display positive self-concepts.

Next, our data sheds light on the (inter-)relations between *perspectives on disability (models)* and different forms of engagement. Those who adopt a social model perspective show two forms of political engagement in particular: they are either active members or have a position in an organisation. In contrast, among those who practise role distance only, less than half are active members. The relations between role distance and non-membership are explicitly highlighted in some interviews. An Irish interviewee with psychosocial difficulties from the 1970s cohort 'follows the work of some organisations but would not have gotten involved for fear of "coming out" as someone with a mental health issue'. Concerning interviewees with an individual model perspective, the level of affiliation is somewhat different. Nearly half of them are active members or occupy positions within an organisation; of this group more persons are active compared to those who distanced themselves from being classified as disabled.

To summarise, we find, first, that persons with positive self-concepts tend to be more politically active than those with negative self-concepts. An exception is inactive members who reveal predominantly positive self-concepts. Second, interviewees with a social model perspective mostly display active forms of engagement, while those who demonstrate role distance exhibit less active forms of engagement. Among those with an individual model approach there seems to be a balance between active engagement and non-affiliation or non-engagement. Overall we find that perspectives on disability are closely related to personal dispositions to becoming affiliated to or engaged in organisations representing persons with disabilities.

Linking collective political participation, life course, identity and socio-demographic variables: A typology

As mentioned above, Schur et al. (2013: 92ff.) conceptualise three typical figures of political activism, distinguishing between fatalists, normalisers and activists. As a third step in our empirical analysis, we adopt this differentiation to develop our own empirically based typology, which aims to link forms of collective political participation with the life course, identity formation and socio-demographic variables. As a result, we distinguish between four different types of (non-)engagement, divided into six subtypes, which correspond to different forms of (non-)affiliation or (non-)engagement (see Table 6.1).

First, we identify the group of *collective activists*, which is characterised by active engagement in an organisation, either as active member or as staff

Table 6.1 (Inter-)relations between collective political participation, life course, identity and socio-demographic variables

Categories	*Collective activists*		*Individual activists*	*Normalisers*	*(Partial) fatalists*	
Collective political participation						
Forms of (non-) engagement	Active member	Staff member or official in disability (rights) organisation	Active, but not a member	Inactive member	Not a member yet, but interested	Non-member
Life course						
Experience with institutions	Less	Less	Less	Less/mixed	Mixed/less	Mixed/more
Experience with the social environment	Discriminatory experience	Discriminatory experience	Discriminatory and/or positive experience	Positive experience	Discriminatory experience	Discriminatory experience
Identity						
Self-concept	Positive	Positive	Positive	Positive	Negative/positive	Positive/negative
Perspective on disability	Individual model/ role distance/social model	Social model	Individual model/ role distance	Role distance/ individual model	Individual model/ role distance	Role distance/ individual model
Socio-demographic variables						
Age group	1950s	1970s	1990s	1950s/1970s	1990s	1990s
Gender	Female	Female/male	Female	Male	Female	Male
Kind of impairments	Mobility/visual	Visual/mobility	Mobility	Visual	Learning/ psychosocial	Learning/ psychosocial

member or official in an organisation. Within our sample, persons with mobility or visual disabilities mostly show this kind of engagement. As regards the life course, collective activists have less experience with institutionalisation and more experience with discrimination, although their narratives contain positive experience as well. Considering their self-concepts, we find that collective activists have predominantly positive self-concepts. However, this group displays two different perspectives on disability (models). The social model perspective is dominant, but is more prevalent among those who are staff members or in an official position, in comparison to active members who adopt the individual model perspective more often or even display role distance. There are further differences as regards gender. Women appear to be more prevalent among active members, while there is an equal balance between men and women among those with official positions in organisations. With regard to age, interviewees in the 1970s cohort are more prevalent among those with staff positions, but the 1950s cohort is more numerous among active members. Many active members trace their organisational engagement back to the availability of more personal time, which is usually typical for retired persons.

Second, *individual activists* are mostly distinguished by their forms of engagement. Their activity is not based on membership or a position in an organisation, but rather takes place independently. Similar to the first type, individual activists have less experience with special institutions and tend to exhibit positive self-concepts. However, in contrast to collective activists, this group mentions positive experience as often as discriminatory experience. The individual activists also differ from collective activists in their perspectives on disability (models). Here, the individual model and distance to being regarded as disabled are more prevalent. Regarding socio-demographic data, women are more frequently represented among individual activists, as are persons with mobility disabilities and the 1990s cohort.

Third, the *normalisers*, for whom inactive membership is characteristic, form a bridge between active forms of engagement and non-engagement. In this group, interviewees exhibit role distance, implying non-identification with the group of disabled persons, possibly in combination with striving for normality. Furthermore, in parallel to our aforementioned individual activists, normalisers exhibit positive self-concepts as well as an individual model or role distance perspective. But we can also observe differences. As regards life courses, we find less or mixed experience with institutions. Interestingly, this type is the only one showing a prevalence of positive experience compared to incidents of discrimination. As regards socio-demographic data, normalisers tend to be male, while females are dominant among collective and individual activists. The 1950s and 1970s cohorts as well as persons with visual disabilities are more frequently found in this group.

Completing the picture, *(partial) fatalists* as the fourth group include two forms of non-engagement. While non-members are characterised by complete non-engagement, there are also interviewees who are not members yet, but interested, i.e. they mention potential interest in affiliation or engagement. Therefore we regard the former as fatalists and the latter as partial fatalists, since they consider the possibility of future engagement. Comparing this type with the previously introduced categories, there are almost no congruencies. As regards the life course, mixed experience with institutionalisation appears more frequently. While those who are not members yet, but interested, have experience with community living, more non-members have experienced special institutions. Considering the aspect of identity, we find differences with regard to self-concept. In contrast to the other types, (partial) fatalists tend to have negative self-concepts nearly as often as positive ones. Further, the perspectives on disability correspond with the individual model approach as well as with role distance. Amongst partial fatalists, persons with learning difficulties or psychosocial difficulties are prevalent as is the 1990 cohort. Again a gender difference emerges in our sample: partial fatalists tend to be female while fatalists are predominantly male.

Discussion of findings

In the remaining section of this chapter we discuss the main findings and connect the results of our study with existing research. In particular, we examine the issues of age, gender and impairment as well as the perspective on disability with regard to the political engagement of persons with disabilities.

With respect to age, our data indicates that the youngest age group is found most frequently among interviewees with non-affiliation. Earlier research has shown that younger people are decreasingly engaged in traditional forms of political participation (Pleyers, 2005). Sandvin (2003) retraces similar differences with regard to age cohorts and generation differences and explains them by drawing on the theory of individualisation (Beck & Beck-Gernsheim, 2002). Accordingly, the younger age groups have more options and at the same time adopt more individual responsibility for their lives. Thus, they are less keen to join organisations that advocate collective interests.

Interestingly, our sample also shows differences between men and women. Female interviewees exhibit more active forms of engagement compared to men, who tend to engage more passively. This finding contrasts with current knowledge, which indicates that men are usually more active politically; this also applies to persons with disabilities (Guldvik et al., 2013; Schur et al., 2003; Waldschmidt, 2009). One possible explanation for our finding is the impact of special institutions; in our sample, female interviewees have less experience with institutionalisation than men. This in turn would reinforce the assumption that special institutions tend to discourage rather than foster political engagement of disabled persons.

A further difference becomes apparent when we consider different kinds of impairments. Interviewees with mobility or visual impairments tend to be more dominant among those with active forms of engagement or inactive affiliation, whereas persons with learning or psychosocial difficulties prevail among the (partial) fatalists. The latter display special features with regard to the three aspects of experience with institutions, experience with the social environment and self-concept. First, (partial) fatalists have more experience with special institutions than collective activists, individual activists or normalisers. This is particularly the case for non-members. Second, experience with discrimination is more frequent among the (partial) fatalists. Third, in contrast to collective activists, who also tend to have experience with discrimination but exhibit positive self-concepts, most (partial) fatalists display negative self-concepts. These results support the works of Anspach (1979) as well as Schur et al. (2003), who suggest that a positive self-concept may encourage active forms of political participation.

Last, our findings emphasise the relevance of perspectives on disability for disability-related engagement. Collective activists refer to a social model perspective more frequently than the other types. This result is in line with theories on group identity, group consciousness and political participation (Acheson & Williamson, 2001; Crenshaw, 1991; Miller et al., 1981; Putnam, 2005; Schur, 1998), contending that the existence of both group identity and group conciousness is a stimulus for political engagement on identity-related topics. In our analysis, the perspective of the individual model corresponds with group identity, while the social model perspective is an indicator for group consciousness. Role distance does not relate to any of the two forms of group belonging. Interestingly, in our sample, those interviewees who adopt a social model perspective are most likely to become politically engaged. Interviewees adhering to an individual model of disability display different but fewer forms of affiliation and engagement. Group identity without group consciousness does not necessarily foster political engagement on disability-related topics, apart from engagement in self-help groups which requires group identity rather than group consciousness. In contrast, persons exhibiting role distance, who are well represented among the normalisers, tend not to become active on behalf of persons with disabilities, but some of them show political engagement on topics unrelated to disability. We assume that the perspective on disability is an indicator of the kind of organisation a person chooses to engage in, whether in impairment-related self-help groups, in advocacy organisations or in cross-disability movement organisations. Unfortunately, we are not able to reconstruct this aspect with the available data.

Conclusion

The aim of this chapter was to investigate different forms of political participation and their relationship to individual life courses and personal identities. The typology (Table 6.1), which we have developed on the basis of our data, offers interesting insights.

First, we can state that the life course – in our study operationalised by experience with institutionalisation and the social environment – matters. If we assume a continuum from active to passive forms of engagement, it seems that the more passive the political engagement is, the more experience with special institutions is prevalent. However, the question of identity is also important. Persons who have experience with community living tend to adopt a positive self-concept. Further, the social model approach, regarded here as equivalent for group consciousness among disabled persons, is more dominant among those with community living experience. Moreover, our typology suggests that de-institutionalisation is an important factor for facilitating the political engagement of disabled persons.

Second, experience with discrimination can have opposing effects. On the one hand, it is linked to negative self-concepts and perspectives on disability which do not promote group consciousness. On the other hand, discriminatory experience may also result in stimulating political engagement. Overall, the picture is complex. Experience with discrimination as such does not necessarily foster political participation; as an additional factor a positive self-concept is required. The latter separates politically engaged persons from those who are not active.

Third, our study emphasises the (inter-)relations between identity formation and political participation. A positive self-concept distinguishes the activists and normalisers from the (partial) fatalists, but both collective and individual activists are notable for following the social model of disability. This finding underlines the relevance of group consciousness, although we cannot determine what comes first, the social model approach or the engagement. Our data indicates that both are possible. The importance of the social model of disability for disabled persons' life courses and their political participation can be traced back to the fact that it provides an opportunity both to identify with a social group and simultaneously to critically reflect this group's position in society.

In terms of structuration theory, we find (inter-)relations between all levels. External structures, operationalised by the categories 'experience with institutionalisation' and 'social environment', are interrelated to both internal structures, i.e. a person's identity, and individual practices. Likewise, internal structures relate to practices of exercising influence in the political field. To come full circle, it can be assumed that these practices in turn influence and eventually change external structures, but further research is needed to verify this supposition. In this chapter, we hope to have shown that in order to present the whole picture it is necessary to consider the interplay between all these levels.

References

Acheson, N. & Williamson, A. (2001). The ambiguous role of welfare structures in relation to the emergence of activism among disabled people: Research evidence from Northern Ireland. *Disability & Society*, *16*(1), 87–102.

Anspach, R. R. (1979). From stigma to identity politics: Political activism among the physically disabled and former mental patients. *Social Science & Medicine*, *13*(A), 765–773.

Beck, U. & Beck-Gernsheim, E. (2002). *Individualization. Institutionalized individualism and its social and political consequences*. London: Sage.

Beckman, L. (2007). Political equality and the disenfranchisement of people with intellectual impairments. *Social Policy and Society*, *6*(1), 13–23.

Crenshaw, K. (1991). Mapping the margins: Intersectionality, identity politics, and violence against women of color. *Stanford Law Review*, *43*(6), 1241–1299.

Goffman, E. (1986 [1963]). *Stigma: Notes on the management of spoiled identity*. New York: Simon & Schuster.

Guldvik, I., Askheim, O. P. & Johansen, V. (2013). Political citizenship and local political participation for disabled people. *Citizenship Studies*, *17*(1), 76–91.

Hahn, H. (1988). The politics of physical differences: Disability and discrimination. *Journal of Social Issues*, *44*(1), 39–47.

Mead, G. H. (1969 [1934]). *Mind, self and society: From the standpoint of a social behaviorist*. Chicago: University of Chicago Press.

Miller, A. H., Gurin, P., Gurin, G. & Malanchuk, O. (1981). Group consciousness and political participation. *American Journal of Political Science*, *25*(3), 494–511.

Oliver, M. (2013). The social model of disability: Thirty years on. *Disability & Society*, *28*(7), 1024–1026.

Pleyers, G. (2005). Young people and alter-globalisation: From disillusionment to a new culture of political participation. In J. Forbrig (Ed.), *Revisiting youth political participation. Challenges for research and democratic practice in Europe* (pp. 133–143). Strasbourg: Council of Europe.

Priestley, M. (2003). *Disability. A life course approach*. Cambridge: Polity Press.

Putnam, M. (2005). Conceptualizing disability: Developing a framework for political disability identity. *Journal of Disability Policy Studies*, *16*(3), 188–198.

Sandvin, J. T. (2003). Loosening bonds and changing identities: Growing up with impairments in post-war Norway. *Disability Studies Quarterly*, *23*(2), 5–19.

Schur, L. (1998). Disability and the psychology of political participation. *Journal of Disability Policy Studies*, *9*(2), 3–31.

Schur, L., Kruse, D. & Blanck, P. (2013). *People with disabilities: Sidelined or mainstreamed?* Cambridge: Cambridge University Press.

Schur, L., Shields, T., Kruse, D. & Schriner, K. (2002). Enabling democracy: Disability and voter turnout. *Political Research Quarterly*, *55*(1), 167–190.

Schur, L., Shields, T. & Schriner, K. (2003). Can I make a difference? Efficacy, employment, and disability. *Political Psychology*, *24*(1), 119–149.

Schur, L., Shields, T. & Schriner, K. (2005). Generational cohorts, group membership, and political participation by people with disabilities. *Political Research Quarterly*, *58*(3), 487–496.

Scotch, R. K. (1988). Disability as the basis for a social movement: Advocacy and the politics of definition. *Journal of Social Issues*, *44*(1), 159–172.

Shah, S. & Priestley, M. (2011). *Disability and social change. Private lives and public policies*. Bristol: Policy Press.

Shakespeare, T. (1996). Disability, identity and difference. In C. Barnes & G. Mercer (Eds), *Exploring the divide. Illness and disability* (pp. 94–113). Leeds: The Disability Press.

Siebers, T. (2013). Disability and the theory of complex embodiment. For identity politics in a new register. In L. Davis (Ed.), *The disability studies reader* (pp. 272–292). New York: Routledge.

Stones, R. (2005). *Structuration theory*. Basingstoke: Palgrave Macmillan.

Voges, W. (Ed.). (1987). *Methoden der Biographie- und Lebenslaufforschung*. Opladen: Leske & Budrich.

Waldschmidt, A. (2009). Politische Partizipation von Menschen mit Behinderungen und Benachteiligungen. In D. Orthmann Bless & R. Stein (Eds), *Lebensgestaltung bei Behinderungen und Benachteiligungen im Erwachsenenalter und Alter*. (Vol. 5, pp. 118–152). Baltmannsweiler: Schneider Verlag Hohengehren.

7 Active Citizenship in using accessible technology

The experiences of three generations

Jennifer Kline, Eilionóir Flynn and Sinéad Keogh

A person born around 1950 has lived to see the introduction of personal computers, mobile phones, and the internet, whereas a person born around 1990 may have lived their whole life with access to all three of those things. The enormous changes in technology over the past 70 years have had a great and lasting impact on people all over the world (Anderson & Tracey, 2001; Castells, 2002). In addition to these advancements, access to assistive technology and the types of assistive technology available have changed greatly as well. This chapter will look at how these changes in information communication technology as well as other technologies may have impacted people with disabilities across Europe. For this purpose, we distinguish between accessible technology and assistive technology. While accessible technology refers to devices that are usable for all end users independent of disability or impairment, assistive technology refers to special devices designed to compensate for a disability or impairment. Although there has been great progress in access and innovations in both assistive technology (AT) and information and communication technology (ICT), many persons with disabilities face barriers in accessing such technologies. This chapter analyses life-course interview data, collected as part of the DISCIT project, and focuses on three major themes relating to the use of accessible technology by people with disabilities:

- the impact of accessible ICT on the lives of persons with disabilities
- the barriers faced by persons with disabilities
- how self-identification as a person with a disability impacts on assistive technology use.

By exploring these themes, we hope to show how AT can facilitate Active Citizenship. The first theme explores how ICT has influenced aspects of Active Citizenship (security, autonomy, influence) for interviewees, with a particular focus on autonomy. The second and the third themes show the exploration of the connection between ICT use and AT use and how Active Citizenship can be limited through both external and internal barriers to accessible technology. External barriers include administrative and financial and can impact the opportunity for full and effective participation in society. How people with disabilities self-identify can create internal facilitators or barriers to accessing accessible technology.

People who do not identify as a person with a disability are less likely to try to involve themselves in discussions around the provision of accessible technology.

The chapter will first set out the methodology for the interviews and analysis of interview data. After the methodology section, the chapter contains a brief literature review of relevant articles and studies that relate to the three themes analysed in this chapter. The following section draws on qualitative data from the DISCIT project to discuss the three thematic sections. This section takes examples from the interview transcripts and summaries to relate the experiences of interviewees with disabilities with accessible technology. The chapter concludes by summarising the findings and identifying policy recommendations and suggestions for further research in these areas.

Methodology: life-course interviews

On the subject of AT and ICT, the topic guide for life-course interviews included three mandatory questions with more optional follow-up questions. How interviewers used the topic guide varied. Some country teams seem to have used the questions verbatim and used the guide as a questionnaire, while others used the

Table 7.1 Extract from the DISCIT topic guide

Foundational questions	*Optional follow-up questions to achieve more elaborated accounts*
6.1 Over the years, have you benefited from any assistive technology in everyday life?	• Have you benefited from any household technology (home devices)? • Has your use of the technologies changed? • If yes, why? • If yes, how did you cope before you got access to these technologies?
6.2 If you think across your life course, to what extent have you used information and communication technology (computers, internet, mobile phones or similar devices)?	• In which contexts (education, work, leisure, communication with others) have you benefited from the devices? • When did you first get access to or were first able to use such devices? • Has your use of such devices changed your life? If yes, how/in what ways? • If yes, how was it before you had access to these technologies?

6.3 Over the years, have you been able to choose or decide what kind of technology you use or would like to use?	• If yes, is there anything or anybody who has been of particular help in this context?
	• If no, what are the main barriers to improving your opportunities to use and benefit from the technologies?
	  • Affordability or accessibility?
	  • Information or knowledge about the devices?
	  • Lack of personal influence on the decision-making?

topic guide as a checklist. In the latter cases the questions may not have been posed if the interviewer felt they were irrelevant.

We analysed the interviews using thematic analysis techniques (Boyatzis, 1998). In analysing the patterns found in the data from the interview summaries, this chapter will focus on three main themes that were identified in the initial analysis of the interview summaries:

1 How has accessible ICT impacted on the lives of people with disabilities?
2 What are the main barriers to AT and ICT and how do those barriers vary across country, generations, gender and disability identity?
3 How was the decision to use accessible technology or AT intertwined with how the interviewee self-identified as a person with a disability?

Brief literature review

Most studies on the use of accessible technology by people with disabilities draw from a narrow population of either one country or one group of disabilities or one type of accessible technology (Abbott, Brown, Evett & Standen, 2014; Dobransky & Hargittai, 2006). Furthermore, there were few cross-generational, cross-country and cross-gender comparisons. Again previous studies have usually focused on just one or two of these (Löfqvistet, Nygren, Széman & Iwarsson, 2005; Steel & Gray, 2009).

Among authors who have written about the use of new technologies, several have looked at the benefits and drawbacks of using ICT to enhance Active Citizenship of people with disabilities. Several have noted issues of accessibility of ICT and other barriers that create a digital divide for various groups of people with disabilities (Blanck, 2014; Dobransky & Hargittai, 2006; Vicente & López, 2010). Dobransky and Hargittai conducted a review of existing literature on ICT use by people with disabilities and found that ICT was beneficial to people with disabilities for communication, social support, and giving them a sense of independence. They also identified common barriers to ICT, in particular incompatibility of AT with ICT, cost and lack of interest in use of the internet (Dobransky & Hargittai, 2006). Vicente and López used an e-user survey that was funded by the European Commission and used in 10 European countries (Vicente & López, 2010). In their analysis of the data, they found that socio-economic barriers were a 'major barrier' to people with disabilities. They also found that many people with disabilities found ICT too intimidating to use.

Others have looked at how ICT has been positively used by various groups of people with disabilities (Söderström, 2009; Stendal, 2012). Söderström examined how young people with disabilities in Norway created social ties through the internet that they were not always able to create in their local environment (Söderström, 2009).

Barriers to accessible technology have been discussed by various authors but usually limited to a single group of people with disabilities such as people with visual disabilities or people with intellectual disabilities. Many articles have looked at the issue of non-use or abandonment of provided AT (Wessels, Dijcks, Soede, Gelde & de Witte, 2003; Zhao & Phillips, 1993). Examinations of the reasons for abandoning use of AT show that a lack of information about how to use a device and inappropriateness of the device predominate (Verza, Carvalho, Battaglia & Uccelli, 2006). Other studies have looked at the psychosocial and cultural reasons for abandonment (Hocking, 1999). Hocking suggested that providers of AT must look beyond the functional purpose of the device and needs of the potential user to consider users' emotional response to the device and the social and cultural context of the disability and the assistive devices. Critiques of European systems of AT provision have noted how user involvement is a critical component in assessing the quality of an AT provision programme (Steele & de Witte, 2011). Steele and De Witte examined changes in the AT service provision systems since the HEART project which studied AT provision systems in 17 countries and made recommendations in 1994. Steele and de Witte's study reported that AT users in 10 of the countries (three of which, Sweden, Italy and Germany, overlap with countries covered by DISCIT) have access to information 'either all of the time or frequently'. The study also stated that only Italy reported infrequent user involvement in decision-making, which contrasts with the experiences with procedural barriers recounted by our interviewees (Steele & de Witte, 2011).

Publications evaluating characteristics of good assistive device provision have often focused on the importance of providers taking into account the personal preferences and individual situations of potential users (Scherer, Craddock & Mackeogh, 2011) and use of a partnership approach (Andrich, Mathiassen, Hoogerwerf & Gelderblom, 2013). There has also been research on how certain groups of people with disabilities have different types of AT needs and on differences in access to AT between different groups. A 2004 study on AT for people with cognitive disabilities (using a definition that would encompass people with intellectual disabilities and people with psychosocial disabilities) catalogued a variety of personal support, assisted care and virtual technologies that could be useful for people with intellectual and/or psychosocial disabilities in overcoming barriers (Braddock, Rizzolo & Thompson, 2004). Several studies looked specifically at barriers to ICT for people with intellectual disabilities. A study in Spain found that 25 per cent of people with intellectual disabilities had parents or caregivers who blocked internet access for the person with the intellectual disability (Rechacha & Cafranga, 2011). Another study found systematic training of people with intellectual disabilities to be effective and beneficial in helping people with intellectual disabilities gain access to computers (Li-Tsang, Yeung, Choi, Chan & Lam, 2006).

Less has been written on the interplay between self-identification as a person with a disability and use of AT. One US study that examined use of AT by different groups of people with disabilities had similar findings, with people with physical and visual disabilities more likely to use AT than people with psychosocial disabilities and intellectual disabilities (Kaye, Yeager & Reed, 2008). The study posited that a lack of awareness of available technology was a reason for lack of use.

This brief overview of the relevant literature demonstrates that the DISCIT study is novel in its approach to understanding the experiences of different generations of people with disabilities across Europe, taking into account how access to technology differs across the life course and by disability type, as well as how it can enhance or pose barriers to Active Citizenship, understood through the dimensions of autonomy, influence and security, as described in Chapter 1.

Operationalising a life-course perspective on Active Citizenship

Before turning to the findings from the life-course interviews on accessible technology, it is important to set out the interpretive lens through which these findings can be analysed. For this research we chose to operationalise the concept of Active Citizenship (see Chapter 1), through a life-course framework, as theories of the life course present a useful framework for analysing the impact of accessible technology on the lives of persons with disabilities and their contributions as active citizens. The idea that welfare states structure the life courses of individuals and groups of citizens, such as persons with disabilities, through law, policy and regulation, for example by regulating access to technology, has been well established in the literature (Mayer & Schoepflin, 1989; Walker & Leisering, 1998; Mortimer & Shanahan, 2003; Yerkes, Peper & Baxter 2013). Much of the existing literature on the life course focuses on the typical life-stages, or 'normal' life course and transitions which individuals experience throughout their lives – for example, from education to employment to retirement. As Priestley notes, 'disability offers the opportunity to question assumptions about the normal life course and to challenge the institutional arrangements that regulate its boundaries' (Priestley, 2003). Furthermore, Priestley notes that the use of life-course analysis 'avoids an over-simplification of disabled people's collective experiences and the marginalisation of issues affecting underrepresented groups' (Priestley, 2003). This provides a useful starting point for our research, as we seek to explore the extent to which access to technology presents barriers or opportunities in navigating life transitions for persons with disabilities.

In analysing the interview data, we draw from Walker and Leisering's approach to life-course analysis which goes beyond an individual, biographical or narrative enquiry, to critically evaluate regimes of policy and practice (particularly in education, social security, employment and pensions) as a means of structuring life-course transitions and the relationships between different generations (Walker & Leisering, 1998). More specifically, in relation to people with disabilities, Shah and Priestley (2011) adopt a methodological approach that combines individual narrative life stories (of three generations of disabled children in Britain) with an analysis of disabling barriers, institutions and relationships. The research conducted for the DISCIT project fits well with this approach, as we combined semi-structured biographical interviews with different generations of people with disabilities with an analysis of existing legislative, policy and practice frameworks in their respective countries. In this context, a life-course analysis will be used as a lens through which the lived experiences of three generations of people with disabilities, and the applicable laws and policies in each country, can be placed in a wider social context.

Access to technology can influence the interactions between people with disabilities and the social institutions that structure and regulate individual lives (especially through health, education and social services). The perceived normal or typical transitions in life, for example from early childhood to education, education to employment and employment to retirement, are also points at which access to technology for people with disabilities can facilitate inclusion and Active Citizenship, or reinforce barriers and contribute to exclusion. The extent to which access to technology influences these transitions and life-stages is discussed in further detail in the following section as we analyse the interview data.

The impact of accessible ICT on the lives of persons with disabilities

The Organisation for Economic Co-operation and Development defines ICT broadly as 'different types of communications networks and the technologies used in them' (OECD, 2014). Draft Comment on Article 9 of the United Nations' Convention on the Rights of Persons with Disabilities (CRPD) drew attention to the importance of accessible ICT:

> Disability laws often fail to include ICT in their definition of accessibility, and disability rights laws concerned with non-discriminatory access in areas such as procurement, employment and education often fail to include access to ICT and the many goods and services central to modern society that are offered through ICT.
>
> (UN Committee on the Rights of Persons with Disabilities, 2013)

Use of ICT was one area in the interviews on accessible technology where users of ICT often spoke clearly about how gaining access to a computer, smartphone or the internet had a positive impact on their lives. Several interviewees credited access to ICT for their education, jobs, advocacy efforts, support and friends. Other studies have tracked the benefits of ICT for people with disabilities (Dobransky & Hargittai, 2006). A few interviewees, however, spoke of their wariness of ICT and some avoided use of ICT completely. Several interviewees specifically discussed how the internet allowed them greater autonomy. Generally, many of the interviewees were enthusiastic about the use of ICT and its impact. A man from Switzerland with a mobility disability born around 1950 described advancements in ICT as 'sensational' and said they made his working and private life much easier. Another man from Switzerland with a mobility disability born around 1970 said ICT was the 'be all and end all' of his life. Several interviewees cited the introduction of ICT as a major turning point in their lives. As one man from the UK said about his phone:

> You know you can just do about anything you want from your handset really. The phones years ago they never used to have internet, they never used to have anything like that, but now you have your smartphone and it does everything I need it to do really. So like my phone is my mini PC. As well as making calls, messaging, it's another world it opens up.
>
> (From an interview with a man from the UK with an intellectual disability born around 1990)

A woman from Italy with a visual disability born around 1970 described the impact of computer access by saying, 'the computer is a window onto the world and knowing it well the blind can do almost everything but above [all] have access to information and culture'. These interviews show the importance of ICT to people with disabilities. This suggests that ICT can play an important role in facilitating Active Citizenship for people with disabilities as will be discussed in more detail below. One woman from the UK said:

> [A] lot of blind people strive to be independent which I believe is a paradigm that is impossible for anybody with a disability. You go shopping as a blind person you need someone to go round the shop and describe. That isn't independence; that is assistive living. For me, the way I get around is if I want to buy clothes, I will do it on the internet. Because with my residual vision and low vision aid, i.e. a magnifier, I am able to see the clothes that I am buying. Likewise, for food shopping, you know, you can get it delivered to your house. That I suppose in a way is assistive living, however it is more mainstream assisted living … able-bodied people get their shopping delivered. Able-bodied people [use] online fashion retail, so it's kind of a half way thing.
>
> (From an interview with a woman from the UK with a visual disability born around 1990)

Use of portable devices such as smartphones and tablets were discussed by many interviewees and were praised for their versatility and ability to help them access a variety of activities.

> I do a lot of things with my phone, even paying bills or shopping, or my tablet, because it is so much easier. Or there's keeping in touch with people because there's carers and things and anything like that so I've got quite a reasonable support network which I can get hold of.
>
> (From an interview with a man from the UK with a psychosocial disability born around 1970)

Another interviewee with a visual disability also discussed how internet access, specifically through portable devices like smartphones and tablets, better enabled her to be independent.

> When you're carrying these things around you have immediate access to the internet. You can find out information, you know, like for me on my phone I have the [tram] app tells me what time the [tram] is at, I've Dublin Bus, I've a train [app], it gives me the information in an accessible format that I can access on my own with relative ease that I wouldn't have had a number of years ago. You know, I find it very hard to see a timetable, so things like that, that's where changes in technology have made a huge impact on my life, you know. You can, you know, you can get so much information on such a small little device now, that has made it, you know, very worthwhile for me.
>
> (From an interview with a woman from Ireland with a visual disability born around 1970)

These experiences suggest that ICT was an important tool for the interviewees to access aspects of Active Citizenship, in particular autonomy. Sometimes use of ICT was helpful in facilitating independence and access to specific areas of life.

Internet and mobile phone technology were useful for some interviewees in facilitating social participation in particular. One woman from the Czech Republic with an intellectual disability born around 1990 said that Skype and Facebook are her main means of interacting with people and making new friends. Another woman from Germany with a psychosocial disability born around 1970 described her social life before access to ICT as 'lonely'; she said, 'if I didn't have internet I sometimes would not have had any contacts to my environment at all (…) Who wants to deal anyhow with a single, unemployed mother?' The internet and social media were also cited by interviewees as a way for people with disabilities to meet and keep in contact with people in disability groups. One man from the UK with a mobility disability born around 1950 spoke about using ICT to keep in touch with a polio self-help group that not only provides social support but shares advice on technologies and medical treatments.

Some interviewees were first introduced to certain types of ICT and learned how to use them in education settings. There were several interviews where the impact of ICT on access to education was clear to the participants because they had stopped education at some point before accessible technology such as computers and voice-to-text software were available, and later returned to education after the use of such technologies had become widespread. One man from Ireland with a visual disability discussed the difference he experienced in accessing education after taking a break in his studies between 2000 and 2011.

> I did all right but what was different was that the reading was far more digital stuff and in [university] they made this stuff much more accessible. So they put a whole load of stuff into Word documents and they'd send them to people by email, so all of a sudden I'd these books and I could read them anywhere at any time, they were coming in through the email on my iPhone. That was the next significant development.
>
> (From an interview with a man from Ireland with a visual disability born around 1970)

Use of ICT as a positive factor in an interviewee's ability to access employment was also discussed. For example, one woman in Germany with a mobility disability (born around 1970) said that ICT was of the utmost importance for her because it allowed her to work and contact people independently. Several interviewees specifically said their current employment would be impossible without ICT. One woman from Switzerland with a psychosocial disability born around 1970 said that she would not be able to undertake her current work in peer counselling without ICT. Another woman from Germany with a mobility disability born around 1970 said ICT enabled her to work independently. Another woman from Switzerland with a mobility disability born around 1950 joked that the computer made her freer since she earned her salary through it.

Interviewees also discussed how accessible ICT sometimes replaced the need for assistive devices. They discussed the positive experience of buying products that worked for them but were not designed solely for people with disabilities (for example tablets and smartphones). One man from Ireland with a visual disability born around 1970 spoke about how he uses a variety of applications on his smartphone now instead of assistive devices: 'Everything's apps now. There used to be a separate thing you'd have to buy for €50 that would do that, and then it'd run out of batteries, you know, but now it's all apps.' Several said that they found the experience of buying accessible ICT as normalising or freeing. One woman discussed her enjoyment of going into a computer store and how she saw accessible ICT as changing the AT landscape.

> But like it's great to be able to just go in like that and see what'll work and make a decision rather than feeling you can only get … I think in a way assistive technology was nearly seen as just for disabled people whereas I think some of the more recent technologies are, I would define them as accessible technologies rather than assistive technologies, where I can use it but you can also use it. And it's the same device. I use it differently but I haven't had to pay anything extra for using it different, so to me that's great, you know, and I think that's the way it has to go that assistive technology shouldn't just be seen for people with disabilities.
>
> (From an interview with a woman from Ireland with a visual disability born around 1970)

What these different experiences show is that for many interviewees access to accessible ICT was an important facilitator for them to become Active Citizens in that the accessible technology often enhanced their autonomy. Accessible ICT was useful for them to become more independent and access social participation, education and employment. The ability to use accessible ICT as opposed to specialised assistive devices was also viewed by interviewees as a positive factor. These benefits are important to consider as we explore in the next section, how the interviewees faced barriers to accessing both AT and accessible ICT.

Barriers faced by persons with disabilities in accessing accessible technology

Barriers to accessing AT

Assistive technology can be defined under the Human Activity Assistive Technology (HAAT) model as 'an enabler for a human doing an activity in context' (Cook & Polgar, 2015). This definition requires the technology to adapt to the person and their particular circumstances rather than the person adapting to the technology (ibid.). The HAAT model is a useful framework for exploring AT in the context of the CRPD and Active Citizenship because of its person-focused approach. The International Organization for Standardization (ISO) defines assistive products under ISO 9999:2016 as:

> any product (including devices, equipment, instruments and software), especially produced or generally available, used by or for persons with disability: For participation; to protect, support, train, measure or substitute for body functions/structures and activities; or to prevent impairments, activity limitations or participation restrictions.
>
> (ISO, 2016, section 2.3)

In addition to these definitions, there are several articles of the CRPD that mention AT (see Chapter 8 in the accompanying Volume 1).

In mapping the different sorts of barriers people with disabilities face in accessing technology, the most common complaints fell into five general categories: availability, informational, procedural, financial and technological. Availability barriers referred to a lack of choice available to the interviewee. This usually occurred in insurance schemes where the interviewee had a limited choice of AT regardless of their particular needs. Technological barriers meant that the AT that the person needed did not exist, or what existed did not work for them. Informational barriers meant that the person did not have enough information to find the AT they wanted or needed. Procedural barriers encompassed rejections by insurance companies, difficulties with the organisation responsible for providing the AT and lengthy waits to receive the technology because of the procedures involved. In several cases, procedural barriers forced the interviewees to buy AT on the private market rather than attempting to access it through public provision. One woman in the UK with a mobility disability (born around 1970) discussed the difficulties she had in getting her stair lift covered.

> [T]hey weren't prepared to let me carry my daughter on my knee 'cos that would be a health and safety issue. So what they said to me is they can put in more care, so I could have more people coming into my home; which again frustrates me because it is intrusive. In the end I said no I will fund my own stair lift.
>
> (From an interview with a woman from the UK with a mobility disability born around 1970)

In discussing financial barriers, a man from Switzerland with a mobility disability spoke about the high cost of AT. He said that the need for AT made 'life with impairments (…) expensive' (Interview with a man from Switzerland with a mobility impairment born around 1950). Availability barriers were often cited and were intertwined with financial barriers as the public provision system had a limited selection of AT and anything additional had to be bought privately by the interviewee. One woman from Switzerland discussed needing a specialised office chair, but the only chair covered by the insurance scheme did not meet her needs so she had to buy her own chair (Interview with a woman from Switzerland with a mobility disability born around 1950).

All of these examples show the difficulties sometimes faced by people with disabilities trying to access AT. It is important to look at the different barriers as AT can be used to overcome barriers in the environment and better enable people with disabilities to live active lives (Scherer & Glueckauf, 2005; Scherer, Craddock & Mackeogh, 2011). Figure 7.1 shows the different barriers discussed by the interviewees according to disability identity.

Very few interviewees with psychosocial or intellectual disabilities discussed barriers to AT use. This is likely to be related to the fact that they often did not mention AT use at all. The non-use of AT by people with psychosocial and intellectual disabilities is consistent with similar previous studies on AT use as compared across disability identities (Kaye et al., 2008). Furthermore, many interviewees with intellectual or psychosocial disabilities interpreted the question on AT use as a question about their physical abilities (see the section on *How self-identification as a person with a disability impacted assistive technology use*).

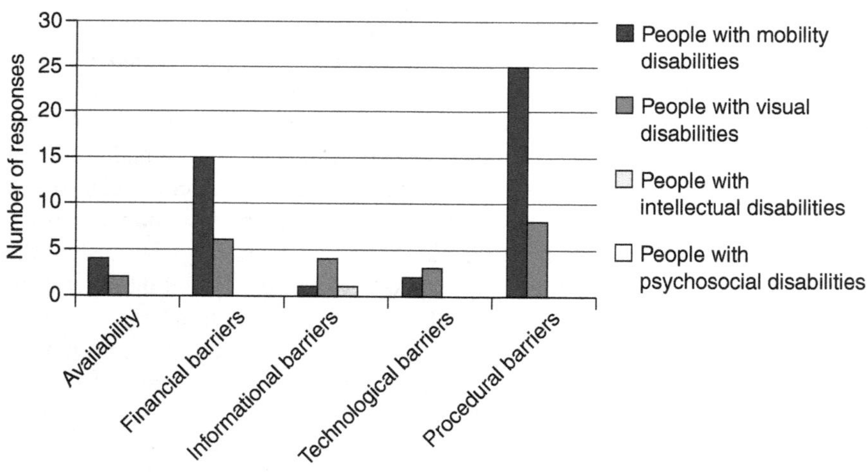

Figure 7.1 Perceived barriers to accessing assistive technology.

Barriers to accessing ICT

Overall, more people discussed the barriers faced in accessing AT rather than ICT. This lack of discussion of barriers to ICT is interesting when compared with earlier research on ICT and disability that predicted over-reliance on ICT would create additional barriers for people with disabilities or that people with disabilities would be excluded from ICT (Sheldon, 2004). That is not to say that there are no barriers to ICT. For example, few interviewees with intellectual disabilities reported internet usage, which suggests that they did experience barriers even if they did not always identify them in the interview. Much has been written about the inaccessibility of ICT to people with intellectual disabilities (Blanck, 2014) as well as barriers to ICT faced by other groups of people with disabilities (Dobranski & Hargittai, 2006). Figure 7.2 shows how many interviewees spoke about barriers they faced in accessing ICT, identified by disability and barrier type.

To the extent that interviewees talked specifically about information and communication technology, a majority mentioned financial barriers. Persons with intellectual disabilities talked more often about informational barriers, while persons with visual disabilities talked more often about technological barriers (Figure 7.2).

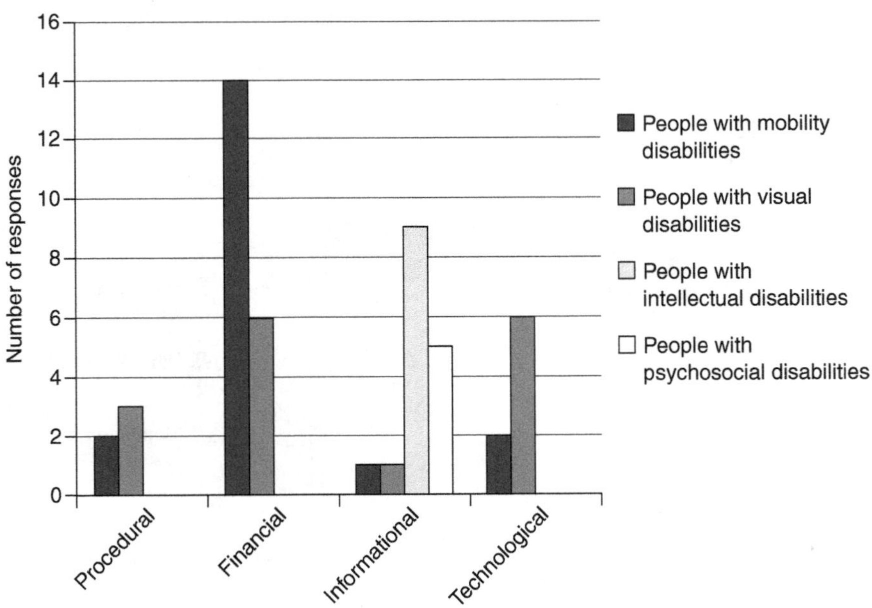

Figure 7.2 Perceived barriers to information and communication technology.

How self-identification as a person with a disability impacted assistive technology use

Although all interview participants knew they were participating in a disability research project, the last question asked in the interview was: 'Do you identify as a person with a disability?' The responses to this question were quite mixed, as illustrated in Figure 7.3. Out of 217 interviewees, 91 positively identified as persons with disabilities, while 67 said they did not identify as a person with a disability. A further 37 interviewees said their views on self-identification as a person with a disability changed over the course of their lives or was complicated, meaning that they neither fully identified as a person with a disability nor fully rejected that identity.

Whether or not someone identified as a person with a disability could impact on whether or not they accessed accessible technology. This is suggested in the data presented in Figure 7.3, which shows AT use among interviewees who did identify as a person with a disability as against those who did not self-identify as a person with a disability. If someone did not identify as a person with a disability in the interview, they may not self-identify for government purposes, thus losing access to public accessible technology provisions programmes.

People with psychosocial disabilities and intellectual disabilities sometimes responded to the question of whether or not they used AT by clarifying that they had no physical disabilities and thus no need. One interviewee with a psychosocial disability said this about accessing disability services:

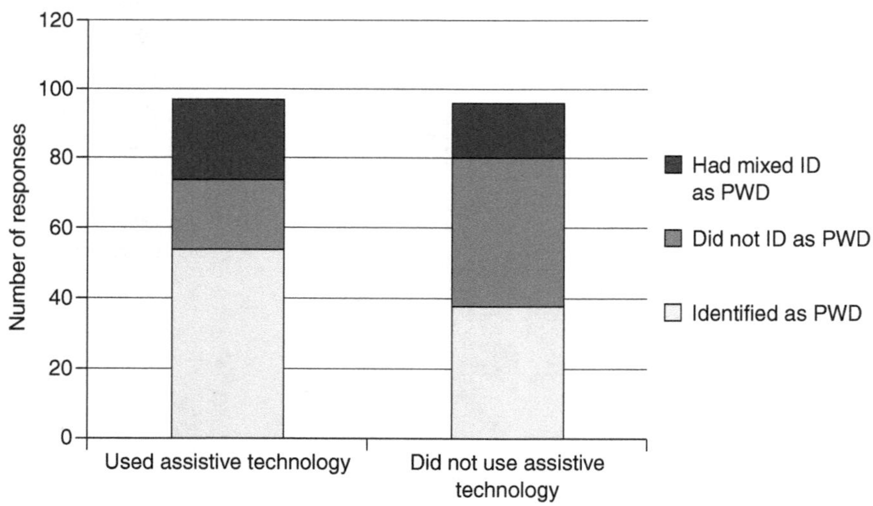

Figure 7.3 Correlation between use and non-use of AT and self-identification as disabled.

Notes

Total numbers. PWD: person with disability. N = 217. There were 17 interviews where the question was not asked or not answered by the interviewee.

> That is the only good that what my first assistant recommended to me that I apply for child …, an identity card for disabled persons (…) although I, erm, did not regard it as necessary …, why do I need an identity card for disabled persons, I just have depression, I'm not disabled I thought. (…) I thought of that as an absurdity that I could obtain one at all … because I cannot imagine in what way depression is a disability for them. I still can walk, I can see, I can hear … and I still ha' all my limbs.
>
> (From an interview with a woman from Germany with a psychosocial disability born around 1970)

These types of response suggest that, while there was a broad awareness of AT for people with physical disabilities, there was a lack of knowledge of existing and emerging AT for people with psychosocial and/or intellectual disabilities. One interviewee in Sweden with an intellectual disability (born around 1990) expressed an interest in AT that would help him remember things. This interviewee's lack of access was surprising given not only the existence of such technology but also the information available on assistive memory devices (e.g. Nordic Centre for Welfare and Social Issues, 2012). In other cases, this lack of knowledge could be related to whether or not government schemes covered AT for such disabilities. For example, the Czech Republic's AT scheme only extends to those with visual or physical disabilities.

AT was sometimes seen as a visual indicator that the interviewee was a person with a disability, and this influenced decisions on use. Several interviewees with visual impairments talked about how they decided whether or not to go out with a white cane in terms of how people reacted to them. One man from Ireland (born around 1970) with partial sight said he felt self-conscious both using and not using a white cane, because he worried that people would think he was faking his disability. Another man from the UK with a visual disability (born around 1970) said he did not use a white cane because it would signal vulnerability and he might get mugged. One woman from Ireland with a visual disability born around 1970 said that for years she had been too embarrassed to use her white cane. A woman from Switzerland with a visual disability (born around 1970) said that people were less friendly to her if she took her cane instead of her guide dog. Guide dogs were praised by several interviewees, not only for their ability to give people greater independence but also because guide dogs decreased the stigma of disability felt by the interviewees. As one interviewee from Ireland with a visual disability (born around 1970) said, they 'humanised the blind person'.

The visibility of AT was also brought up by interviewees with mobility disabilities. One woman with a mobility disability spoke about transitioning to a wheelchair and how she feared that would lead to greater social exclusion:

> And everything that I thought would be so bad, because I had heard from many that when you get a wheelchair people stop talking to you. And I have no such experiences! And I think it's about you and how you are. For

> example, I am used to defend my own rights and needs, I do not expect them to talk with those who are with me if it's me they should have an answer from. I feel that many have negative experiences with using a wheelchair, but I have only had positive experiences. It has expanded my radius of action, and I got back the energy and the motivation.
>
> (From an interview with a woman from Norway with a mobility disability born around 1950)

All of these examples illustrate how social stigmas influence the choices made for and by people with disabilities in their AT choices.

As this section shows, whether or not a person with a disability self-identifies or wishes to publically present as a 'person with a disability' can sometimes influence their use of AT. In some cases, not identifying as a person with a disability meant interviewees did not consider AT as a tool for them. In other cases, interviewees did not use visible AT as they did not want to appear disabled as they navigated public spaces. This issue of AT as stigmatising also applies to the use of accessible ICT especially with interviewees who preferred accessible ICT to assistive devices because it was the same technology everyone else around them was using.

Conclusion

The DISCIT project's approach to technology and disability was unique in a number of ways. One was that it used the term 'accessible technology' which encompassed ICT, AT and universal design. This broad focus allowed us to look both at how people with disabilities use accessible ICT and AT and at many other aspects of Active Citizenship. This broad remit allowed for the analysis of three broad and interrelated themes: (1) use of accessible ICT; (2) barriers to accessible technology; and (3) disability identity and AT use. These themes were chosen to highlight how use of accessible technology sometimes shaped the trajectories, transformations and turning points in interviewees' lives.

What we found throughout the interviews is that, for many people, access to ICT facilitated Active Citizenship in many areas of their lives from education to work to social participation to independent living. However, interviewees sometimes faced barriers in accessing ICT. This was especially true for people with intellectual disabilities who, for a variety of reasons, often had no access to or experience with the internet or computers or even in some cases mobile phones. Interviews with people with intellectual disabilities who did have access generally attested to positive experiences with such technology. This suggests that countries should look at how to increase access to ICT for people with disabilities, whether through increased information, financial subsidies, grants or computer classes.

While interviewees generally spoke of experiences with and access to ICT in positive terms, comments on access to AT were mixed. Many interview participants discussed in critical terms the experience of accessing AT through public provision systems. They complained of a lack of choice (availability) and procedural barriers which were often the result of unyielding bureaucratic systems or administrators who did not adequately listen to the needs and concerns of the interviewee who would ultimately use the device. This suggests that changes to the public provision system that increase the influence and autonomy of people with disabilities are needed. More respect for and involvement of people with disabilities in the AT provision systems in general would do much to remove many of the barriers described by interviewees. More specifically, changes that could be beneficial include:

- better training of accessible technology providers on human rights and the rights of persons with disabilities;
- amendments to the service systems that give the person with the disability better choice and control over what sort of AT they receive;
- recognition in the service system that the person with the disability is an expert in his or her own body and experience and, as such, should be respected; and
- assistive technology providers employing and consulting with end users of AT in procurement, setting of lists (for insurance companies) or any stage that determines the availability of AT in the system.

With regard to financial barriers, governments must realise the importance of accessible technology in the lives of people with disabilities and how it is sometimes integral to the ability of people with disabilities to live active and full lives. Providers of AT should consider the needs not only of people with physical disabilities but also of people with intellectual and psychosocial disabilities. Such groups do not always identify as persons with disabilities, so systems that predicate access to AT on identification as a person with a disability (i.e. through use of disability cards) should perhaps be examined. More information on types of AT also needs to be published and made available to people with psychosocial and intellectual disabilities so that such groups have the option of accessing it. It is also important that more work is done in society to reduce societal stigmatisation of disability, which sometimes impacted on whether a person with a disability accessed or publicly used the necessary AT.

This chapter has highlighted just a few ways in which accessible ICT and AT impact on Active Citizenship. The accounts of interviewees on the use of accessible ICT and the barriers they encounter show the promise of ICT for people with disabilities in different areas of their lives as well as the disparities in terms of access that still exist for people with disabilities. The accounts of how people access AT highlighted the barriers to access. Identifying the different types of barriers shows the need not only for targeted actions aimed at the systems of provision themselves in their general delivery but also for a nuanced approach to provision that takes into account the diversity within the identity of disability. This research shows the significance of accessible technology and AT as a tool that enables Active Citizenship as well as the importance of discussing and listening to people with disabilities about their accessible and assistive technology needs. Without better involvement of people with disabilities in assistive and accessible technology policies, the systems of provision will continue to contain barriers to access, thereby limiting the Active Citizenship of people with disabilities.

References

Abbott, C., Brown, D., Evett, L. & Standen, P. (2014). Emerging issues and current trends in assistive technology use 2007–2010: Practising, assisting and enabling learning for all. *Disability and Rehabilitation: Assistive Technology*, *9*(6), 453–462.

Anderson, B. & Tracey, K. (2001). Digital living: The impact (or otherwise) of the Internet on everyday life. *American Behavioral Scientist*, *45*(3), 456–475.

Andrich, R., Mathiassen, N., Hoogerwerf, E. & Gelderblom, G. J. (2013). Service delivery systems for assistive technology in Europe: An AAATE/EASTIN position paper. *Technology & Disability*, *25*(3), 127–146. doi: 10.3233/TAD-130381.

Blanck, P. (2014). The struggle for Web eQuality by persons with cognitive disabilities. *Behavioral Sciences & The Law*, *32*(1), 4–32.

Boyatzis, R. E. (1998). *Transforming qualitiative information. Thematic analysis and code development.* Thousand Oaks, CA: Sage Publications.

Braddock, D., Rizzolo, M. C. & Thompson, M. (2004). Emerging technologies and cognitive disability. *Journal of Special Education Technology*, *19*(4), 49–56.

Castells, M. (2002). Local and global: Cities in the network society. *Tijdschrift voor economische en sociale geografie*, *93*, 548–558. doi: 10.1111/1467-9663.00225.

Cook, A. M. & Polgar, J. M. (2015). *Assistive technologies. Principles & practices* (4th ed.) St. Louis, MI: Elvesier.

Dobransky, K. & Hargittai, E. (2006). The disability divide in internet access and use. *Information, Communication & Society*, *9*(3), 313–334.

Hocking, C. (1999). Function or feelings: Factors in abandonment of assistive devices. *Technology & Disability*, *11*(1/2), 3.

International Organization for Standardization and International Electrotechnical Commission. (2016). *Assistive products for persons with disability – Classification and terminology.* (ISO 9999:2016). Geneva: ISO.

Kaye, H., Yeager, P. & Reed, M. (2008). Disparities in usage of assistive technology among people with disabilities. *Assistive Technology*, *20*(4), 194–203.

Li-Tsang, C. W. P., Yeung, S. S. S., Choi, J. C. Y., Chan, C. C. H. & Lam, C. S. (2006). The effect of systematic information and communication technology (ICT) training programme for people with intellectual disabilities. *The British Journal of Development Disabilities*, *52*(1), 3–18.

Löfqvist, L., Nygren, C., Széman, Z. & Iwarsson, S. (2005). Assistive devices among very old people in five European countries. *Scandinavian Journal of Occupational Therapy*, *12*(4), 181–192.

Mayer, K. U. & Schoepflin, U. (1989). The state and the life course. *Annual Review of Sociology*, *15*, 185–209.

Mortimer, J. T. & Shanahan, M. J. (Eds). (2003). *Handbook of the life course*. New York: Springer.

Nordic Centre for Welfare and Social Issues. (2012). *Assistive technology for support of mental function when living with mental illness*, 6–9. Retrieved from www.sjukra.is/media/notendaleidbeiningar/assistive_technology.pdf.

OECD. (2014). *Communication spending* (indicator). doi: 10.1787/316a8ef1-en (accessed on 13 January 2016).

Priestley, M. (2003). *Disability: A life course approach*. Bristol: Policy Press.

Recacha, P. G. & Cafranga, A. M. (2011). Las personas con discapacidad intelectual ante las TIC. *Comunicar*, *18*, 173–180.

Scherer, M. J. & Glueckauf, R. (2005). Assessing the benefits of assistive technologies for activities and participation. *Rehabilitation Psychology*, *50*(2), 132–141. http://dx.doi.org/10.1037/0090-5550.50.2.132.

Scherer, M. J., Craddock, G. & Mackeogh, T. (2011). The relationship of personal factors and subjective well-being to the use of assistive technology devices. *Disability and Rehabilitation*, *33*(10), 811–817. doi: 10.3109/09638288.2010.511418.

Shah, S. & Priestley, M. (2011). *Disability and social change: Private lives and public bodies*. Bristol: Policy Press.

Sheldon, A. (2004). Changing technology. In J. Swain & S. French (Eds), *Disabling barriers – Enabling environments 155* (2nd ed.). London: SAGE Publications.

Söderström, S. (2009). Offline social ties and online use of computers: A study of disabled youth and their use of ICT advances. *New Media Society*, *11*, 709–727.

Steel, D. M. & Gray, M. A. (2009). Baby boomers' use and perception of recommended assistive technology. *International Journal of Therapy and Rehabilitation*, *16*(10), 546–556.

Steel, E. & de Witte, L. P. (2011). Advances in European assistive technology service delivery and recommendations for further improvement. *Technology and Disability*, *23*(3), 131–138. doi: 10.3233/TAD-2011-0321.

Stendal, K. (2012). How do people with disability use and experience virtual worlds and ICT: A literature review. *Journal for Virtual Worlds Research*, *5*(1). doi: http://dx.doi.org/10.4101/jvwr.v5i1.6173.

UN Committee on the Rights of Persons with Disabilities. (2013). General comment N. 9 on accessibility. Retrieved from www.ohchr.org/EN/HRBodies/CRPD/Pages/DGCArticles12And9.aspx.

Verza, R., Carvalho, M. L., Battaglia, M. A. & Uccelli, M. M. (2006). An interdisciplinary approach to evaluating the need for assistive technology reduces equipment abandonment. *Multiple Sclerosis Journal 12*(1), 88–93. doi: 10.1191/1352458506ms1233oa.

Vicente, M. R. & López, A. J. (2010). A multidimensional analysis of the disability digital divide: Some evidence for internet use. *The Information Society*, *26*(1), 48–64. doi: 10.1080/01615440903423245.

Walker, R. & Leisering, L. (Eds). (1998). *The dynamics of modern society: Poverty, policy and welfare*. Bristol: Policy Press.

Wessels, R., Dijcks, B., Soede, M., Gelderblom, G. J. & De Witte, L. (2003). Non-use of provided assistive technology devices: A literature overview. *Technology and Disability*, *15*(4), 231–238.

Yerkes, M. A., Peper, B. & Baxter J. (2013). Welfare states and the life course. In B. Greves (Ed.), *The Routledge handbook of the welfare state*. Oxford: Routledge.

Zhao, H. & Phillips, B. (1993). Predictors of assistive technology abandonment. *Assistive Technology: The Official Journal of RESNA*, *5*(1), 36–45.

8 How do persons with psychosocial disabilities experience and practise Active Citizenship in education and work?

Marie Sépulchre, Rafael Lindqvist, Victoria Schuller and Kjetil Klette Bøhler

Mental health has become a main concern in the European policy landscape. It is now widely recognised that mental illness reduces the wellbeing of individuals and their families and has an important economic cost (Scarpetta & Colombo, 2016; WHO, 2015). However, these issues tend to be studied from a medical perspective, and Morrow and Weisser (2012) observed that 'the social and structural aspects of mental health continue to be marginalised as do the voices of people with lived experience of mental distress' (p. 30).

This chapter adopts a relational approach to mental health and recognises that experiences of psychosocial disabilities take place in a social, structural and historical context (Morrow & Weisser, 2012; Mulvany, 2000; Ramon & Williams, 2005; WHO, 2012). We also acknowledge that psychosocial disabilities are not permanent conditions but evolve during the life course and can be different from one day to another (Thoits, 2006; WHO, 2012). Drawing on life-course interviews with persons with psychosocial disabilities, this chapter explores pathways and practices of Active Citizenship. The scope of this chapter does not permit the treatment of all aspects of Active Citizenship. We focus on Active Citizenship in relation to education and work. Education is an important means by which individuals become citizens (Marshall, 1992) and it is through paid and unpaid work that individuals contribute to society. It is important to note that this chapter adopts a broad understanding of education and work; education is considered both as formal education and as life-long learning, and work is considered as paid and unpaid contributions to society.

The chapter is structured in the following way: the first part discusses Active Citizenship for persons with psychosocial disabilities and delineates the conceptual framework. The second part presents the methodology used for collecting and analysing the data. The third part turns to the empirical analysis and discusses informants' experiences of Active Citizenship in education and work. The fourth part sets the findings in a life-course perspective, and finally the chapter concludes by summarising the main findings.

Active Citizenship for persons with psychosocial disabilities

Active Citizenship is far from a given for persons with psychosocial disabilities. People labelled unreasonable and mentally ill have been excluded from society, treated in psychiatric hospitals, subjected to compulsory treatments and forced sterilisation, and denied the right to vote and to decide about their personal finances (Carey, 2003; Rogers & Pilgrim, 1989; Sayce, 2000; Sépulchre & Lindqvist, 2016; Ware, Hopper, Tugenberg, Dickey & Fisher, 2007). Although many large segregated psychiatric hospitals have been closed down over the past few decades and although the rights of persons with psychosocial disabilities are increasingly being recognised, the evidence indicates that persons with psychosocial disabilities still face stigma, discrimination, compulsory treatment, economic hardship, unemployment, and unequal access to healthcare, education and work (Eurofound, 2003; Kozma & Petri, 2012; Link & Phelan, 2001; Sayce, 2000; Thornicroft, 2006; Whitley & Campbell, 2014; WHO, 2005). It follows that they risk being marginalised and excluded from participation in society (Nelson, Lord & Ochocka, 2001; Parr, 2008; Sayce & Curran, 2007; Ware et al., 2007).

This chapter draws on the theoretical framework elaborated for the DISCIT project (see Chapters 1 and 2). In the project, the concept of Active Citizenship operationalises the notion of 'full and effective participation in the community' of the United Nations Convention on the Rights of Persons with Disabilities (CRPD) (UN, 2006). The DISCIT framework considers that practices of Active Citizenship are shaped by the extent to which individuals have the opportunity to enjoy a minimum level of security (financially and in terms of health), to make choices concerning their lives and to participate in decisions concerning their community and society in general. These different dimensions of Active Citizenship – which we refer to as security, autonomy and influence – are interrelated and equally important (see also Waldschmidt, 2013). This chapter examines the life-course narratives of persons with psychosocial disabilities and the factors that enhanced or hampered their practices of Active Citizenship (see Table 8.1).

With regard to factors hampering Active Citizenship, we distinguish between barriers and risks. We define *barriers* as personal, socio-economic or environmental factors which restrict an individual's ability to be an active citizen in a given situation. Examples of barriers are psychosocial problems, difficult family relations, poverty, high educational fees and discriminatory practices in the labour market. *Risks*, on the other hand, are circumstances that may lead to a

Table 8.1 Four types of factors influencing Active Citizenship

	Present	*Future*
Encourages Active Citizenship	Facilitator	Opportunity
Restricts Active Citizenship	Barrier	Risk

reduced level of Active Citizenship in the future. Risks are, for example, uncertain development of psychosocial disabilities, fragile relationships with friends and family and unstable economic situations. Individuals manage these uncertainties during the life course according to socio-structural contexts (Apitzsch, 2010; Reiter, 2010).

In this chapter, we refer to a reduced level of Active Citizenship as Restricted Citizenship to indicate instances where practices of Active Citizenship are restricted by various factors. We prefer the notion of Restricted Citizenship to the notion of Passive Citizenship, because the latter is commonly understood in the literature as passive membership in a state (Turner, 1990) or as passive reception of welfare provision (Giddens, 1998; Rosanvallon, 1995). Hence, in this chapter we use the notion of Restricted Citizenship because we do not look at passive membership in general but seek to examine how a series of barriers and risks restricts the interviewees' practices of citizenship.

This chapter also takes into account factors that enhance full and effective participation in society, thereby distinguishing between *facilitators* and *opportunities*. We understand *facilitators* as factors at the personal, socio-economic and environmental level which are readily available to enhance Active Citizenship. An academic degree, vocational training, welfare benefits and 'key persons' – i.e. persons who provide support and enhance a person's Active Citizenship – can constitute facilitators. By contrast, *opportunities* are factors that imply changes and the creation of new possibilities leading to Active Citizenship in the future. Examples of opportunities are the development of user-associations, personalised welfare services and anti-discrimination legislation. Drawing on the capability approach, Ware and colleagues (2007) developed a framework to define social integration of persons with psychiatric disabilities. They noted the importance of opportunities provided by social environments because these 'offer opportunities for individual competency to be developed and exercised' (p. 469). We use the capability approach to understand how internal and external structures are linked with the agency of persons with disabilities (see Chapter 2).

As with the distinction between barriers and risks, opportunities and facilitators are distinguished in terms of time relations. In short, we understand barriers and facilitators as factors that have a direct impact in the present, and risks and opportunities as being related to potential practices of Active Citizenship in the future (see Table 8.1). It should be noted that a particular factor, such as a piece of legislation or contact with a social worker, cannot be qualified as barrier, risk, facilitator or opportunity per se. Rather, its effect can only be measured in relation to an individual's lived experience of citizenship. Drawing on the capability approach, we can say that one factor can become a risk, barrier, opportunity or facilitator, depending on its meaning within a specific context and depending on personal, social and environmental conversion factors that will enable the conversion of means into capability sets and functioning (Robeyns, 2005). Take, for example, high educational expectations in the family. These expectations may be a factor enabling a person to take up education in the present (facilitator) or contribute to making this a possibility for employment in the future (opportunity).

However, if the individual struggles with her studies, these expectations may increase her psychosocial difficulties and decrease her possibilities for Active Citizenship at present (barrier) or in the future (risk).

Data and methods

The data for this chapter consists of the interview summaries of 52 life-course interviews with persons with psychosocial disabilities living in the Czech Republic, Germany, Ireland, Italy, Norway, Serbia, Sweden, Switzerland and the United Kingdom. The sample is diverse in terms of gender (25 women and 27 men) and age (17 interviewees were born around 1950, 18 were born around 1970 and 17 were born around 1990). Although the interviewees varied in many respects, such as type of psychosocial difficulties, self-identification as a person with disabilities, gender, age and country of residence, all had experienced long-term psychosocial difficulties during their life courses and many interviewees had received support from the welfare system (for details about the methodology, see Chapter 3).

The first step in the analysis was to read and code the interview summaries. We coded the persons' experiences in the different areas covered by the interviews and used the concepts of barriers, risks, opportunities and facilitators to highlight the factors that seemed to influence the experiences mentioned in the interview summaries. As a second step of the analysis, we examined the factors coded as barriers, risks, facilitators and opportunities and sought to understand the mechanisms leading into and out of Active Citizenship in education and work. Drawing on life-course methods, we paid special attention to factors marking turning points and transitions in individual life trajectories (Carlsson, 2011, p. 3; see also Chapter 2). The third step of the analysis was to consider the complexity and dynamic aspects of Active Citizenship. While we had mainly focused on particular events and short-term experiences of Active Citizenship up to this point, in the final part of the analysis we introduced a life-course perspective and explored the varying degrees to which interviewees were able to participate in society during their lives. The empirical analysis revealed a diversity of Active Citizenship experiences, which we tried to capture in an ideal-typical model (Weber, 2011, p. 90ff.) of four pathways leading into and out of Active Citizenship. The following section presents the results of the empirical analysis. It starts by discussing the experiences and practices of Active Citizenship of persons with psychosocial disabilities in education and then turns to the realm of work.

Experiences of (Active) Citizenship through education

Education is a central area for Active Citizenship in the sense that it provides knowledge and skills that can be used in everyday life (such as literacy and numeracy), knowledge about the functioning of society and the world, and knowledge about citizenship rights and duties (Lawton, Cairns & Gardner, 2000;

Marshall, 1992). It also includes training for a job and provides educational qualifications, which are often requested by employers. Education is protected by Article 24 of the CRPD that recognises the right of persons with disabilities to education and lifelong learning. Education is typically provided through schooling during the first part of the life course but, in this chapter, we also look at self-education and adult education. To give a quick overview of the empirical data (52 interviews in total): 45 interviewees had participated in mainstream education, two interviewees had only attended special education and five had experienced both mainstream and special education. Regarding tertiary education, 22 interviewees had started higher education and 14 had completed higher education.

Barriers and risks relating to education

Many interviewees had come across barriers to receiving the education they desired. The family situation could be a barrier to education, and several interviewees reported that their parents had psychosocial difficulties, drinking problems or mood swings. This was the case for a Swiss man (born around 1970). Due to continuing fights with his mother – who was later diagnosed with schizophrenia – his father left the family when the participant was seven. When his older sister also moved out, he lived alone with his mother and he experienced the same difficulties with her as his father and his sister had before him. This situation resulted in fatigue and anxieties, and the interviewee spoke of lacking the energy to participate in school. While he had been a good student before his sister moved out, his grades now started to drop and he described feeling increasingly overwhelmed by regular school tasks. Moreover, he was harassed by the other students due to his mother's condition and because he was perceived as weak.

Practical barriers could also prevent education. A Serbian woman (born around 1990) reported that she could not continue at school after her primary education because her parents did not have the time to drive her to the nearby city where the secondary school was located. Another type of barrier was informal work in the family and gendered expectations. A Swiss woman (born around 1950) could not participate in secondary education because she had to take care of her younger siblings. Later, she was forced by her father to study home economics (as many women of her generation did) and then train as a salesperson, although she wanted to study further and be a nurse (see also Chapter 10).

Social isolation was often mentioned in the interviews. Many interviewees reported experiences of being alone, having very few friends, being bullied and fighting with their peers during their years of schooling. Barriers to social inclusion could be environmental factors such as prejudice about mental ill health and different behaviour, but many interviewees also believed that their social isolation was caused by personal factors such as episodes of psychosocial distress (e.g. during periods of depression) or by their personality as 'loners'. Some interviewees remembered their psychosocial difficulties as starting during primary school and having a negative impact on their education. A man from Sweden (born around 1990) explained that his parents sent him to a psychologist because they were worried that he did not have any friends. He received a psychiatric diagnosis but he did not receive any additional support and remained isolated from his peers. Another example is a Norwegian woman (born around 1990) who sought support from a teacher in secondary school. One day, when she was 17, she felt deeply depressed and contacted the teacher for a meeting, which she described as follows:

> I felt that it was enough, too many negative feelings to deal with, so I asked her if I could talk to her, and then it all ran out of me, and I understand that she was very scared because I said bluntly that I didn't want to live anymore and that I had tried to kill myself. So she took this very seriously and wanted to help me, and contacted the psychiatric clinic for adolescents, and they decided to place me at an institution for psychiatric patients, because they feared I would kill myself.
>
> (From an interview with a Norwegian woman with psychosocial impairment born around 1990)

Following this meeting, the interviewee described how she was taken out of school and had to stay in a closed psychiatric clinic until the age of 23, which prevented her from finishing upper secondary school and qualifying for higher education. This narrative suggests that teachers were ill equipped to deal with psychosocial difficulties and that the long period of hospitalisation was a barrier to education. The disclosure of psychosocial difficulties can be interpreted as a turning point which drastically changed her educational trajectory.

Similarly, various interviewees recalled previous hospital stays as traumatic experiences, because they had been hospitalised without their consent, had been isolated from their families for an extended period of time and/or had not received helpful treatments. Such experiences were more likely to be found in the narratives of persons born around 1950 but could even be found in the narratives of people born around 1990 living in countries where large psychiatric institutions still exist (notably the Czech Republic and Serbia). Interviewees also pointed to the side-effects of the psychiatric medication, which hampered their intellectual faculties, their ability to concentrate and their interest in music and art.

For those who dropped out of education or who wanted to learn new skills later in life, adult education was a possibility. Financial barriers could, however, stand in the way of such plans. An English man (born around 1970) explained that he wanted to become a teaching assistant, helping people with learning difficulties in the area of informatics and he enrolled in a course to realise this goal. However, a policy change introduced by the new government saw funding taken away and fees introduced for such adult training courses. This marked a turning point for the interviewee because he could not afford to pay these fees, which sent him back into a downward spiral of depression. From then on, he remained unemployed and only attended activities for people with mental health problems.

These findings echo the results of studies about the experiences of persons with psychiatric disabilities in education. In a study about higher education, Megivern, Pellerito and Mowbray (2003) found that psychiatric symptomatology, lack of integration on campus (e.g. difficulties making and keeping friends), competing responsibilities (e.g. family responsibilities), conflictual relationships with family members and financial problems constituted barriers in higher education. To that list of barriers, Belch (2011) added the stigma attached to mental health, which also appeared as a factor in the life-course interviews.

Facilitators and opportunities relating to education

In addition to negative experiences, the interviewees also reported positive experiences in education and their life-course narratives suggest that 'key persons', i.e. persons who provided support in various ways, were important facilitators in educational trajectories. For instance, after he had left school at the age of 16, an Irish man (born around 1970) received special attention and support from a social worker who saw his potential and encouraged him to continue in education. The interviewee reported that, thanks to this support, he was now finishing a PhD in psychology. The importance of support and connectedness for active participation in life has been highlighted by other studies about the experiences of persons with psychosocial disabilities (Belch, 2011; Ridgway, 2001; Ware et al., 2007). Discussing the situation of persons with psychosocial disabilities in higher education, Belch (2011) concluded that 'one fundamental goal of higher education is to create and sustain campus communities that are welcoming, supportive, understanding and caring' (p. 89).

Some interviewees pointed to the importance of making their own choices about education independently of what their family wanted. An example is a Norwegian woman (born around 1950) who had struggled to find out what she wanted to study in higher education before embarking on teacher training:

> It was an experimental, alternative and really exciting [teaching] school. A completely new way of thinking about teaching, it became such a period of blossoming for me. It was kind of my own arena, because my siblings had taken higher university degrees in chemistry and the like. And I chose something completely different. And I loved the teaching school: it was enjoyment and play from morning to night. So this was kind of an important turning point for me. I was able to use my own creativity, and I started in the theatre, and I started to think about pedagogical methods for children in theatre, with dance and movements and things like that … And then I worked as a teacher from 1972 to 2000.
>
> (Interview with a Norwegian woman with psychosocial disabilities born around 1950)

This quote suggests that the teacher education was a turning point in the interviewee's life and that it created an opportunity that helped her access different dimensions of Active Citizenship later in life. First, working for almost 30 years as a teacher provided her with a stable financial situation and seems to have improved her mental health (security). Second, teaching initiated 'a period of blossoming' that helped her define the life she wanted to live and to choose work based upon her own interests (autonomy). And finally, through her engagement in the school and her focus on arts and creativity, she participated in shaping her society (influence). Likewise, an Irish woman (born around 1950) found that she had received the education she wanted because she had had a good quality education, lots of choices regarding school subjects and some very good teachers. Moreover, the process of learning and reflecting seemed to be a facilitator for coping with psychosocial difficulties. For example, a British man (born around 1990) described writing a book both as an educational journey and as personal therapy; he declared that 'the book is about paths and self-teaching really, because that is what got me through life'.

Experiences of Restricted and Active Citizenship in work

Work is a central area of Active Citizenship in the sense that it provides financial income, social status in society and a network of colleagues (Evans & Repper, 2000; Jahoda, 1982; Leff & Warner, 2006; Warr, 1987). In contrast, Stuart (2006) observed that unemployment and the lack of valorised social roles put persons with psychosocial disabilities 'in a position of double jeopardy; on the one hand, being stigmatized because of their mental disorder (making it harder to gain competitive employment) and on the other hand, being stigmatized for their lack of occupation' (p. 522). Article 27 of the CRPD protects the right to work, 'including the right to the opportunity to gain a living through work freely chosen or to be accepted in a labour market and work environment that is open, inclusive and accessible to persons with disabilities'.

To give a quick overview of the data (52 interviews in total): 36 interviewees had exclusively participated in the regular labour market (among these, 22 interviewees reported having had mainly short-term contracts), 4 interviewees had worked in sheltered employment, 8 interviewees had worked in both regular and sheltered employment, 2 interviewees had helped out in the family business (without formal work contracts) and 2 interviewees had only participated in unpaid traineeships. Fourteen interviewees had faced severe financial problems and 42 interviewees had received welfare benefits for some periods of their lives. Apart from paid work in the regular labour market, the notion of work used in this chapter includes informal work in the family, in the community and in voluntary organisations. Twenty-two interviewees had worked as volunteers, 29 had participated in peer-support groups and 11 had been involved in politics. Activities in the labour market, voluntary and informal work were not mutually exclusive, however, and many interviewees spoke of activities in different types of work throughout their life course.

Barriers and risks relating to work

Many interviewees characterised the mainstream labour market as extremely competitive, and young interviewees in particular explained how they struggled to find meaningful jobs or traineeships. Some interviewees reported that they were not able to live up to society's expectation of having a full-time job and being active in the mainstream labour market. Too much pressure was often viewed as a barrier in the workplace, leading to sick leave and hospitalisation. A Czech woman (born around 1950) explained that her workload increased so much after a period of corporate restructuring that she had to finish her work at home in the evenings. She did not complain because she was afraid of losing her job but, after months of hard work, she had a nervous breakdown and was hospitalised. This period of hospitalisation marked a turning point in her work trajectory and was followed by a period of unemployment and psychosocial difficulties.

Psychosocial difficulties often include fluctuating work abilities, which form an important barrier to Active Citizenship in the labour market. Barriers may be created by employers who refuse to accommodate special needs. For example, a Swiss man (born around 1970) reported that he was dismissed because his employer lacked understanding about his unpunctuality. Barriers may also be created by the personal consequences of psychosocial disabilities. For example, a Swedish woman (born around 1990) explained that it was impossible to work during some periods because depression 'knocked her off course'. In a similar vein, a German man (born around 1970) said that his psychosis had forced him to retire at the age of 35.

Many interviewees felt trapped in low-paid jobs or in the welfare system. After a period of inactivity, an Italian man (born around 1970) got a job in the kitchen of a social cooperative, where he received a very small salary. He had to wash dishes, serve food and clean the yard. The interviewee said that he would rather have prepared the food but that this was not possible because he did not know how to cook. He concluded that it was hard to find work in his situation. Another example is a Swedish man (born around 1990) who tried to find a position in the labour market. After he had experienced difficulties in a number of supported traineeships, the Employment Agency transferred him to the Social Insurance Agency and he obtained sickness benefits. He regretted that he had very little money to live on but was afraid of losing these benefits if he looked for a job or returned to education. He felt trapped by the rules of the welfare system. Various interviewees believed that vocational rehabilitation measures would be facilitators to finding a job after a period of hospitalisation but regretted the limited availability of such support at psychiatric hospitals and employment agencies. In other cases, the interviewees did not think that they could benefit from any kind of support; they believed that they were not capable of being active in the labour market because of their psychosocial disabilities.

Negative attitudes and discrimination were pointed to as barriers in the workplace and many interviewees feared the stigma of mental health so strongly that they refrained from disclosing their psychosocial difficulties to their employers and relatives. This is in line with the findings of Whitley and Campbell (2014) who observed that, although their participants did not commonly experience stigma and discrimination, they perceived stigma and discrimination as potential problems and took preventive measures to avoid such problems. The life-course interviews suggest that the choice not to disclose psychosocial disabilities can be interpreted as one such preventive measure. However, although the decision not to disclose psychosocial disabilities limited the risk of stigmatisation, it led to other problems; the interviewees did not receive the support they needed and had to take sick leave or quit their job when their personal situation became overwhelming.

Some interviewees had to retire early and were on disability pensions. They sometimes found other meaningful occupations, but a Swedish man (born around 1970) expressed the opinion that receiving a disability pension was not the same as having a 'real job'. Although he explained that he would prefer to have a job and earn a proper salary, he believed that paid employment was not an option because of his depression and psychosis. He had, however, found a meaningful occupation at a sheltered workshop. Moreover, several interviewees recalled that the decision to retire early had been made in moments of mental distress when they felt incapable of working and that retiring had not always been voluntary. Some interviewees would have preferred to continue working. For example, a German woman (born around 1970) explained that she was forced to retire although she had applied for a place on a retraining programme:

> I did not apply for a pension at all. I applied for retraining because of my spine … Yes, then I was examined by a general practitioner who said that I could work, then also by a psychologist. And she said: 'No. People who have depression do not have to work, do not need any work because they can't work anyway.' That's why I got a pension instead of retraining.
>
> (From an interview with a German woman with psychosocial disabilities born around 1970)

At the same time, the process of obtaining social or disability benefits was sometimes very complicated and many interviewees explained that they had struggled – and sometimes even gone to court – before receiving welfare benefits. In countries with low welfare payments, the interviewees tried to earn additional income by taking extra jobs (reported, for example, in the Czech Republic), or were fully dependent on their relatives (reported, for example, in Italy and Serbia). Even in the Scandinavian countries, which are known for their generous welfare benefits, interviewees reported that they had very little money to live on, struggled to obtain or keep benefits and felt trapped because taking a paid job would mean losing their benefits. Overall, the interviews suggest that being outside the labour market implied a series of risks. An obvious but central concern was that interviewees risked living in poverty and having limited access to quality (mental) health care, alternative forms of therapy (e.g. art and theatre), housing, participation in civil society, leisure activities and technology. For example, a Swedish woman (born around 1990) said that she could only afford to go to the cinema when she received money from her father. This example demonstrates the consequences of low incomes for social inclusion, since activities such as going to the cinema are not only private leisure activities but can also be part of communal activities with friends.

Facilitators and opportunities relating to work

The interviews suggest that participation in a meaningful occupation is an important element of inclusion in society. The story of a Norwegian woman (born around 1990) provides an illustration. She reported that, after seven years in a psychiatric institution, during which she was given the wrong diagnosis and treatment, she moved back to the community and took up sports. She explained that this improved her mental strength and confidence and that as a result she decided to become a personal trainer. Through work, she felt included in the community and achieved a stable financial situation.

Interviewees pointed to the importance of financial support through social welfare programmes during transition periods, such as periods of unemployment or hospitalisation. Likewise, services such as re-integration programmes and support from mental health care professionals created opportunities to return to work. For some interviewees, the availability of sheltered jobs near their homes was an important facilitator. A Swedish woman (born around 1970) explained that she had a good relationship with her work colleagues and bosses at the sheltered workshop. She enjoyed being in a work environment with other people who faced psychosocial difficulties, although she specified that they never spoke about mental health problems in the workplace.

Similar to education, key persons were mentioned as important facilitators for work. A Czech woman (born around 1950) explained that the support of her husband had enabled her to remain in a job, because he had helped her when she had to finish her work at home. Key persons could also be employers. A German woman (born round 1950) reported that her boss gave her flexibility when she had a 'bad week'. She appreciated that he accommodated her without treating her as inferior to her colleagues. In general, flexible working arrangements seemed to be an important facilitator for active participation in work. For example, a Czech woman (born around 1990) who had difficulties keeping a job because of her psychosocial problems explained that working from home as a self-employed teacher suited her needs.

Besides paid work, interviewees were engaged in informal work in their families or in the community. The life-course interviews suggest that such activities provided a space for social recognition and security. For example, an English man (born around 1990) volunteered as an 'ambassador' for people with mental health problems. He described how being on this project gave him a sense of purpose and how he contributed to raising awareness about the issue of psychosocial disabilities through his participation in advocacy work throughout the country. Similarly, other interviewees stated that their participation in peer support groups and organisations of various kinds enabled them to learn new skills, meet people and cope with their psychosocial problems. Many interviewees who had been through periods of mental distress were actively engaged in self-help groups or worked as peer counsellors. They explained that they had chosen this activity because they wanted to share their experiences and help people with similar difficulties.

Active Citizenship from a life-course perspective: four pathways

The empirical analysis suggests that practices of Active Citizenship are restricted when people lack education, are financially and emotionally dependent on their relatives, experience psychosocial disabilities, are socially isolated or have a vulnerable position in the labour market. By contrast, Active Citizenship is enhanced by facilitators such as key persons, meaningful activities, flexible working arrangements and welfare benefits. In our analysis of the life-course interviews, we observed that experiences of Active Citizenship are sometimes followed by periods of Restricted Citizenship, and vice-versa. Four ideal-typical pathways can be sketched on the basis of our empirical data (see Table 8.2).

Before presenting the four pathways, it is, however, important to note that these ideal-typical categories do not aim to explain or include all details of the life-course interviews. Rather, ideal-types give a simplified picture of a complex phenomenon and highlight some salient characteristics (Weber, 1949).

Pathway 1: experiencing multiple facilitators and using opportunities

Pathway 1 refers to the situation of persons who described themselves as successful students and who found that they had received the education they wished for, i.e. a situation of (more or less) permanent Active Citizenship. Their education turned out to be a facilitator for securing paid work, obtaining a job that they liked, achieving a recognised social status and enjoying financial security. Although these persons had experienced difficulties related to their psychosocial

Table 8.2 Four ideal-typical pathways of citizenship

	Followed by Active Citizenship	*Followed by Restricted Citizenship*
Active Citizenship	Experiencing multiple facilitators and using opportunities (Pathway 1)	Experiencing facilitators and opportunities, followed by barriers and risks that become a reality (Pathway 2)
Restricted Citizenship	Experiencing barriers and risks, then getting access to facilitators and using opportunities (Pathway 3)	Experiencing multiple barriers and risks that become a reality (Pathway 4)

disabilities, the availability of welfare programmes, key persons and other types of facilitators supported and encouraged their Active Citizenship.

The story of a Swedish woman (born around 1950) illustrates this pathway. Although not a very good student and challenged by episodes of psychosocial difficulties, she managed to finish her education and worked for 30 years as an assistant nurse in a hospital. She had to retire early but was happy with her life and the friends she met in an organisation for persons with psychosocial disabilities.

Pathway 2: experiencing facilitators and opportunities, followed by barriers and risks that become a reality

Pathway 2 includes persons who practised Active Citizenship at a certain point in their lives but who, following a series of difficulties, became marginalised and had problems participating actively in society, i.e. found themselves in a vicious circle or downward spiral of decreasing levels of Active Citizenship. This is, for example, the case for interviewees who experienced stress in the workplace and had to quit their jobs. Consequently, they found that they could not take on a full-time position and wanted a part-time job, which proved difficult to find. Hence, they relied on financial help from relatives or on meagre welfare benefits, struggled to find a meaningful occupation and faced increased psychosocial disabilities. This pathway led to situations of Restricted Citizenship, implying financial problems, inactivity and social isolation.

This pathway can be illustrated by the story of an Italian man (born around 1950) who successfully finished his education, was politically active and worked as a lawyer for a few years. He married but then divorced and developed depression. He was hospitalised and received electroshocks and drug treatments. Then he met another partner, but she died shortly afterwards and his psychosocial disabilities worsened again. At the time of the interview, he was working in a social cooperative, but was dissatisfied because he found that this occupation was not commensurate with his level of education.

Pathway 3: experiencing barriers and risks, then getting access to facilitators and using opportunities

Pathway 3 refers to the experience of persons who started from a situation of Restricted Citizenship but had the opportunity to increase their participation in society later in life, i.e. entered a virtuous circle of interdependent mechanisms that faciliated more Active Citizenship. For example, some interviewees grew up with family members experiencing psychosocial difficulties, had multiple periods of hospitalisation in psychiatric hospitals, dropped out of school and felt that they did not engage in any worthwhile activity for some time. Meeting a key person at a psychiatric hospital, being enrolled in an educational programme at a charity or an organisation, being introduced to a peer support group and doing voluntary work were examples of opportunities that could lead interviewees from Restricted to Active Citizenship. However, it is noteworthy that, although these forms of social engagement can be seen as examples of the autonomy and influence dimensions of Active Citizenship, interviewees engaging solely in unpaid work were often deprived of Active Citizenship in relation to financial security. The empirical data indicated that this situation could be compensated for by adequate financial support from welfare systems.

The story of a Czech woman (born around 1990) is an example of this pathway. The interviewee had a difficult and lonely childhood following the divorce of her parents, during which she had to support her mother emotionally. After the death of her father, she attempted to commit suicide and was subsequently hospitalised. Later, she successfully finished her tertiary education and started working as a kindergarten teacher. At the time of the interview, she was happily married and on maternity leave to take care of her little girl.

Pathway 4: experiencing multiple barriers and risks that become a reality

Pathway 4 refers to persons who for the most part faced barriers throughout their life courses and for whom risks related to psychosocial disabilities became a reality, i.e. remained in a situation of more or less permanent exclusion from Active Citizenship. For example, some interviewees were bullied, did not receive adequate support in school or the workplace, dropped out of school, were forced to retire early, experienced many periods of mental distress or struggled to obtain adequate support from family and welfare organisations. Typically, in this pathway persons were offered a disability pension which gave them rudimentary material security but little autonomy or influence. The interviews suggested that the persons ran the risk of being 'archived' in the social security agency with little prospect of being offered psychosocial rehabilitation, a meaningful occupation or social contacts after becoming entitled to a disability pension. This, in turn, put them at risk of being locked into a situation of Restricted Citizenship.

The story of a German woman (born around 1970) provides an illustration of this pathway. The interviewee did not get the education she wanted, she experienced several periods of financial insecurity, had difficulties keeping a job and had to accept early retirement although it was not her preference. Asked to narrate important changes and turning points in her life, she said that they were all 'crap'.

These four ideal-typical pathways into and out of Active Citizenship shed light on the diverse life-course narratives found in the empirical data. The life-course perspective highlights the influence of factors over the long term. This influence is not visible in the analysis of cross-sectional snapshots of the interviewees' lives that only show the situation at a particular point in time.

Conclusion

Drawing on life-course interviews with women and men with psychosocial disabilities, this chapter has analysed their practices of Active Citizenship – with a particular focus on education and work – and sought to identify various types of factors (personal, socio-economic and environmental) that influenced these practices. In contrast to studies focusing on the impact of mental ill-health, this chapter analysed the interviewees' experiences from a socio-structural perspective and described the interplay between psychosocial disabilities and other factors, including relationships with family and peers, financial situations, fear of stigma and discrimination, mental health treatments and flexible working arrangements. Inspired by the capability approach, we emphasised that the social environment must offer opportunities in order for Active Citizenship to develop. Furthermore, as this chapter drew on life-course interviews with persons with psychosocial disabilities, the data covered their experiences of education and work over a long period of time. This enabled us to see that practices of Active Citizenship vary throughout the life course, which we conceptualised as four ideal-typical pathways into and out of Active Citizenship.

The overall findings of our empirical analysis are in line with previous studies about persons with psychosocial disabilities that called attention to the fact that, although the deinstitutionalisation of psychiatric care has created opportunities for inclusion and participation in the community, Active Citizenship is at risk when individuals do not have access to adequate mental health services and welfare provisions, reasonable accommodation in educational and work settings, meaningful occupations and social networks (Knapp, McDaid, Mossialos & Thornicroft, 2007; Nelson et al., 2001; Parr, 2008; Sayce & Curran, 2007). On this basis, we argue that policies aimed at improving the Active Citizenship of persons with psychosocial disabilities need to adopt a life-course perspective and strengthen a wide range of facilitators and opportunities that encourage all three dimensions of Active Citizenship – security, influence and autonomy. A life-course perspective is important as it shows that the opportunities for exercising Active Citizenship change over time. Persons who are socially isolated and out of paid work at one point in time can be integrated into a social network and engaged in an occupation of their choice a few months later.

References

Apitzsch, B. (2010). Informal networks and risk coping strategies in temporary organizations: The case of media production in Germany. *Forum: Qualitative Social Research, 11*(1).

Belch, H. A. (2011). Understanding the experiences of students with psychiatric disabilities: A foundation for creating conditions of support and success. *New Directions for Student Services, 134*, 73–94. http://doi.org/10.1002/ss.

Carey, A. C. (2003). Beyond the medical model: A reconsideration of 'feeblemindedness', citizenship, and eugenic restrictions. *Disability & Society, 18*(4), 411–430. http://doi.org/10.1080/0968759032000080977.

Carlsson, C. (2011). Using 'turning points' to understand processes of change in offending: Notes from a Swedish study on life courses and crime. *British Journal of Criminology, 52*(1), 1–16. http://doi.org/10.1093/bjc/azr062.

Eurofound. (2003). *Illness, disability and social inclusion.* Dublin: European Foundation for the Improvement of Living and Working Conditions.

Evans, J. & Repper, J. (2000). Employment, social inclusion and mental health. *Journal of Psychiatric and Mental Health Nursing, 7*, 15–24.

Giddens, A. (1998). *The third way. The renewal of social democracy.* Cambridge: Polity Press.

Jahoda, M. (1982). *Employment and unemployment: A social-psychological analysis.* Cambridge: Cambridge University Press.

Knapp, M., McDaid, D., Mossialos, E. & Thornicroft, G. (2007). *Mental health policy and practice across Europe. The future direction of mental health care.* Berkshire: Open University Press.

Kozma, A. & Petri, G. (2012). *Mapping exclusion. Institutional and community-based services in the mental health field in Europe.* Brussels: Mental Health Europe.

Lawton, D., Cairns, J. & Gardner, P. (2000). *Education for citizenship.* London: Continuum.

Leff, J. P. & Warner, R. (2006). *Social inclusion of people with mental illness.* Cambridge: Cambridge University Press.

Link, B. G. & Phelan, J. C. (2001). Conceptualizing stigma. *Annual Review of Sociology, 27*, 363–385. http://doi.org/10.1146/annurev.soc.27.1.363.

Marshall, T. H. (1992). Citizenship and social class. In T. H. Marshall & T. Bottomore (Eds), *Citizenship and social class* (pp. 3–51). London: Pluto Press.

Megivern, D., Pellerito, S. & Mowbray, C. (2003). Barriers to higher education for individuals with psychiatric disabilities. *Psychiatric Rehabilitation Journal, 26*(3), 217–231.

Morrow, M. & Weisser, J. (2012). Towards a social justice framework of mental health recovery. *Studies in Social Justice, 6*(1), 27–43.

Mulvany, J. (2000). Disability, impairment or illness? The relevance of the social model of disability to the study of mental disorder. *Sociology of Health and Illness, 22*, 582–601. http://doi.org/10.1111/1467-9566.00221.

Nelson, G., Lord, J. & Ochocka, J. (2001). *Shifting the paradigm in the community mental health.* Toronto: Toronto University Press.

Parr, H. (2008). *Mental health and social space. Towards inclusionary geographies.* Oxford: Blackwell.

Ramon, S. & Williams, J. E. (2005). Towards a conceptual framework: The meanings attached to the psychosocial, the promise and the problem. In J. E. Williams & S. Ramon (Eds), *Mental health at the crossroads. The promise of the psychosocial approach* (pp. 13–24). Aldershot: Ashgate.

Reiter, H. (2010). Context, experience, expectation, and action – Towards an empirically grounded, general model for analyzing biographical uncertainty. *Forum: Qualitative Social Research, 11*(1).

Ridgway, P. (2001). Restoring psychiatric disability: Learning from first person recovery narratives. *Psychiatric Rehabilitation Journal, 24*(4), 335–343.

Robeyns, I. (2005). The capability approach: A theoretical survey. *Journal of Human Development, 6*(1), 93–117. http://doi.org/10.1080/146498805200034266.

Rogers, A. & Pilgrim, D. (1989). Mental health and citizenship. *Critical Social Policy, 9*, 44–55. http://doi.org/10.1177/026101838900902604.

Rosanvallon, P. (1995). *La Nouvelle Question Sociale: Repenser l'Etat-Providence.* Paris: Seuil.

Sayce, L. (2000). *From psychiatric patient to citizen. Overcoming discrimination and social exclusion.* Basingstoke: Palgrave Macmillan.

Sayce, L. & Curran, C. (2007). Tackling social exclusion across Europe. In M. Knapp, D. McDaid, E. Mossialos & G. Thornicroft (Eds), *Mental health policy and practice across Europe – The future direction of mental health care* (pp. 34–59). Maidenhead: Open University Press.

Scarpetta, S. & Colombo, F. (2016). Stepping up to tackle mental ill-health. Retrieved 13 April 2016, from http://oecdinsights.org/2016/04/13/stepping-up-to-tackle-mental-ill-health/.

Sépulchre, M. & Lindqvist, R. (2016). Enhancing active citizenship for persons with psychosocial disabilities. *Scandinavian Journal of Disability Research*, *18*(4), 316–327. http://doi.org/10.1080/15017419.2015.1105288.

Stuart, H. (2006). Mental illness and employment discrimination. *Current Opinion in Psychiatry*, *19*, 522–526. http://doi.org/10.1097/01.yco.0000238482.27270.5d.

Thoits, P. A. (2006). Self, identity and mental health. In C. S. Aneshensel & J. C. Phelan (Eds), *Handbook of sociology of mental health* (pp. 345–368). London: Springer.

Thornicroft, G. (2006). *Shunned. Discrimination against people with mental illness.* Oxford: Oxford University Press.

Turner, B. S. (1990). Outline of a theory of citizenship. *Sociology*, *24*(2), 189–217. http://doi.org/10.1177/0038038590024002002.

United Nations. (2006). *Convention on the rights of persons with disabilities* (resolution adopted by the General Assembly, 24 January 2007, A/RES/61/106).

Waldschmidt, A. (2013). *The relevance of Active Citizenship for persons with disabilities. Active Citizenship for persons with disabilities – Current knowledge and analytical framework – A Working Paper*. DISCIT.

Ware, N. C., Hopper, K., Tugenberg, T., Dickey, B. & Fisher, D. (2007). Connectedness and citizenship: Redefining social integration. *Psychiatric Services*, *58*(4), 469–474.

Warr, P. (1987). *Unemployment and mental health*. Oxford: Clarendon Press.

Weber, M. (1949). 'Objectivity' in social sciences and social policy. In E. A. Shils & H. A. Finch (Eds), *The methodology of the social sciences* (pp 49–112). New York: The Free Press.

Weber, M. (2011 [1903–1917]). *Methodology of the social sciences.* London: Routledge.

Whitley, R. & Campbell, R. (2014). Stigma, agency and recovery amongst people with severe mental illness. *Social Science & Medicine*, *107*, 1–8. http://doi.org/10.1016/j.socscimed.2014.02.010.

WHO. (2005). *Mental health: Facing the challenges, building solutions: Report from the WHO European Ministerial Conference*. Copenhagen: WHO Regional Office for Europe.

WHO. (2012). *Risks to mental health: An overview of vulnerabilities and risk factors. Background Paper*. Geneva: World Health Organization.

WHO. (2015). The European mental health action plan 2013–2020. Retrieved 13 April 2016, from www.euro.who.int/en/publications/abstracts/european-mental-health-action-plan-20132020-the.

9 The role of the family in structuring the opportunities for exercising Active Citizenship among persons with disabilities

Mario Biggeri, Caterina Arciprete, Rita Barbuto, Federico Ciani and Giampiero Griffo

The opportunity to enjoy full and effective participation in society is at the heart of what it means to live in a democratic society. The right of persons with disabilities to participate in society on an equal basis with others is grounded in the United Nations Convention on the Rights of Persons with Disabilities (CRPD). The debate on the factors that enable or prevent persons with disabilities from fully participating in society, including the notion of Active Citizenship, has recently intensified (Forsyth, Colver, Alvanides, Woolley & Lowe, 2007; Heah, Case, McGuire & Law, 2007). The main factors that can influence the opportunity of persons with disabilities to exercise Active Citizenship include physical and environmental characteristics, social norms, and institutional and domestic settings. Among these factors, the role of the family is still a relatively underexplored issue.

The notion of Active Citizenship is quite complex and is based on three integrated aspects: security, autonomy and influence (see Chapter 1). These three elements are strongly complementary and can be influenced by many factors. They play a central role in our wellbeing and inclusion in society when we are both young adults and older adults, and they play a central role in our capacity to be active citizens. The capacity to be an active citizen does not begin as individuals turn 18, but it starts to be shaped, nurtured and to evolve during childhood and adolescence when families and caregivers play a central role (Ballet, Biggeri & Comim, 2011).

The CRPD leaves no doubt that the opportunity to flourish for a person (and in particular a child) with disabilities is strongly influenced by the capacity of the family to cope with such a challenge. It also acknowledges that the realisation of the rights of a person with disabilities is closely interconnected with the multidimensional wellbeing of family members. Thus, the CRPD incorporates the right of families to contribute to the realisation of the rights of the person with disabilities. This right is clearly established in the Convention, which states: 'Persons with disabilities and their family members should receive the necessary protection and assistance to enable families to contribute towards the full and equal enjoyment of the rights of persons with disabilities' (Preamble of the CRPD). In addition, the Convention implicitly recognises that the family has extra responsibilities in many other domains such as education and health (UN, 2006, Art. 24–25).

Furthermore, by equating children with disabilities with other children, the United Nations Convention on the Rights of the Child (UNCRC) asserts their right to '(…) grow up in a family environment, in an atmosphere of happiness, love and understanding' (Preamble of the UNCRC, 1989).

Thus, even if the focus of the CRPD is the person with disabilities, the Convention recognises the crucial role played by the family with particular reference to the flourishing of children with disabilities. Moreover, the Convention highlights that the family should also be considered as a stakeholder potentially impacted by disabilities.

When discussing the role of the family, some clarification is required. Indeed, the concept of 'family' is complex and evolving and it varies across cultures and over time. Despite this, as this is a central concept for this chapter, a working definition can be useful. Following Emerson (2014, p. 420), we refer to family as 'all forms of family grouping across the life course of the person with disabilities'. Of course, the perimeter of family can be defined differently from case to case according to the relations that are relevant for the person at a given moment (childhood, adolescence, adulthood, old age) and for a given domain of one's wellbeing (e.g. housing, economic security, etc.). While dealing with the importance of the family for the full participation of persons with disabilities in society, we focus mainly on the family of origin. Although we do not explicitly address it in this chapter, we are fully aware of the importance of the family that the person with disabilities sets up when he or she grows up. Indeed, having a partner and experiencing sexuality, relationships and caring roles are fundamental to wellbeing.

In the literature, there is wide consensus on the relevance of families in contributing to the participation of members with disabilities in society. The nature of this contribution has been found to be both positive and negative: for instance, there is much discussion concerning 'overprotection' (Holmbeck et al., 2002) as well as clear evidence of the ability of families to cope with the shortcomings of welfare systems and to provide unique forms of support (Palmer, 2013).

The main aim of this chapter is to investigate the role played by the family context in supporting or hampering the full participation of persons with disabilities in society through the analysis of life-course interviews.

The methodology used in this chapter follows the life-course interviews method outlined in Chapter 3. A large quantity of life-course interviews was collected in nine European countries covering different types of disability and three different cohorts of adults with disabilities. Life-course interviews were analysed in order to capture disabling or enabling factors in the family and their interaction with the environment and institutional settings. The results were then interpreted in a simple and systematic way in order to produce some informative statistics.

The role of the family: literature review

A healthy family environment is a prerequisite for fostering the individual's cognitive and non-cognitive development from early childhood. Children who grow up in the absence of love, care and stimulation are more likely to have lower cognitive scores than their counterparts and to suffer from psychosocial problems when they become adults (Heckman, Pinto & Savelyev, 2012). For children with disabilities, the attitude of the family is even more determinant in fostering (or hampering) the child's future integration within society (Comim, 2011; Forsyth et al., 2007). Families are the primary caregivers and a critical source of support for their sons and daughters with disabilities (Rimmermann, 2015). Indeed, unpaid family carers tend to meet most of the needs of persons with disabilities (WHO, 2012). When individuals develop complex needs, non-professional family members play a critical role in meeting a wide range of care needs, typically without recognition or entitlement to support themselves (Barret, Hale & Butler, 2014, 149; WHO, 2011).

The social framework of the family is often co-responsible for the potential stigmatisation of the child with disabilities. Indeed, when the disability condition becomes apparent, the families are usually unprepared psychologically and do not know how to behave. In order to mitigate anxieties and guilt, parents and family caregivers tend to concentrate their efforts on trying to erase the problem, often with no results: they persist with the illusion of a possible cure for their children, consulting the best experts in the biomedical field and, in a worst-case scenario, asking the advice of untrustworthy people.

The salience of the family in influencing the life courses of children with disabilities is not constant across cohorts and countries. In general, in countries characterised by weaker social protection systems, the role of the family is stronger as family members tend to self-produce or to buy on the market the services that public institutions do not provide (Emerson, 2014). On the other hand, in countries with strong and effective welfare systems, the economic and non-economic characteristics of the family are less determinant in influencing the life course of the individual with disabilities. The creation of a services system capable of weakening the linkage between the family of origin and the capability set enjoyed by the individual has been pursued as an explicit goal by Nordic welfare systems, in particular for persons with disabilities (Esping-Andersen, 2002).

The same argument holds for cohorts. Indeed, the salience of the family is greater for people born during periods in which the welfare state is weak or dismantled, than for people born during decades of a strong welfare state. In any case, it is worth remembering that services (e.g. care) self-produced by the family are not perfect substitutes for services provided by public social protection systems or by services bought on the market. In this sense, structured welfare states should unburden families from material extra-care to allow them to concentrate on other kinds of task centred around the relationship among family members rather than on the care burden (Kozlowski, Matson, Horovitz, Worley & Neal, 2011).

Thus, families remain inevitably responsible for providing the bulk of support to sons and daughters with disabilities, at least until they reach adulthood.

It is well documented that being able to cope well with a disability is crucial for the wellbeing of the child with disabilities. Indeed, the reduction of parenting stress is paramount in the enhancement of a child's family life and in the child's ultimate integration within society (Trute & Hiebert-Murphy, 2002). Families raising a son or daughter with disabilities represent the whole spectrum of society with all the differences, contradictions and interactions among different factors. Indeed, sharing such a relevant common experience (i.e. having a child with disabilities) is not sufficient to create a homogeneous category. Therefore, while some families can cope well with a challenge such as the disabilities of a child, others do not have the financial, social, cultural or psychosocial resources that are needed to build resilience and cope well with a child's disabilities.

The extent to which the inclusion of a person with disabilities within society is dependent on the assistance offered by family members varies across contexts, types of disability, degrees of severity and the age of the persons with disabilities. At one end of the spectrum, there is a family with a very young child with severe disabilities living in a country where no assistance is provided to persons with disabilities. At the other end of the spectrum, there is a family whose son or daughter has a moderate disability, living in a society that provides persons with disabilities with all the medical, financial and technological assistance that is needed to achieve independent living. Between the two ends of the spectrum are the majority of circumstances, where the family remains critical in coping with the shortcomings of welfare systems and providing unique forms of support (Palmer, 2013; Trani, Bakhshi & Biggeri, 2011).

As was pointed out before, the common experience of having a child with disabilities is not sufficient to make these families a homogeneous group. However, there are some commonalities among them: families supporting children with disabilities, including children with intellectual disabilities, have on average a lower level of wellbeing, primarily due to their increased rates of exposure to poverty-associated environmental adversities (WHO, 2012; Emerson, 2014; Olsson, Larsman & Hwang, 2008).

Given this complex situation, it is crucial to understand both the circumstances that allow these families to contribute positively to the child's integration within society and the circumstances in which families constitute a further barrier to the wellbeing of the person with disabilities.

Research prior the 1980s assumed that the onset of a disability in a member of a family would inevitably lead to family dysfunction and pathological reactions. Families whose son or daughter has a disability were found to be more likely to experience negative influences such as reduced social and leisure activities, higher stress levels and depression, financial problems, and generally a pervasive negative impact on family functioning (Conoley & Sheridan, 1996).

However, the evidence to support these findings is not clear and in the following years it was increasingly demonstrated that the presence of a child with disabilities within the family can, in some cases, contribute positively to the wellbeing of family members, despite the psychological adjustment that family members have to face. Having a child with disabilities can unleash positive influences in the family by leading to psychological growth, increasing happiness, fulfilment and family cohesion, in addition to strengthening solidarity and openness towards the community (Connell et al., 1995; Hawley & DeHann, 1996; Schumacher, Stewart & Archbold, 1998; Stainton & Besser, 1998).

Overall, families adopt different coping strategies, differentiated by life-stage, type and severity of disability and gender, and by the structure and characteristics of the family.

In relation to age and life-stage, studies find that parents whose child has had a developmental disability since early childhood have a better pattern of resilience. These parents have been shown to accommodate their child's needs by making changes in family routines (e.g. reduced participation of mothers in the labour force and redistribution of child-care responsibilities among family members). As a result, they demonstrate positive coping and adaptation skills (Glidden, 1989; Krauss, Simeonsson & Ramey, 1989; Turnbull et al., 1993). On the other hand, parents who face the onset of disabilities during mid-life (e.g. mental disability during their child's adolescence) find it more difficult to accommodate the child's needs (Mailick Seltzer, Greenberg, Floyd, Pettee & Hong, 2001) and are more likely to be exposed to life disruption and altered life trajectories.

In order to avoid the fallacy of a paternalist approach when talking about the effects of family wellbeing on the ability of the person with disabilities to flourish, it must be acknowledged that the relationship is one of interdependence rather than of dependence. This implies that we cannot focus solely on the dyadic relationship between caregiver and the person with disabilities, neglecting the broader context that may involve other informal and formal carers (Barrett et al., 2014).

As illustrated above, positive family adaptation in response to the stressors (economic, psychological) associated with raising a child with disabilities can be defined as household resilience (McConnell, Savage & Breitkreuz, 2014). It follows that children growing up in resilient families are more likely to have positive outcomes. So what are the conditions that are needed for families to develop resilience? A consistent body of research focuses on child-specific factors, namely child behaviours, producing evidence that, as behavioural problems increase, so too does the risk of dysfunctional outputs in the family (Emerson, 2014). However, the evidence is not entirely consistent (McConnell et al., 2014).

When an ecological approach is adopted, the results seem to be more convincing. These theories posit that a family's resilience is determined on the one hand by the characteristics of the family (such as socio-economic conditions, parent–carer optimism, internal locus of control) and on the other by the characteristics of society. McConnell et al. (2014) find that families with low levels of social support and high levels of financial hardship typically struggle with positive adaptation, while families with sound socio-ecological resources are likely to perform well even in the presence of severe stressors.

Overall, the literature demonstrates that the family environment has a strong influence on the inclusion of the person with disabilities within society. This influence is likely to be stronger in the case of children with disabilities who need even more support and guidance than other children. Some families are able to cope well with having a son or daughter with disabilities and this results in increased wellbeing of the person and of the whole family. Other families find it hard to adapt to a situation characterised by an increased financial burden and psychological stress. When families are unable to cope well, persons with disabilities find it even harder to develop agency, self-esteem and trust towards the community, i.e. all the factors that will enable her or him to be an active citizen.

The literature providing explanations for the different coping strategies adopted by families is still quite limited. This chapter attempts to contribute to this literature by combining a sound theoretical framework with analysis of qualitative data.

Disability and family as conversion factor for Active Citizenship

In order to identify the potential channels through which family can influence the exercise of Active Citizenship, we refer both to structuration theory and to the capability approach as a joint theoretical framework (see also Chapter 2).

The structuration theory framework (O'Reilly 2012; Stones, 2005) underlines the dynamic relationship between individual conversion factors (internal structure), societal environmental conversion factors (the external structure) and the dynamics between outcomes and practical actions (see Figure 2.1, Chapter 2).

The capability perspective shifts the primary attention away from means to the ends that people have reason to pursue (Sen, 1999, p. 90). This perspective gives salience to 'opportunity freedoms' (capabilities) and 'process freedoms' (rights, entitlements and empowerment) as well as the individual's and the communities' experiences, values and participation.

The central insight of the capability approach is the notion of capabilities as the opportunities a person has to lead a valuable life. Individuals are not equally capable of transforming commodities into capabilities due to conversion factors. Sen (1990) distinguishes three different types of conversion factor: social, personal and environmental. Biggeri and Ferrannini (2014) add territorial functionings in recognition of the fact that the changing properties of the immediate settings in which people live and interact shape their capability space. Conversion factors are all dynamic, meaning that they can change throughout a person's life.

Active Citizenship is constituted by three main pillars: security, autonomy and influence (Chapter 1). These three components are not alternatives but are rather strongly complementary; in fact it is not possible to achieve Active Citizenship in the absence of one of these three constituents (see Chapter 1).

Becoming an active citizen, that is, one who has achieved the relevant functionings, depends on several elements. These elements, when combined, shape the process of capability expansion or reduction (see also Robeyns, 2005; Trani, Bakhshi, Noor & Mashkoor, 2009).

Based on this framework, the research question can now be framed as follows: how does the family act as a conversion factor and influence the capability 'to exercise Active Citizenship' and its associated achieved functionings (security, autonomy and influence)?

First, families can influence the security component of the person with disabilities directly or indirectly. On the one hand, the financial means of the family clearly sets the degree of financial assistance that the persons with disabilities will need from the state. On the other hand, the family's capacity to deal with the public social welfare system will influence the opportunity for persons with disabilities to receive benefits from the state. Such influence can be determinant in countries where high levels of bureaucracy make it difficult to exercise rights. Parents who have a considerable degree of knowledge, have a positive attitude to public services and have expectations around the autonomy of the child with disabilities will be able to narrow the distance between the person with disabilities and the social protection system.

Second, families can influence the autonomy component of the person with disabilities by nurturing awareness that persons with disabilities can be independent from childhood. Children, especially those with disabilities, are too often portrayed as passive recipients of care and as lacking in self-determination. Instead, they should be considered as autonomous agents, able to express their points of view, values and aspirations (Ballet et al., 2011). Autonomous individuals possess qualities of independence, self-direction, self-determination, self-governance and self-care. Autonomy cannot be considered as a 'developmental endpoint, synonymous with psychological maturity and personal fulfilment either for nondisabled or disabled children' (Vaicekauskaite, 2007, p. 32), but rather autonomy evolves over time and must be nurtured from childhood (Ballet et al., 2011). Thus, families can be either autonomy supportive (e.g. giving an internal frame of reference, providing a meaningful rationale, allowing choices, encouraging self-perspective) or controlling (e.g. exerting pressure to behave in specific ways) (Ballet et al., 2011; Comim, 2011).

Third, families can have an impact on the influence component of active citizenship for the person with disabilities. Indeed, in order to have influence, persons with disabilities must not only be free from those constraints over which parents usually have little control (e.g. lack of information, physical barriers to access the political arena), but must also go through a process of empowerment that starts within the individual. In other words, one can have an influence on society as long as one feels worthy of doing so. More generally, one can do something only if one feels worthy of desiring it. Thus, by influencing the degree of self-esteem and agency of the person with disabilities, the family greatly influences the opportunity for the person to claim his or her rights and to have an influence on the surrounding society.

Thus, family members, if proactive, can stimulate the active citizen component of the family member with disabilities in several ways: they can open up opportunities, help to shape positive and proactive attitudes, help the children through their preference formation, fight against stigmatisation and lobby for the rights of persons with disabilities, e.g. through collective actions as organisations of persons with disabilities demonstrate.

The environment in which the child grows up has a significant influence on his or her capacity to be active and proactive (Ryan & Deci, 2000), and family members can greatly contribute to enabling the child (including those with disabilities) to aspire, to be secure, to be autonomous and to be the agent of his or her life (Biggeri, Ballet & Comim, 2011).

Description of the role of the family through the analysis of life-course interviews

Methodological issues

We have analysed the role of the family as a factor in hampering or supporting the full participation of persons with disabilities in society by systematising the information collected through the life-course interviews according to the interpretative framework presented above.

In particular, our unit of interest is composed of the relevant events which occur over the life course of the person and of the role played by family in these events. Following the research methodology adopted by the DISCIT research project (Chapter 3), we have identified two broad classes of relevant events: transitions and turning points. Transitions are defined as 'changes in status and role which are generally known about and prepared for – such as from being single to being married, or from student to full-time worker' (Green, 2010, p. 25). Turning points are changes 'in the direction of the life course, with respect to a previously established trajectory, that has the long-term impact of altering the probability of life destinations' (Wheaton & Gotlib, 1997, p. 5).

Both transitions and turning points may be defined as positive or negative. They are considered positive if the event tends to increase the person's degree of participation in society. On the other hand, they are negative if they increase the distance from full enjoyment of citizenship rights and duties.

As regards the role of the family, we have defined it as positive if it enhances the impact of a positive event or diminishes the impact of a negative event. The contrary is true in the case of a negative role. In both cases, the role of the family is defined as non-neutral. The role of the family may also be neutral if it has not been relevant in defining the direction and size of the event's impact.

We analysed 211 life-course interviews. Among them, we identified 1,212 relevant events (744 turning points and 468 transitions).

We have organised the information as follows. Starting with the interview reports, we have identified each event (according to the self-detection of the interviewee) and merged two different sets of information in the data set. The first consists of information at the level of the individual (such as gender, age, country of residence, kind of impairment etc.). The second set is composed of event-level information (direction of the event, domains involved in the event, etc.).

To clarify, let us suppose that a person reports having received a good job offer from a firm based in another town and that his or her family have convinced the person to refuse the offer because the parents do not have enough confidence in his or her ability to live autonomously in a new town. Suppose also that, as a result, the person internalises the stigmatisation relating to his or her ability to work. In this case, we have a negative turning point primarily involving professional life on which the family has had a negative influence.

Data analysis

Confluent families

The first aspect that emerges from the interviews is that families have a relevant role in influencing the opportunities of persons with disabilities throughout their lives. However, referring to the family as if it were a unique component is per se a simplification. Indeed, it is not possible to interpret the relationship between the person with disabilities and the family as dyadic. In fact, families never constitute a homogeneous entity, but include different caregivers with different, and sometimes conflictual, roles. Parents themselves are likely to have different views on what is best for their sons and daughters and often perceive their role as ambiguous.

When parents do not represent a reliable source of care, interviewees are likely to look for material and non-material care from other family members such as grandparents, siblings or cousins. According to a Czech man with mobility disability (born around 1990): 'The only person who understands me is my uncle, my mother's brother. He is the only person I trust and if I need to talk about something I turn to him.' Members of the extended family are of vital importance for most interviewees. However, their role is more precarious: grandparents are likely to die when the person with disabilities is still young, and the other members (e.g. cousins) may stop exercising their role for a variety of reasons (financial constraints, moving out, new problems etc.).

Negotiations with family

The kind of impact that the family can have on the flourishing of the person with disabilities can vary widely: as expected, there are cases where the family is a catalyst for the autonomy-building process, and others where the family acts as an obstacle. Throughout the interviews, families are heterogeneous in the way that they deal with the disability. Some of them are overprotective, some families are supportive and autonomy enhancing, while others are so disintegrated that they are not able to pursue their children's wellbeing.

Families play a meaningful role throughout the lives of persons with disabilities through several mechanisms. First of all, they influence the self-identity of the person with disabilities and his or her view on disability. They further influence the person's life by providing economic support, by setting the distance with public institutions, by encouraging their offspring to pursue what they value, and by teaching them the value of autonomy and rights. Some tension commonly arises between the parents' desire to protect their sons and daughters, and the desire of individuals with disabilities to be autonomous:

> my father and mother (…) brought me to a Friary and (…) I started walking. So I'm walking from that day to this thanks to God. […] When my mother seen me, God love her she got, you know, she got very sad when seen me learning how to walk. I remember it well, I came back and I was walking around by the table and I fell, and I could stand up for a few minutes now, and I got up and that's my miracle.
>
> (From an interview with an Irish woman with intellectual disability, born around 1950)

Usually persons with disabilities negotiate with their parents over a number of decisions, such as whether to buy a wheelchair, or whether or not to enter mainstream education.

Country differences in the role of the family

The relevance of the family varies according to the national context (see Table 9.1). In Italy, for example, the family plays a non-neutral role in more than half of the events, while in other countries this proportion is substantially lower. This picture highlights a strong heterogeneity. It seems sensible to hypothesise that culture and traditions, the presence of weaker or stronger social protection systems, and the social perceptions of disability are all determinants. However, the available information does not allow for an exhaustive explanation.

It is also important to consider the typology of the domain in which the relevant event occurs. Certain domains are more likely to be impacted by the family than others (see Table 9.2). In the case of housing, for example, the family is involved in 71.78 per cent of cases (positive in 51.92 per cent). In other domains, the involvement is much less pervasive (e.g. participation).

Table 9.1 Relevant events and the role of the family (per cent)

Country	*Neutral*	*Non-neutral*
Total	55.45	44.55
Czech Republic	53.49	46.51
Germany	51.41	48.59
Ireland	55.78	44.22
Italy	47.68	52.32
Norway	59.06	40.94
Serbia	59.23	40.77
Sweden	68.85	31.15
Switzerland	46.15	53.85
United Kingdom	61.62	38.38

Table 9.2 Domains of life and the role of the family (per cent)

Domain	*Neutral*	*Positive*	*Negative*
Education	56.86	32.77	10.36
Work	74.27	19.22	6.51
Social relations	53.57	34.00	12.44
Family	9.39	60.50	30.11
Housing	28.22	51.92	19.86
Participation	76.34	23.21	0.45
Technology	75.00	20.00	5.00
Assistance	68.67	23.33	8.00
Health	67.11	21.10	11.79

The most consistent finding across cohort, gender and type of disability is the importance attributed by persons with disabilities to moving out and gaining independence.

> Because at a certain point, I wanted to live on my own and the *only* reason was: I wanted to have the thrill: What is it really like to live on my own? Do I get along? Do I mess up completely? Or, do I not get along? And so on and so forth. But apparently, it looks different.
>
> (From an interview with a German woman with intellectual disability, born around 1970)

In this sense, the presence or absence of a supportive family is highly relevant: to gain housing autonomy thanks to or despite the family of origin is not devoid of consequences for the life course of the person. The decision to move out is not an easy one, because individuals often need special living arrangements and some assistance, in addition to the financial means to afford private rent when no public housing is available. Notwithstanding these difficulties, a large majority of the interviewees refer to the decision to move out on their own as the most meaningful and positive choice they have ever made.

Functional alternatives to family

If we take into consideration both housing and other domains of life, although families play a meaningful role in determining the opportunities of their sons and daughters, their role should not be idealised. When persons with disabilities lack family support, they are found to be capable of enacting compensatory measures that allow them to achieve their objectives. Having a caring family can undoubtedly help children to grow up with a positive attitude; however, families do not necessarily represent an irreplaceable source of love and economic support. Although families have an important role in some cases, this is not always the case, and many interviewees have a flourishing life even when the family of origin is disintegrated and unsupportive. In many cases, this is possible thanks to the role played by persons external to the family. Thus, it is the quality of the relationship rather than its source that represents an irreplaceable asset. Most of the time, that role is taken by the partner. According to a Czech women with intellectual disabilities (born around 1970): 'The most important turning point in my life was to be together with my partner'. At a younger age it can also be a friend or teacher.

Disability-specific experiences

Another non-neutral factor in determining the role of the family in the life of persons with disabilities is the kind of disability experienced by the person.

The interviews show that the relation between the person with disabilities and his or her family is much more complicated in the case of psychosocial disabilities than in other cases.

Table 9.3 shows that the family played a negative role in more than one quarter of the relevant events of interviewees' lives.

What is stressed in the interviews is the existence of a circular relationship between the problems of the family context and the onset of psychosocial disabilities. Persons with psychosocial disabilities are more likely to live in disintegrated families (e.g. due to alcohol, violence or divorce). For instance, a German woman with psychosocial disability (born around 1990) said: 'I left home due to violence and beating'. The disruption of the family often appears to be a cause rather than a consequence of the onset of psychosocial disabilities. At the same time, the presence of a family member with psychosocial disabilities tends to erode the strength and quality of relationships within the family.

As Table 9.4 shows, the case of psychosocial disabilities is the most critical one, irrespective of the domain involved in the transition or turning point. The family played a negative role in more than half of cases for persons with psychosocial disabilities, while the proportion is much lower for all other categories.

Moreover, there is evidence that disruptive relations within the family of origin are reproduced outside: for example, those who have grown up in a violent context tend to replicate in a new family the same type of relationships, confirming the findings of the literature (see, for example, Kolbo, Blakely & Engleman, 1996).

Gender also tends to be non-neutral: the family plays a negative role in 14 per cent of relevant events experienced by women (as against 10 per cent for men).

Table 9.3 Category of impairment and the role of the family (per cent)

Impairment	*Neutral*	*Positive*	*Negative*
Visual	58.41	34.25	7.34
Mobility	52.01	40.25	7.74
Intellectual	56.83	33.45	9.71
Psychosocial	54.58	19.37	26.06

Table 9.4 Impairment, role of the family and domain involved in the transition or turning point (per cent)

Domain	*Visual*			*Mobility*			*Intellectual*			*Psychosocial*		
	Neutral	*Positive*	*Negative*	*Neutral*	*Positive*	*Negative*	*Neutral*	*Positive*	*Negative*	*Neutral*	*Positive*	*Negative*
Education	52.43	39.81	7.77	51.96	42.16	5.88	62.65	28.92	8.43	63.77	13.04	23.19
Work	68.67	26.51	4.82	83.08	15.38	1.54	74.03	22.08	3.90	73.17	12.20	14.63
Social relations	55.56	36.11	8.33	51.88	42.50	5.63	56.96	33.54	9.49	49.65	22.70	27.66
Family	10.42	72.92	16.67	5.95	76.19	17.86	7.41	66.67	25.93	12.87	30.69	56.44
Housing	24.05	64.56	11.39	23.61	63.89	12.50	33.85	46.15	20.00	32.39	30.99	36.62
Participation	80.43	19.57	0.00	65.67	32.84	1.49	80.28	19.72	0.00	82.50	17.50	0.00
Technology	86.21	12.07	1.72	64.81	25.93	9.26	57.14	42.86	0.00	100.00	0.00	0.00
Assistance	75.76	19.70	4.55	61.02	32.20	6.78	63.27	27.55	9.18	73.53	13.73	12.75
Health	77.78	17.36	4.86	57.66	34.31	8.03	69.41	21.18	9.41	64.38	13.13	22.50

This difference may signal a problem of intersectional discrimination within the family. Among the factors underlying this phenomenon, there is a much higher prevalence of violence against women with disabilities than against men, even within the family, and in particular for women with psychosocial disabilities (Mays, 2006).

Finally, no systematic relation is found between the family's role and cohort. This does not imply that family attitudes towards disability have not changed over the decades, but our qualitative data does not provide clear evidence for this. In terms of age, rather than cohort, the family of origin plays a more important role when the person is young. This role is later assumed by the new family. When the person with disabilities has not formed a new family, he or she remains dependent on parents who are now old and care dependent. These situations are common and particularly deleterious for the wellbeing of all members of the family.

Even if the important role played by the family is acknowledged with all its complexity, it would be a mistake to consider the family as an all-absorbing factor in the lives of persons with disabilities. Their lives are influenced by several actors, and often the role played by the family in a relevant event of the life course (i.e. a transition or a turning point) is neutral, as the family has no influence on its ultimate impact in fostering or hampering the Active Citizenship of the person.

Conclusions and policy implications

The analysis of the interviews has outlined an extremely complex picture. By affecting the availability of goods and services, and by influencing personal history, psychology and aptitude, the family has a massive influence on the process of capability evolution and on the capacity to be an active citizen. Furthermore, the exercise of Active Citizenship is not constant throughout the life of an individual but varies depending on the interaction between internal and external structures. The meso-level structures, such as organisations, are also important, affecting collective agency and individual aspirations.

While the lack of key information (such as the socio-economic status of the family) makes it difficult to paint a complete picture, it is still possible to highlight some aspects.

First, this chapter confirms the relevant role of families in influencing the life chances of children with disabilities. This role varies by dimension, with families having less influence on the employment opportunities of their children with disabilities, and more influence on social relations. In terms of whether the influence is positive or negative, we found strong heterogeneity among families. Such heterogeneity is reflected in the ambivalent attitudes that persons with disabilities have towards their family of origin.

Second, we find that persons with psychosocial disabilities, especially women, and their families are most vulnerable. Most of the time, they and their caregivers are trapped in a vicious circle with little chance of gaining continuous support from external authorities.

The third finding is that most of the interviewees cited 'moving out' as the most positive, helpful and meaningful turning point of their lives. Thus, the capacity of family members to be supportive in such a decision can be extremely relevant in facilitating the process of independence and autonomy of persons with disabilities.

Fourth and finally, it is worth highlighting that the role of the family is heterogeneous across countries, with some countries, such as Italy, presenting a higher percentage of families demonstrating a non-neutral impact on the child's well-being. This partly confirms the hypothesis that culture and traditions, the presence of weaker or stronger social protection systems, and social perceptions of disabilities are all factors that play a significant role.

Overall, these findings allow us to consider some implications, in particular for the relationship between the family and policies aimed at the development of Active Citizenship among persons with disabilities.

In terms of policies, recognising that the family has such a critical role in the fulfilment of the rights of persons with disabilities leads to a mainstreaming of the family dimension in all policies addressing disability. The most illustrative example of these types of policies is household tax exemptions. Non-material support is also needed; there is strong empirical evidence for the effectiveness of services such as interventions aimed at improving parenting skills for parents of children and adolescents with disabilities and at providing psychological support (Emerson, 2014).

These statements should not be taken as a justification for a shift from the person with disabilities to the family as the unit of concern in policies addressing disability. There are at least four aspects that must be taken into account.

First, we must consider that the principle of self-determination of people with disabilities is also realised through a process of gradual emancipation from the family of origin. Family ties, albeit critical in the development of a child, might become a burden for a person with disabilities as he or she grows up. Phenomena such as 'overprotection' are common and can hamper individual realisation. Parents can have a detrimental effect on individual self-realisation by replacing the child's wishes with their own will. As Morris (1993) points out, interpreting persons with disabilities as 'dependent people' can lead to overprotective attitudes on the part of professionals and families. The emphasis on the role of the family might lead to a perception of the disabled person as powerless and dependent on family members (Barnes, 2000; Morris, 1993, 1997, 2004). This is why the set of organisations commonly labelled the 'Independent Living Movement' claim that what is needed is more empowerment rather than more care. Their concern is that policies should provide direct payment so that the person who needs help can determine him or herself how much help is needed, and can have control over the way care is delivered. This, in turn, sets family members free from the obligations of caring, thus allowing for more equal and reciprocal relationships within the family (Barnes, 2000; Morris, 1993, 1997, 2004; Pinto, 2011). Consequently, empowering families (and only indirectly the person with disabilities) is often seen as an indicator of a paternalistic approach to disability.

Second, from a social justice perspective, an excessive reliance on family as the centre of policies for persons with disabilities may foster the reproduction of inequality across generations. In fact, if inequality in access to economic and material resources can be mitigated by distributive policies, the lack of access to cultural and relational resources can hardly be solved by focusing on the family rather than on persons with disabilities.

Third, from a policy-making point of view, an excessive focus on families might hide a lack of commitment by public institutions to providing universal access to sustainable, appropriate and good quality services. Moreover, even if there is clear evidence that families of persons with disabilities are more likely to experience discrimination, poverty and social exclusion, policy makers should never neglect the fact that (1) supporting a 'fragile' family and (2) fostering the full participation in society of a person with disabilities are two different (even if interlinked) policy goals.

Fourth, while recognising that families caring for children with disabilities experience significant challenges in terms of psychosocial equilibrium, financial burden and curtailed employment opportunities, any political measure must recognise the autonomy of both caregivers and care recipients and challenge the divide between the carer and the cared for (Pinto 2011).

In conclusion, the complexity of the family as a system and the complexity of the relations and interactions between the family and the person with disabilities do not permit a reliance on the family as an automatic transmission belt for policies. The involvement of the family in policies aimed at fostering the wellbeing and Active Citizenship of persons with disabilities must be individualised and tailored. Indeed, the best way to support family empowerment is through peer-to-peer counselling model projects (Barbuto, Biggeri & Griffo, 2011; Bellanca, Biggeri & Marchetta, 2011). For example, one positive aspect of the Italian educational inclusion system is the practice of involving children with disabilities and their families, working together on a daily basis for disability rights protection in society. Consideration of the family as a key part of the social inclusion of children with disabilities is still lacking in many EU member states.

Only through the deep personalisation of interventions will it be possible to structure the interventions to exploit synergies between the systems of services provision and the family. Standardised ways of including the family in disability policies risk being structured on hypotheses that may work in general (e.g. a more educated parent is more effective in promoting the Active Citizenship of the child) but may not be inclusive. Finally, this chapter has shown that, besides financial resources, social relations are important for the wellbeing of children and their families. Social relations boost self-esteem, confidence and aspirations. Thus, peer counselling for both children and their caregivers can be effective tools for encouraging the development of awareness as well as for developing support and knowledge of resources and services (Barbuto et al., 2011). Finally, it is important to recognise that the temporal dimension in the design of social work interventions is crucial for the wellbeing of the child with disabilities and his or her caregivers.

References

Ballet, J., Biggeri, M. & Comim, F. (2011). Children's agency and the capability approach: A conceptual framework. In J. Ballet, M. Biggeri & F. Comim, *Children and the capability approach* (pp. 22–45). New York: Palgrave Macmillan.

Barbuto, R., Biggeri, M. & Griffo, G. (2011). Life project, peer counselling and self-help groups as tools to expand capabilities, agency and human rights. *ALTER-European Journal of Disability Research/Revue Européenne de Recherche sur le Handicap*, *5*(3), 192–205.

Barnes, C. (2000). A working social model? Disability, work and disability politics in the 21st century. *Critical Social Policy*, *20*(4), 441–457.

Barnes, C. (2007). Direct payments for personal assistants for disabled people: A key to independent living? *Background notes to a verbal presentation at the Centre for Independent Living*, Dublin, Conference 'Independent Living 2007, Croke Park Conference Centre, Dublin, 5 June 2007.

Barrett, P., Hale, B. & Butler, M. (2014). *Family care and social capital: Transitions in informal care*. Dordrecht: Springer.

Bellanca, N., Biggeri, M. & Marchetta, F. (2011). An extension of the capability approach: Towards a theory of dis-capability. *ALTER-European Journal of Disability Research/Revue Européenne de Recherche sur le Handicap*, *5*(3), 158–176.

Biggeri, M. & Ferrannini, A. (2014). *Sustainable human development: A new territorial and people-centered perspective*. New York: Palgrave Macmillan.

Biggeri, M., Ballet, J. & Comim, F. (Eds). (2011). *Children and the capability approach*. New York: Palgrave Macmillan.

Comim, F. (2011). Developing children's capabilities: The role of emotions and parenting style. In M. Biggeri, J. Ballet, F. Comim (Eds), *Children and the capability approach*. New York: Palgrave Macmillan.

Connell, J. I., Kubisch, A. C., Schorr, L. B. & Weiss, C. H. (Eds). (1995). New approaches to evaluating community initiatives. Washington DC: The Aspen Institute.

Conoley, J. C. & Sheridan, S. M. (1996). Pediatric traumatic brain injury challenges and interventions for families. *Journal of Learning Disabilities*, *29*(6), 662–669.

Emerson, E. (2014). Families supporting a child with intellectual or developmental disabilities: The current state of knowledge. *Journal of Applied Research in Intellectual Disabilities*, *27*(5), 420–430.

Esping-Andersen, G. (2002). *Why we need a new welfare state*. Oxford: Oxford University Press.

Forsyth, R., Colver, A., Alvanides, S., Woolley, M. & Lowe, M. (2007). Participation of young severely disabled children is influenced by their intrinsic impairments and environment. *Developmental Medicine & Child Neurology*, *49*(5), 345–349.

Glidden, L. M. (1989). Parents for children, children for parents. Washington, DC: American Association on Mental Retardation.

Green, L. (2010). *Understanding the life course*. Cambridge: Polity Press.

Hawley, D. R. & DeHann L. (1996). Toward a definition of family resilience: Integrating lifespan and family perspectives. *Family Process*, *35*(3), 283–298.

Heah, T., Case, T., McGuire, B. & Law, M. (2007). Successful participation: The lived experience among children with disabilities. *Canadian Journal of Occupational Therapy*, *74*(1), 38–47.

Heckman, J., Pinto, R. & Savelyev, P. (2012). Understanding the mechanisms through which an influential early childhood program boosted adult outcomes. *The American Economic Review, 103*(6), 2052–2086.

Holmbeck, G. N., Johnson, S. Z., Wills, K. E., McKernon, W., Rose, B., Erklin, S. & Kemper, T. (2002). Observed and perceived parental overprotection in relation to psychosocial adjustment in preadolescents with a physical disability: The mediational role of behavioral autonomy. *Journal of Consulting and Clinical Psychology, 70*(1), 96.

Kolbo, J. R., Blakely, E. H. & Engleman, D. (1996). Children who witness domestic violence: A review of empirical literature. *Journal of Interpersonal Violence, 11*(2), 281–293.

Kozlowski, A. M., Matson, J. L., Horovitz, M., Worley, J. A. & Neal, D. (2011). Parents' first concerns of their child's development in toddlers with autism spectrum disorders. *Developmental Neurorehabilitation, 14*(2), 72–78.

Krauss, M. W., Simeonsson, R. & Ramey, S. (1989). Special issue on research on families. *American Journal of Mental Retardation, 94*(3).

Mailick Seltzer, M., Greenberg, J. S., Floyd, F. J., Pettee, Y. & Hong, J. (2001). Life course impacts of parenting a child with a disability. *American Journal on Mental Retardation, 106*(3), 265–286.

Mays, J. M. (2006). Feminist disability theory: Domestic violence against women with a disability. *Disability & Society, 21*(2), 147–158.

McConnell, D., Savage, A. & Breitkreuz, R. (2014). Resilience in families raising children with disabilities and behavior problems. *Research in Developmental Disabilities, 35*(4), 833–848.

Morris, J. (1993). *Independent lives? Community care and disabled people*. London: Macmillan Press.

Morris, J. (1997). Care or empowerment? A disability rights perspective. *Social Policy & Administration, 31*(1), 54–60.

Morris, J. (2004). Independent living and community care: A disempowering framework. *Disability & Society, 19*(5), 427–442.

Olsson, M. B., Larsman, P. & Hwang, P. C. (2008). Relationships among risk, sense of coherence, and well-being in parents of children with and without intellectual disabilities. *Journal of Policy and Practice in Intellectual Disabilities, 5*(4), 227–236.

O'Reilly, K. (2012). *International migration and social theory*. New York: Palgrave Macmillan.

Palmer, J. (2013). The convention on the rights of persons with disabilities: Will ratification lead to a holistic approach to postsecondary education for persons with disabilities? *Seton Hall Law Review, 43*(2), 552–593.

Pinto, P. C. (2011). Family, disability and social policy in Portugal: Where are we at, and where do we want to go? *Sociologia On Line*, 2(4) 39–60.

Rimmermann, A. (2015). *Family policy and disability*. Cambridge: Cambridge University Press.

Robeyns, I. (2005). The capability approach: A theoretical survey. *Journal of Human Development, 6*(1), 93–117.

Ryan, R. M. & Deci, E. L. (2000). Self-determination theory and the facilitation of intrinsic motivation, social development, and well-being. *American Psychologist, 55*(1), 68–78.

Schumacher, K. L., Stewart, B. J. & Archbold, P. G. (1998). Conceptualization and measurement of doing family caregiving well. *Image: The Journal of Nursing Scholarship, 30*(1), 63–70.

Sen, A. (1990). Justice: Means versus freedoms. *Philosophy & Public Affairs*, 111–121.

Sen, A. K. (1999). *Development as freedom*. Oxford: Oxford University Press.

Stainton, T. & Besser, H. (1998). The positive impact of children with an intellectual disability on the family. *Journal of Intellectual and Developmental Disability, 23*(1), 57–70.

Stones, R. (2005). *Structuration theory*. New York: Palgrave Macmillan.

Trani, J. F., Bakhshi, P. & Biggeri, M. (2011). Rethinking children's disabilities through the capability lens: A framework for analysis and policy implications. In J. F. Trani, P. Bakhshi & M. Biggeri, *Children and the capability approach* (pp. 245–270). New York: Palgrave Macmillan.

Trani, J. F., Bakhshi, P., Noor, A. A. & Mashkoor, A. (2009). Lack of a will or of a way? Taking a capability approach for analysing disability policy shortcomings and ensuring programme impact in Afghanistan. *European Journal of Development Research, 21*(2), 297–319.

Trute, B. & Hiebert-Murphy, D. (2002). Family adjustment to childhood developmental disability: A measure of parent appraisal of family impacts. *Journal of Pediatric Psychology, 27*(3), 271–280.

Turnbull, A. P., Patterson, J. M., Behr, S. K., Murphy, D. L., Marquis, J. G. & Blue-Banning, M. J. (1993). Cognitive coping, families, and disability. In *Based on a participatory research conference on cognitive coping in families who have a member with a developmental disability: Theoretical and empirical implications and directions, held in Lawerence, KS, June 1991*. Paul H. Brookes Publishing.

UN. (2006). *Convention on the rights of persons with disabilities*. New York: United Nations.

UNCRC. (1989). *Convention on the rights of the child*. New York: United Nations.

Vaicekauskaite, R. (2007). Parents' perspectives on social exclusion and the development of psychological autonomy in children with disabilities. *Illinois Child Welfare, 1*(3), 30–40.

Wheaton, B. & Gotlib, I. H. (1997). Trajectories and turning points over the life course: Concepts and themes. In I. H. Gotlib (Ed.). *Stress and adversity over the life course: Trajectories and turning points* (1–25). Cambridge: Cambridge University Press.

World Health Organization. (2011). *World report on disability*. Geneva: World Health Organization.

World Health Organization. (2012). *Better health, better lives: Research priorities*. Geneva: World Health Organization.

10 Gendering Active Citizenship

Experiences of women with disabilities

Marie Sépulchre, Victoria Schuller, Jennifer Kline and Anna M. Kittelsaa

Persons with disabilities do not have equal opportunities to participate in society because of poverty, discrimination, violence and inaccessibility (WHO, 2011). This is especially true of women with disabilities who experience gender discrimination as well as disabling barriers (WHO, 2011). The United Nations Convention on the Rights of Persons with Disabilities (CRPD) recognises in its preamble 'that women and girls with disabilities are often at greater risk, both within and outside the home, of violence, injury or abuse, neglect or negligent treatment, maltreatment or exploitation' (UN, 2006). Yet, despite a range of barriers and glass ceilings, many women with disabilities play active roles in their families, communities and in society at large (EDF, 2014). However, little is known about the involvement of women with disabilities as citizens. A scoping review showed that many studies on citizenship and disability discuss citizenship in terms of access to social rights – leaving aside persons with disabilities' contributions to society – and treat 'persons with disabilities' as a homogeneous category (Sépulchre, 2016). This chapter addresses this research gap and explores the lived experiences of Active Citizenship of women with disabilities in various social settings.

Our starting point is that both disability and citizenship are gendered. Disability is gendered, as it does not have the same consequences for men and women (Barron, 2008; Gerschick, 2000; Meekosha & Dowse, 1997; Morris, 1991; Thomas, 1999; Traustadóttir, 2006). In a study about the transition from adolescence to adulthood, Barron (1997) observed that, apart from obstacles that may affect the everyday lives of disabled young people in general, some obstacles were related to gendered social practices, in which individuals were expected to conform to ideals of physical beauty and to assume carer responsibilities. However, being a woman should not only be considered in terms of disadvantages, but as a dimension that influences women's lived experiences in general. Thomas (1999), who collected stories of women with disabilities, found that they spoke of many feminine issues such as:

> Becoming, being or wanting to be a mother; being a single parent; being a grandmother; being a wife; having a male partner or boyfriend (sometimes in very happy relationships, sometimes not); being an unpaid carer of others;

> managing the emotions of others in families and personal relationships (emotional labour); disadvantages in education and in paid work associated with being female; concerns about appearance, beauty, attractiveness; experiencing sexual abuse, harassment and domestic violence; matters of financial or material independence and dependence.
>
> (p. 85)

All these topics have been discussed in feminist research, but Thomas (1999) concluded that living with disability gives 'new twists' to these experiences.

Citizenship is also gendered or, more specifically, the traditional understanding of citizenship is masculine (Fraser & Gordon, 1994; Lister, 2003; Orloff, 1993; Walby, 1994). It is masculine because, on the one hand, women have formally been excluded from citizenship from classical Greece – where only a few 'great men' were deemed worthy to be active citizens (Burchell, 2002) – until the 20th century, where women fought for and finally gained full citizenship rights in many Western countries. On the other hand, citizenship has been related to traditionally masculine activities taking place in the public sphere – such as participation in politics, in paid work and in the army. Until recently, women were second-class citizens; their agency as citizens was not recognised and they lived under the 'cover' of their husbands who, as head of household, enjoyed the status of citizenship (Fraser & Gordon, 1994; Lister, 2003). The conceptualisation of citizenship as both a status and a practice (Lister, 2003) is important for women, because it highlights that, although many women have now obtained formal citizenship rights, in practice they still face unequal opportunities and discrimination on the basis of gender (Lister, 2003; UNDP, 2015). Feminist scholars criticised the narrow definition of citizenship limited to the labour market and the realm of official politics, because it disregards women's agency in informal labour and civil society (Lister, 1997; Sevenhuijsen, 2000). They also criticised traditional theories of citizenship that disregard the importance of care, gender and sexuality. Sevenhuijsen (2000) argued that care is not confined to private interactions, but that it should be placed at the centre of the debates about rights, obligations and responsibilities. Finally, acknowledging Plummer's (2001) notion of 'intimate citizenship', Lister (2002, p. 199) argued that citizenship does indeed include intimate and sexual issues and observed that these are objects of citizenship struggles.

The evolution of persons with disabilities' citizenship presents similarities to women's citizenship, because both groups were long held outside the realm of citizenship and are still fighting to be truly accepted in the community of citizens. An important difference, however, is that being a woman is not as closely tied to experiences of stigmatisation and discrimination as being disabled (Waldschmidt, 2014). Indeed, while women were confined to the private sphere, persons labelled as disabled have been conceived of as a burden for society and as having neither domestic nor familial responsibilities nor public presence (Meekosha & Dowse, 1997).

Drawing on life-course interviews with women with disabilities, this chapter investigates their experiences of Active Citizenship. By the term 'women with disabilities' we understand women who 'have long-term physical, mental, intellectual or sensory impairments which in interaction with various barriers may hinder their full and effective participation in society on an equal basis with others' (CRPD, Art 1). Hence, we adopt a relational understanding of disability (Thomas, 2004). In this chapter, after explaining our intersectional perspective on Active Citizenship, we describe our data and methodology. The following section presents women with disabilities' experiences of Active Citizenship in education, intimate relationships, family care, labour market participation and participation in politics and civil society. Finally we summarise the main findings of this study and suggest directions for future research.

Active Citizenship – an intersectional perspective

This chapter adopts an intersectional approach to study the experiences of Active Citizenship of women with disabilities. The term intersectionality was coined by Kimberlé Crenshaw (1989), who argued for the need to explore the multidimensionality of black women's experiences instead of treating 'race and gender as mutually exclusive categories of experience and analysis' (p. 139). Likewise, feminist disability scholars called attention to the situation of disabled women who were largely neglected by both feminist and disability research (see e.g. Keith, 1992; Morris, 1993).

McCall (2005) distinguished three ways of studying intersectionality: anti-categorical, intra-categorical and inter-categorical. In contrast to the anti-categorical perspective that questions the use of any categories, and in contrast to the inter-categorical approach that compares different groups of people, this chapter applies an 'intra-categorical perspective'. This means that we focus on the variety of experiences of Active Citizenship of individuals located at the intersection of the dimensions 'womanhood' and 'disability'. In other words, we do not assume that being a woman and having disabilities automatically leads to double discrimination (for a critique of the 'double discrimination' approach. see e.g. Barron, 2008; Morris, 1993; Stuart, 1993; Traustadóttir, 2006; Waldschmidt, 2014) but we look at the complexity of narratives and at the 'new twists' that womanhood and disability give to Active Citizenship.

The concept of Active Citizenship highlights the importance of practices. Being an active citizen implies enjoying a basic level of security and wellbeing, deciding about matters concerning one's own life and influencing decisions concerning one's society. These three dimensions are referred to as security, autonomy and influence (see Chapter 1). In this chapter, we focus on how practices of Active Citizenship are influenced by internal and external factors. Drawing on the capability approach (Sen, 1993), we underline the fact that individuals who are in similar situations do not necessarily achieve the same outcomes in terms of Active Citizenship, and that such achievement depends on whether given conditions ('conversion factors') are enabling or disabling. Moreover, we use a life-course perspective to investigate: (1) the expectations, rights and obligations relative to participation in different life-course stages, (2) the social processes that shape the experience of women with disabilities in these life-course stages, and (3) the way women with disabilities cope with dominant expectations relative to participation over the life course (see Chapter 2). Although we focus mostly on adulthood, the life-course perspective highlights that individuals are expected to take on various roles during their lives. Assuming a new role – such as starting university or becoming a mother – can be viewed as a transition or turning point in a life trajectory and is linked to social expectations.

When relevant, we relate the accounts of our informants to external structures: e.g. gender specific social expectations, stereotypes about persons with disabilities, social services and networks of significant others (O'Reilly, 2012; Stones, 2005). We focus in particular on the relationship between different roles and highlight the interdependencies, hierarchy or conflicts between the women's various responsibilities (Stones, 2005).

Data and methodology

The empirical data for this chapter consists of the summaries of life-course interviews with 104 women with disabilities living in the nine countries covered by DISCIT (for details about the methodology, see Chapter 3) and full interview transcripts from Ireland, Norway, Sweden and Switzerland (which are the home countries of the authors of this chapter). We started the analysis by defining different social roles that are particularly relevant for discussing the gendered aspects of Active Citizenship of women with disabilities. Based on the work of Thomas (1999, see quote above) and on feminist citizenship literature, we identified the following social roles: as student/pupil, as partner/wife, as care-giver in the family, as labour market participant and as participant in politics and civil society. An important limitation of our data is that the life-course interviews did not include questions about motherhood, family life, romantic relationships, sexuality, care or informal work inside the family. Nevertheless, these topics can be found in our data because they were raised by some interviewees.

Women's experiences of Active Citizenship in different social settings

This section discusses women with disabilities' experiences of Active Citizenship in different social settings. We focus on situations where the dimensions of womanhood and disability were particularly salient.

Active Citizenship in education

Women have lacked – and continue to lack – equal access to education and have often been relegated to traditionally 'feminine' areas of study (Bradley, 2000; Moore, 1987; UNICEF, 2015). Similarly, people with disabilities often encounter barriers in accessing education (Fuller, Healey, Bradley & Hall, 2004; Shevlin, Kenny & Neela, 2004). Education is crucial for participation in society and the CRPD Article 24 protects the right to education for persons with disabilities. However, some interviewees reported that they did not receive the level of school or vocational education that they would have wished for themselves. For instance, a woman from Switzerland with psychosocial disabilities (born around 1950) could not enter secondary school because she had to do many household chores and was expected to care for her younger siblings. Her father denied her the opportunity to obtain a secondary school degree even though she had the grades to pursue this education:

> My father then, eh, exercised his 'violence' as I would call it today and, eh, did not let me do it. I would also have liked to train as a nurse, and I already knew that with the middle school it would not be enough, that one needed three years of secondary school for that. And so I then had to, first I wanted to train as a hairdresser. My father then compelled me to train as a salesperson for groceries.
>
> (From an interview with a woman from Switzerland with psychosocial disabilities born around 1950)

This quote suggests that not only was the interviewee denied secondary education but she was also not allowed to choose the vocation she would train in. Her alternative choice to secondary school would have been to become a hairdresser, but her father forced her to become a salesperson. Furthermore, the interviewee explained that, after middle school and prior to starting vocational training, she had to do a year of home economics training to become 'a good housekeeper', like many women of her generation (Lebeaume, 2014). Later in life, the interviewee changed her career through repeated retraining to better fit her interests. At the time of the interview, she worked as a peer counsellor for persons with psychosocial problems. From a life-course perspective, this example indicates that, although gendered expectations and her responsibilities as carer for her younger siblings prevented the interviewee from studying nursing when she was younger, she had the opportunity to study and get a job that she liked when she was older. The interview also suggests that the interviewee's experience of disability had an influence on her choice of profession, since she became a peer counsellor for persons with psychosocial disabilities.

A woman from Norway with visual impairment (born around 1950) also seemed to have been influenced by society's expectations towards both women and persons with disabilities, as she married early and worked as a telephonist at the Association of the Blind, which was a typical job for visually impaired persons at that time (Scadden, 1992). However, after a few years of marriage she divorced, realised that she wanted to be a teacher and went back to education. She said that she did not go to college earlier because she did not consider herself to be good enough. She added: 'I did not have the courage [to study]. And then I thought that it must be wonderful to get married'. She eventually completed her studies to become a teacher and went on to become a special education teacher because she wanted to teach children with visual impairments.

This example suggests that, while gendered norms seem to have influenced the interviewee's decision to marry early, having a visual impairment seems to have influenced her career, as she first worked at the Association of the Blind and then as a special education teacher for children with visual impairment.

In other cases, women with disabilities were pushed into pursuing education because of the assumption that their disability would prevent them from establishing their own family and carrying out care responsibilities. For example, a woman from Sweden with mobility impairment (born around 1950) explained how her mother did not believe that she would ever meet a partner and have children. Therefore, her mother encouraged her to continue her education so that she would find a good job and be financially independent. Barron (2008) observed the same phenomenon in her study about women with mobility impairment and argued that the higher level of education of these women could not be interpreted as a sign of feminine emancipation but as a lack of choice. The Swedish interviewee explained, however, that she did not listen to her mother and had a child directly after secondary education. A few years later, she obtained a university degree.

Relationships with peers were also named as a factor that influenced women's experiences in education. An interviewee from Switzerland completed her primary education in a school for children with cerebral palsy and then transferred to a mainstream grammar school. Her difficulty, she said, was that she had been socialised in a way that did not fit the all-girls class she suddenly found herself in:

> It was a shock because in, in the cerebral palsy school we had been a very small class with seven students. And there I had been the only girl. That is, myself and six other [male] students. [...] In grammar school, there were then suddenly 28 girls, right? That was a hell of a shock. Because I couldn't, I was not in their world. I did not know what to talk about. I only talked about football and, and about some, yes, just boys' topics, right? The others were completely, completely 'from the moon' for me, right?
>
> (From an interview with a woman from Switzerland with mobility impairment born around 1950)

This quote suggests that her disability posed less of a barrier to fitting in at her new school than her allegedly 'atypical' gender behaviour. Her disability, however, seems to have played a role during her days at grammar school, namely in terms of romantic relationships. She explained that this was the only time in her life where she really felt disabled:

> ...during adolescence, I felt disabled when it came to relationships and so on, right? Then, my co-, my co-students had partners or boyfriends or so, and I, I, well actually my best friend from grammar school and I, we, we were the only ones who were single. And then I indeed thought, yes, that's

> because of the impairment. But it could have been just as well that this was not the case, but I did feel disabled at that point. Eh, it was also the time when higher heels were popular, right? And then the mini-skirts, and I couldn't have either of that. It would have looked ridiculous, if I had tried to move in, eh, in such high heels, right.
>
> (From an interview with a woman from Switzerland with mobility impairment born around 1950)

Feeling disabled in the context of romantic relationships in adolescence was also found in a study of three generations of women with disabilities in Sweden (Helmius, 1999). Referring to Barron (1997), Helmius (1999) concluded that these difficulties are part of 'the bumpy road to womanhood' experienced by women with disabilities because of stereotypical assumptions concerning disability. Our data suggest that experiences of education are influenced by both gendered expectations and expectations towards persons with disabilities. However, although some women could not go to college when they were young, the interviews suggest that some women found the opportunity to pursue their education later in life, and that difficulties in finding romantic partners during adolescence did not necessarily mean the interviewees were single as adults.

Active Citizenship in intimate relationships

Article 23 of the CRPD requires persons with disabilities to be protected from discrimination related to marriage, family, parenthood and relationships. Yet, women with disabilities are often not seen as appropriate holders of care responsibilities or not deemed able to live up to expectations as wife, partner and girlfriend (Barron, 2008; Bonnie, 2014; Keith, 1992; Traustadóttir, 1990) and are often victims of violence and sexual harassment (Crawford & Ostrove, 2003; Curry et al., 2009; Ortoleva & Lewis, 2012).

Among the interviewees with intellectual impairments, only one woman from Norway (born around 1950) said that she was married. Her wedding seems to have been an important and happy event, as it was the first thing she discussed in the interview. In contrast, a woman from the Czech Republic with intellectual disabilities (born around 1990) said that she used to have a girlfriend but that she broke up with her because her parents told her they were not a good couple. The parents' disapproval may have been related to the fact that women with disabilities, and in particular women with intellectual disabilities, are not expected to be in a sexual/romantic relationship, but it could also be that the parents did not want their daughter to have a homosexual relationship (for a discussion about how people with intellectual disability are encouraged to have 'an ordinary sexual life', see Brown (1994)).

The lack of expectations for women with disabilities to engage in romantic relationships was, however, not limited to women with intellectual disabilities. A woman from Ireland with mobility impairment (born around 1990) explained that when she travelled with her boyfriend, they were often given two single beds.

> Like a lot of the time for instance in hotel rooms, even if I request a double room, we'll get a twin room and it'll just be like, 'Why? I asked you for a double room for a reason,' you know, and like I'm just lucky with the man that I'm with that he gets it as well, so we just laugh about it but that mightn't have been the case when he knew me first and that might have scared him off, 'OK, well if this is going to happen to us every time we go to a hotel room, I don't want to.' You know, where you have to go down and go, 'Actually, I did order a double room, I meant it.' You know, you don't want to be screaming about your personal life, so that's a big issue.
>
> (From an interview with a woman from Ireland with mobility impairment born around 1990)

This quote suggests that the interviewee felt discriminated against because of the default assumption that her relationship with her boyfriend was not sexual, and that she found it embarrassing to have to spell that out for the hotel. Similarly, Crawford and Ostrove found that the negative social constructions of people with disabilities as 'incompetent and helpless, intellectually challenged, super-capable and asexual' (2003, p. 190) deeply affected women with disabilities' interpersonal relationships.

Some interviewees also spoke about the important role their partners played in their lives and the support they derived from them. A woman from Italy with psychosocial disabilities (born around 1990) said that having a boyfriend pushed her to explore the possibility of living on her own and achieving more autonomy. Similarly, a woman from Switzerland with intellectual disabilities (born around 1970) pointed out how much self-confidence she had been able to gain through her partner.

Living with a partner or spouse is, however, not always a positive experience. Domestic abuse perpetrated against women with disabilities is a well-documented issue (see e.g. Curry et al., 2009; Ortoleva & Lewis, 2012) that also appeared in our empirical data. A woman from Switzerland with psychosocial disabilities (born around 1950) identified the separation from her first husband as an important turning point in her life, because he had been controlling her every move and did not allow her any freedom. Another woman from Sweden with an intellectual disability (born around 1950) spoke about a partner who had physically abused her and had taken her money. Financial control by an abusive husband was also described by a woman from Germany with a psychosocial disability (born around 1970), who concluded that her marriage had been 'only violence, humiliation and misery'. We collected similar stories about abuse and harassment in Norway.

The interviewees' experiences indicate that engaging in intimate relationships is expected of women in general but not always of women with disabilities. Being a partner or a wife is related to Active Citizenship because it provides a social status that is valued in adulthood and is part of 'normal sexuality' (Helmius, 1999). Intimate relationships also influence agency in other social spheres. The interviews suggest that the sense of autonomy and security increased for women who experienced happy relationships but was restricted for women in violent or controlling relationships.

Active Citizenship in care for the family

CRPD Article 23 specifically protects the right of women with disabilities to become mothers. This provision seems pertinent in light of the attitudinal and practical barriers faced by women with disabilities who wish to become mothers (Conley-Jung & Olkin, 2001; Grue & Lærum, 2002; Traustadóttir, 1990). A woman from Ireland with mobility impairment (born around 1990) said that she had no idea where to access information about the specific issues she might face as a pregnant woman with a physical disability. Similarly, a woman from the Czech Republic with psychosocial disabilities (born around 1990) spoke of trying to get information from her psychiatrist about how her disability and medication would affect her ability to parent. The psychiatrist told her that he did not deal with 'these kinds of gendered topics' and that she needed to ask someone else to what extent her condition could be hereditary and whether she would be able to raise her children. The answer of the psychiatrist illustrates two important barriers that women with disabilities face when they decide to have children: the assumptions that they are not capable of being 'good mothers' and the assumption that their children will be impaired (Grue & Lærum, 2002; Mayes, Llewellyn & McConnell, 2006). These barriers are particularly relevant for women with intellectual and psychosocial disabilities who have been – and often still are – denied their reproductive and sexual rights (Carey, 2003; McConnell & Llewellyn, 2002; Tilley, Walmsley, Earle & Atkinson, 2012). In our data, none of our female interviewees with intellectual disabilities had children, and three women with psychosocial disabilities – among a total of 11 women who reported having children – had their children taken away from them. No women with mobility impairments reported such experiences, but one woman from the Czech Republic with a visual impairment (born around 1950) said that her daughter, who had severe disabilities, was taken into care. It is unclear whether this was her choice or if the interviewee was considered unable to take care of her daughter because of her own visual impairment.

Social services can be a great help in performing one's role as a mother, but these are not always available to women with disabilities. A woman from Sweden with mobility impairment (born around 1950) recalled how complicated it was to convince the home care staff to help her with the care of her baby. She described the introduction of personal assistance in the 1990s in Sweden as a tremendous improvement because it gave her much more freedom to organise the care she needed. In the same vein, a woman from Germany with visual impairment (born around 1950) said that it would have been helpful to have received support to help her children with their homework. And a woman from Norway with visual impairment (born around 1970) spoke about the challenge of accessing support when she was raising her children. She was told that 'with visual impairments one should expect some difficulties'.

Some mothers spoke of how important their children were to them. Several women explicitly said that having children constituted a significant turning point in their lives. For example, a woman from Serbia with a visual impairment (born around 1950) described her life as successful thanks to her three children. The interviews suggest that having children had a significant impact on professional careers, as the interviewees explained that they took maternity leave, reduced their working hours and/or had to change jobs when their children were young. A woman from the United Kingdom with mobility impairment (born around 1970) spoke of arranging her part-time work schedule so that she was able to take her children to school. Another example was a woman from the Czech Republic with psychosocial difficulties (born around 1950) who got her first job as an operator at a computer centre with morning and night shifts. When she was single and childless, she did not mind working night shifts. Then she had her child and asked to only work morning shifts, but the company did not fulfil this request and the interviewee had to quit her job. She quickly found a new job, but was soon dismissed because she was frequently absent from work to take care of her son who was often sick. After staying home with her child for some time, she found a new job but said it was stressful to manage both her responsibilities as a mother and as a worker. Because of the conflict between these responsibilities, she eventually quit her job and decided to stay home until her son started school. Similarly, a woman from Switzerland also explained that she stopped working when she had her first child. Although she did some voluntary work in between, she only returned to paid employment when her children were in their final years of school. About her decision to be a full-time mother, she said:

> Before, I worked and then I was basically just at home with the children. But I always did this with pleasure and I also did not have the feeling that this was inferior. I enjoyed doing it, I had a couple of girlfriends and we were out and about with the kids a lot. Actually, yes, I never missed working life.
>
> (From an interview with a woman from Switzerland with visual impairment born around 1950)

These two examples are similar, in that both women faced difficulties combining the responsibilities of a mother and a worker, and interrupted their professional careers when their children were young, but only the latter interviewee described this experience as a period of her life she truly enjoyed. The interview data does not allow for an explanation of the reasons for these contrasting experiences but suggest that gendered expectations – rather than expectations relating to having a disability – influenced the decision to stay home with the child. From earlier research we know that cross-national divergences in work–life balance policies make a difference for women's participation in working life (e.g. Lister et al., 2007; Siim, 2000).

Apart from the role as mothers, we looked at the whole range of practices undertaken by women with disabilities in relation to their family members. As such, we adopted a relational understanding of care (Fine & Glendinning, 2005; Keith, 1992; Morris, 1991; Orme, 1998; Rummery & Fine, 2012; Sevenhuijsen, 2000) and called attention to the practices of care undertaken by women with disabilities (Keith, 1992). For example, an interviewee from Ireland said:

> I would give a certain amount of care to my brother who has an intellectual disability or like I babysit children in the family and I just think that a lot of people assume that because somebody has a physical disability that they don't contribute to family life or to those kind of things as much as others would. I mightn't do it in a physical way, sometimes I do like, but say for instance if my mother needs to look after my brother for something in particular, like he's sick or something ... Like there'll always be something that I can do to contribute to the situation and I just think sometimes that people think that people with disabilities are sitting at home being the ones cared for all the time but a lot of us are in reciprocal relationships with our families and contributing as much to the household as everyone else.
>
> (From an interview with a woman from Ireland with mobility impairment born around 1990)

In this quote, the interviewee criticised the stereotypical ideas about persons with disabilities and drew attention to her actual practices of care. Similarly, a woman with an intellectual disability spoke about her contributions to her family. For example, in talking about money, she said:

> Money in our family isn't really a thing, like I'd no money the other day and I had to get cream but I didn't have enough money, my sister gave me the money. Say like, my mam might need a lend of money and give something – she wouldn't pay me back but she'd give it to me when I needed it.
>
> (From an interview with a woman from Ireland with intellectual disability born around 1990)

The interviewee pointed at relations of interdependence inside the family, where family members help each other when needed. Similarly, a woman from Serbia with mobility impairment (born around 1950) spoke of how she provided financial support for her family by buying her family's home and paying for 24-hour assistance when her mother was ill. The interviews suggest that taking care of one's elderly parents could be an important responsibility that could influence life choices. For example, a woman from Italy with mobility impairment (born around 1970) explained that she had always lived at her parents' house in Naples. At the moment of the interview, she expressed how she had recently been thinking about living on her own but moving out would be a complicated decision because, although she had the financial means, she could not bring herself to leave her parents alone.

These examples suggest that women with disabilities are actively engaged in practices of care for their children and family members in general, although they were not always expected to have children or be carers. It also suggests that gendered expectations were salient for the women who had children and stayed at home with them.

Active Citizenship in labour market participation

A recent report of the International Labour Organisation (ILO, 2010) showed a continuing gender disparity, both in terms of opportunities and of quality of employment; nearly one fourth of women are unpaid family workers and many women work in segregated sectors with precarious working arrangements and low salaries. This appeared in our data, and a woman in the United Kingdom, for example, said she had been discouraged from employment because of her gender:

> In those days a lot of women didn't work after they were married. I was just normal, go along with the flow … You weren't given choices in my day. You were told what to do, and so I didn't ask what I should be.
>
> (From an interview with a woman from the UK with mobility impairment born around 1950)

In the previous section we discussed how having children impacted on the professional career of some of the interviewees. Another aspect that came out of the analysis is that women with disabilities struggled to find a job that they liked because of society's preconceptions about what they should do and because they did not get adequate support and help to deal with their impairments and/or family responsibilities (see also González, 2009). For example, a woman from Germany with a visual impairment (born around 1950) explained that she started working as a shorthand typist at the age of 18. She did not like it but this profession was her parents' choice and a typical job for blind women at that time. About a year later, she got married and had her first child. She continued working part-time but, after the birth of her second child, she quit her job and stayed at home with her children. Then she wanted to get back to work, but not as a shorthand typist. She started to study informatics but could not complete her programme because the material was not accessible for persons with visual impairment and because of her responsibilities as a mother. The interviewee went back to the labour market later, but worked mainly as a telephone operator.

In the section about education, we gave examples of interviewees who could not choose their career because of gendered expectations and family responsibilities. However, some women were able to access further education and find a job they liked later in life. There was also the example of a woman who was encouraged to pursue further education because of the assumption that she would never get married. Overall, these narratives suggest that being a woman and having disabilities influenced the interviewees' experiences and opportunities in the labour market.

Active Citizenship in participation in politics and civil society

From a feminist perspective, participation in the community is particularly important for women because it 'represents the area in which women are most often able to act as citizens' (Lister, 2003, p. 84). With regard to persons with disabilities, Roker, Player and Coleman (1998) found that many young adults with disabilities participate in voluntary activities and help out in the community, contrary to misconceptions that people with disabilities only receive help from others. In a similar way, Balandin, Llewellyn, Dew, Ballin and Schneider (2006) found that older people with disabilities had positive attitudes towards volunteering and that many participated in such activities. Yet, they called attention to the fact that persons with disabilities do not have the same possibilities of engaging in voluntary activities and may need some support to participate in such activities.

As the DISCIT project recruited many interviewees through disability organisations (see Chapter 3), it was not surprising that many interviewees participated actively in such organisations (see Chapter 6). Many interviewees were also involved in political parties, cultural organisations, and charities and these experiences were sometimes gendered. For example, a woman from Sweden with visual impairment (born around 1970) became international secretary for a disability organisation. She recalled that it was not so easy to be the only woman in a male environment.

> There were only men and it used to be called the gentlemen's club because we had meetings twice a year for what was called [name of the organisation] … it was only men until I arrived … [but] when I understood that they listened to what I said that they, like, listened to my opinions and my comments, like, agreed with me then I got a real kick upwards, that I remember and I became much stronger, but in the beginning I was a little like: 'Okay, what shall little I do here?'
>
> (From an interview with a woman from Sweden with visual impairment born around 1970)

This quote suggests that, at first, the interviewee was uncomfortable being the only woman in these meetings, but that it was a positive experience because she felt valued by her male colleagues who listened to her. The experience of this interviewee resonates with the findings of Hugemark and Roman (2007), who pointed at gender inequality in Swedish disability organisations. It also resonates with the more general observation that women with disabilities tend to be marginalised in both disability and feminist organisations (Meekosha, 2002). As a reaction to this situation, Hugemark and Roman (2007) noticed that women with disabilities built their own organisation to create a feminine arena within the disability movement. Likewise, the empirical analysis suggests that some interviewees were active in organisations of women with disabilities. For example, a woman from Italy with mobility impairment (born around 1970) who had been active in various disability organisations for a long time was elected the representative of women with disabilities in a federation of disability organisations. She worked to raise awareness of the specific situation of women with disabilities and enhance their inclusion in society.

Engagement in politics could be a gendered experience. A woman from Norway with mobility impairment who had been politically active for a long time explained that she resigned when the party decided not to support the educational needs of a girl with disabilities. Further, she found it very difficult to continue supporting her party when it decided to vote in favour of prenatal screening after 11 weeks. This was especially tough because the interviewee had previously been advised to abort following a test showing that there was a 50 per cent chance that her child would have a disability.

Overall, the life-course interviews shed light on some gendered aspects of participation in civil society and political life relative to personal experiences or to being a woman in a male-dominated setting.

Conclusion

This chapter drew on life-course interviews with women with disabilities to analyse Active Citizenship from an intersectional perspective. We considered women with disabilities first and foremost as women (Barron, 1997; Mayes et al., 2006) and looked at the influence of disability on the 'normal stuff' of contemporary women's lives (Thomas, 1999). Inspired by feminist critiques of traditional conceptions of citizenship, we highlighted the dimensions of care and intimacy, and the interdependency of public and private roles. This approach complemented the conceptualisation of Active Citizenship around the dimensions of security, autonomy and influence with aspects of gender, sexuality, care and interdependency. We found that the interviewees' experiences and practices of Active Citizenship were influenced by expectations relative to both disability and womanhood. Moreover, in contrast to studies focusing on one societal arena, this chapter analysed women with disabilities' Active Citizenship in different social settings. We highlighted the diversity of women's agency, their experiences of disability and the challenges relative to combining multiple responsibilities (e.g. as mothers and as workers). The chapter called attention to the fact that women who could not participate in the labour market could be active in civil society organisations or in the family. Furthermore, the life-course perspective adopted in the chapter suggested that women who were limited in their practices of Active Citizenship at one point (e.g. during adolescence or in an abusive marriage) could experience Active Citizenship later in life (e.g. due to retraining, a supportive partner or self-help groups).

We encourage further studies to build upon our findings and continue the analysis of the 'new twists' that womanhood and disability give to Active Citizenship. There is also a need to analyse the Active Citizenship of men with disabilities and look at how manhood intersects with disability and influences expectations and experiences of disabled men's participation in society (Thomas,

2006). Finally, there is a need for inter-categorical studies which compare the experiences of women and men with disabilities and the experience of women with different backgrounds.

References

Balandin, S., Llewellyn, G., Dew, A., Ballin, L. & Schneider, J. (2006). Older disabled workers' perceptions of volunteering. *Disability & Society*, *21*(7), 677–692. http://doi.org/10.1080/09687590600995139.

Barron, K. (1997). The bumpy road to womanhood. *Disability & Society*, *12*(2), 223–240. http://doi.org/10.1080/09687599727344.

Barron, K. (2008). Kön och funktionshinder [Gender and disability]. In L. Grönvik & M. Söder (Eds), *Bara funktionshindrad? Funktionshinder och intersektionalitet [Only disabled? Disability and intersectionality]* (pp. 28–46). Malmö: Gleerups.

Bonnie, S. (2014). Disabled people, disability and sexuality. In J. Swain, S. French, C. Barnes & C. Thomas (Eds), *Disabling barriers – Enabling environments* (pp. 125–132). London: Sage.

Bradley, K. (2000). Higher education: Sociology of education. *Sociology of Education*, *73*(1), 1–18. http://doi.org/10.2307/2673196.

Brown, H. (1994). 'An ordinary sexual life?' A review of the normalisation principle as it applies to the sexual options of people with learning disabilities. *Disability & Society*, *9*(2), 123–144. http://doi.org/10.1080/09687599466780181.

Burchell, D. (2002). Ancient citizenship and its inheritors. In E. F. Isin & B. S. Turner (Eds), *Handbook of citizenship studies* (pp. 89–104). London: Sage.

Carey, A. C. (2003). Beyond the medical model: A reconsideration of 'feeblemindedness', citizenship, and eugenic restrictions. *Disability & Society*, *18*(4), 411–430. http://doi.org/10.1080/0968759032000080977.

Conley-Jung, C. & Olkin, R. (2001). Mothers with visual impairments who are raising young children. *Journal of Visual Impairment & Blindness*, *95*(1), 14–29.

Crawford, D. & Ostrove, J. M. (2003). Representations of disability and the interpersonal relationships of women with disabilities. *Women & Therapy*, *26*(3–4), 179–194. http://doi.org/10.1300/J015v26n03.

Crenshaw, K. (1989). Demarginalizing the intersection of race and sex: A black feminist critique of antidiscrimination doctrine, feminist theory, and antiracist politics. *University of Chicago Legal Forum*, *1989*(8), 139–168.

Curry, M. A., Renker, P., Hughes, R. B., Robinson-Whelen, S., Oschwald, M., Swank, P. R. & Powers, L. E. (2009). Development of measures of abuse among women with disabilities and the characteristics of their perpetrators. *Violence against Women*, *15*(9), 1001–1025. http://doi.org/10.1177/1077801209340308.

EDF. (2014). *Alternative report to the UN committee on the rights of persons with disabilities*. Brussels: EDF.

Fine, M. & Glendinning, C. (2005). Dependence, independence or inter-dependence? Revisiting the concepts of 'care' and 'dependency'. *Ageing and Society*, *25*(4), 601–621. http://doi.org/10.1017/S0144686X05003600.

Fraser, N. & Gordon, L. (1994). Civil citizenship against social citizenship? In B. van Steenbergen (Ed.), *The condition of citizenship* (pp. 90–107). London: Sage.

Fuller, M., Healey, M., Bradley, A. & Hall, T. (2004). Barriers to learning: A systematic study of the experience of disabled students in one university. *Studies in Higher Education*, *29*(3), 303–318. http://doi.org/10.1080/0307507041000l682592.

Gerschick, T. J. (2000). Toward a theory of disability and gender. *Signs*, *25*(4), 1263–1268.

González, M. L. (2009). Getting to know reality and breaking stereotypes: The experience of two generations of working disabled women. *Disability & Society*, *24*(4), 447–459. http://doi.org/10.1080/09687590902879056.

Grue, L. & Lærum, K. T. (2002). 'Doing motherhood': Some experiences of mothers with physical disabilities. *Disability & Society*, *17*(6), 671–683. http://doi.org/10.1080/0968759022000010443.

Helmius, G. (1999). Disability, sexuality and sociosexual relationships in women's everyday life. *Scandinavian Journal of Disability Research*, *1*(1), 50–63. http://doi.org/10.1080/15017419909510737.

Hugemark, A. & Roman, C. (2007). Diversity and divisions in the Swedish disability movement: Disability, gender, and social justice. *Scandinavian Journal of Disability Research*, *9*(1), 26–45. http://doi.org/10.1080/15017410600979553.

ILO. (2010). *Women in labour markets: Measuring progress and identifying challenges*. Geneva: ILO.

Keith, L. (1992). Who cares wins? Women, caring and disability. *Disability, Handicap & Society*, *7*(2), 167–175. http://doi.org/10.1080/02674649266780191.

Lebeaume, J. (2014). *L'Enseignement Ménager en France. Sciences et Techniques au Féminin, 1880–1980*. Rennes: Presses Universitaires de Rennes.

Lister, R. (1997). Dialectics of citizenship. *Hypatia*, *12*(4), 6–26.

Lister, R. (2002). Sexual citizenship. In I. F. Engin & B. S. Turner (Eds), *Handbook of citizenship studies* (pp. 191–207). London: Sage.

Lister, R. (2003). *Citizenship feminist perspectives* (2nd ed.). Basingstoke: Macmillan.

Lister, R., Williams, F., Anttonen, A., Bussemaker, J., Gerhard, U., Heinen, J., … Gavanas, A. (2007). *Gendering citizenship in Western Europe: New challenges for citizenship research in a cross-national context*. Bristol: Policy Press.

Mayes, R., Llewellyn, G. & McConnell, D. (2006). Misconception: The experience of pregnancy for women with intellectual disabilities. *Scandinavian Journal of Disability Research*, *8*(2–3), 120–131. http://doi.org/10.1080/15017410600774178.

McCall, L. (2005). The complexity of intersectionality. *Signs*, *30*(3), 1771–1800. http://doi.org/10.1163/_afco_asc_2291.

McConnell, D. & Llewellyn, G. (2002). Stereotypes, parents with intellectual disability and child protection. *Journal of Social Welfare and Family Law*, *24*(3), 297–317. http://doi.org/10.1080/09649060210161294.

Meekosha, H. (2002). Virtual activists? Women and the making of identities of disability. *Hypatia*, *17*(3), 67–88. http://doi.org/10.1353/hyp. 2002.0064.

Meekosha, H. & Dowse, L. (1997). Enabling citizenship: Gender, disability and citizenship in Australia. *Feminist Review*, *57*, 49–72.

Moore, K. M. (1987). Women's access and opportunity in higher education: Toward the twenty-first century. *Comparative Education*, *23*(1), 23–34. http://doi.org/10.1080/0305006870230104.

Morris, J. (1991). *Pride against prejudice: Transforming attitudes to disability*. Philadelphia, PA: New Society Publishers.

Morris, J. (1993). Feminism and disability. *Feminist Review*, *43*, 57–70. http://doi.org/10.2307/1395069.

O'Reilly, K. (2012). *International migration and social theory.* Basingstoke: Palgrave Macmillan.
Orloff, A. S. (1993). Gender and the social rights of citizenship: The comparative analysis of gender relations and welfare states. *American Sociological Review, 53*(3), 303–328.
Orme, J. (1998). Community care: Gender issues. *The British Journal of Social Work, 28,* 615–622.
Ortoleva, S. & Lewis, H. (2012). Forgotten sisters – A report on violence against women with disabilities: An overview of its nature, scope, causes and consequences. *Northeastern Public Law and Theory Faculty Research Paper Series* (Vol. 104).
Plummer, K. (2001). The square of intimate citizenship: Some preliminary proposals. *Citizenship Studies, 5*(3), 237–253. http://doi.org/10.1080/1362102012008522.
Roker, D., Player, K. & Coleman, J. (1998). Challenging the image: The involvement of young people with disabilities in volunteering and campaigning. *Disability & Society, 13*(5), 725–741. http://doi.org/http://dx.doi.org/10.1080/09687599826489.
Rummery, K. & Fine, M. (2012). Care: A critical review of theory, policy and practice. *Social Policy & Administration, 46*(3), 321–343. http://doi.org/10.1111/j.1467-9515.2012.00845.x.
Scadden, L. A. (1992). The effect of new technology on the employment of blind and visually impaired persons in four Western European countries. In H. A. Hunt & M. Berkowitz (Eds), *New technologies and the employment of disabled persons* (pp. 39–56). Geneva: International Labour Office.
Sen, A. (1993). Capability and well-being. In M. Nussbaum & A. Sen (Eds), *The quality of life* (pp. 30–54). Oxford: Oxford Scholarship Online. http://doi.org/10.1093/0198287976.003.0003.
Sépulchre, M. (2016). Research about citizenship and disability: A scoping review. *Disability & Rehabilitation.* http://doi.org/http://dx.doi.org/10.3109/09638288.2016.1172674.
Sevenhuijsen, S. (2000). Caring in the third way: The relation between obligation, responsibility and care in third way discourse. *Critical Social Policy, 20*(1), 5–37. http://doi.org/10.1177/026101830002000102.
Shevlin, M., Kenny, M. & Neela, E. (2004). Access routes to higher education for young people with disabilities: A question of chance? *Irish Educational Studies, 23*(2), 37–53. http://doi.org/10.1080/0332331040230206.
Siim, B. (2000). *Gender and citizenship. Politics and agency in France, Britain and Denmark.* Cambridge: Cambridge University Press.
Stones, R. (2005). *Structuration theory.* Basingstoke: Palgrave Macmillan.
Stuart, O. (1993). Double oppression: An appropriate starting-point? In J. Swain, V. Finkelstein, S. French & M. Oliver (Eds), *Disabling barriers – Enabling environments* (pp. 93–100). London: Sage.
Thomas, C. (1999). *Female forms.* Buckinghamshire: Open University Press.
Thomas, C. (2004). How is disability understood? An examination of sociological approaches. *Disability & Society, 19*(6), 569–583. http://doi.org/10.1080/0968759042000252506.
Thomas, C. (2006). Disability and gender: Reflections on theory and research. *Scandinavian Journal of Disability Research, 8*(2–3), 177–185. http://doi.org/10.1080/15017410600731368.
Tilley, E., Walmsley, J., Earle, S. & Atkinson, D. (2012). 'The silence is roaring': Sterilization, reproductive rights and women with intellectual disabilities. *Disability & Society, 27*(3), 413–426. http://doi.org/10.1080/09687599.2012.654991.

Traustadóttir, R. (1990). Obstacles to equality: The double discrimination of women with disabilities. Retrieved 20 April 2016, from www.independentliving.org/docs3/chp1997.html#overview.

Traustadóttir, R. (2006). Disability and gender: Introduction to the special issue. *Scandinavian Journal of Disability Research*, *8*(2–3), 81–84. http://doi.org/10.1080/15017410600831341.

UN. (2006). *Convention on the rights of persons with disabilities.* Retrieved 20 April 2016, from www.un.org/disabilities/convention/conventionfull.shtml.

UNDP. (2015). *Human development report.* New York: United Nations.

UNICEF. (2015). *Girls' education and gender equality.* Retrieved 11 April 2016, from www.unicef.org/education/bege_70640.html.

Walby, S. (1994). Is citizenship gendered? *Sociology*, *28*(2), 379–395. http://doi.org/10.1177/0038038594028002002.

Waldschmidt, A. (2014). Jenseits der doppelten Diskriminierung? Disability, gender und die Intersektionalitätsdebatte. In M. Löw (Ed.), *Vielfalt und Zusammenhalt Verhandlungen des 36. Kongresses der Deutschen Gesellschaft für Soziologie in Bochum und Dortmund 2012* (pp. 871–883). Frankfurt: Campus.

WHO. (2011). *World report on disability. The World Health Organization.* Geneva: The World Health Organization. http://doi.org/10.1016/S0140-6736(11)60844-1.

11 Transitions to Active Citizenship for young persons with disabilities

Virtuous and vicious cycles of functionings

Rune Halvorsen and Kjetil Klette Bøhler

Young adults are at a critical stage in adjusting to dominant life expectations. According to Wyn and White (1997, p. 4) 'youth is most productively conceptualized as a *social process* in which the meaning and experience of becoming adult is socially mediated'. Transition to adulthood and the efforts to become active citizens are interrelated, in that youth are 'citizens in the making' (Marshall, 1950, p. 25). Young adults above the legal age are by default recognised as full citizens, in the sense that they are granted legal rights and obligations on an equal level with other adults. Yet, they are only at the stage of realising their potential to participate as full members of society.

To investigate the transition to adulthood for young persons with disabilities, we have examined under which conditions young adults with disabilities are most likely to achieve the dimensions of Active Citizenship, i.e.

- *security* (enjoying social protection against illness, poverty, violence);
- *autonomy* (exercising freedom to choose the life and daily activities one has reason to value and avoiding unwanted dependence or interference from others); and
- *influence* (participating in discussions and decisions affecting one's own life and society at large) (see Chapter 1, this volume).

To answer this question we have sought to identify barriers and facilitators that young adults with disabilities experience in the transition from education to the labour market. In particular, we examine the interrelationship between how young adults cope with the dominant expectations of achieving regular employment, developing a firm self-identity, and navigating the challenges of defining and living the life they have reasons to value, including participation in leisure activities and interaction with peers.

The transition to adulthood is especially critical for youth with disabilities as they experience more severe barriers to become active citizens, e.g. inaccessible transport, buildings and information, inflexible organisation of education and working life, and stereotypes about the working capacity and skills of persons with disabilities (Amsterdam, Knoppers & Jongmans, 2015; Coleman-Fountain, 2016; Waldschmidt, 2017; Worth, 2013). To an even greater extent than youth *without* disabilities, disabled youth have to make active choices about who they want to be, and how they are to realise their aspirations about how to contribute to or involve themselves in society. Yet, disabled youth has occupied a marginal position in youth research (MacIntyre, 2014). To the extent that earlier research has examined the lived experiences of disabled youth, it has largely examined factors that make the lived experience of disabled youth special or unique (e.g. Amanda, 2016; Grue & Heiberg, 2000; Tuffrey, Bateman & Colver, 2013). Links to youth research in general have been less developed. In contrast, this chapter argues that the experiences of disabled youth may serve as a magnifier of many of the processes that young adults go through today, independent of disabilities or not.

Confronted with dominant beliefs about the normal life-course, youth with disabilities have to make active choices. Dominant expectations about the normal life-course have not only included expectations about what people ought to achieve in life (regular employment, economic self-sufficiency, independent household, a life-partner and children). Disabled youth are also confronted with expectations about when important life events should take place (Hagestad & Neugarten, 1985) and expectations about the normal duration of events (Merton, 1984). Disabled youth are often forced to develop new and innovative ways of coping and organising their lives. They have to consider which activities they want to involve themselves in but also realistically will be able to participate in, given their health condition or impairment, the resources they have access to, and the social and attitudinal barriers to participation that they face.

To examine these dynamics, we have drawn on the Capability Approach (Nussbaum, 2000; Sen 1992, 1999, 2009). Empirically, we have analysed life-course interviews with disabled youth in Norway conducted in 2014. Narrowing down the focus to Norway allows us to analyse in greater detail the dynamics at micro level; i.e. the social processes that impinge on the Active Citizenship of young adults at the individual level, with the same socio-political legacies and current disability policy system as context.

First, we provide an overview of what we know from earlier research about the opportunities for exercising Active Citizenship among young adults with disabilities in Norway. Second, we present a model for more dynamic conceptualisation of the transitions to Active Citizenship. Third, we compare the lived experiences of youth with mobility, visual, intellectual and psychosocial disabilities in their efforts to enter the labour market in Norway. Fourth, we conclude by discussing how development of analytic models derived from data about disabled youth may contribute to improved understanding of what it means to be young in contemporary society.

Earlier research on the Active Citizenship of young adults with disabilities (in Norway)

In the 2000s, Norway spent more public funds on income maintenance and support in cash or in kind for persons with disabilities than most other European countries (Halvorsen, Hvinden, Bickenbach, Ferri & Guillén Rodriguez, 2017). The risk of poverty rate among persons with disabilities has also been lower than in most other European countries. However, despite the uncertainties related to the reliability and comparability of available employment statistics (Tøssebro & Hvinden, 2017), there can be no doubt that young adults with disabilities have experienced greater difficulties in achieving paid work than their non-disabled peers and stronger exclusion from gainful employment. To the extent that they have been employed, they more often have had marginal positions, e.g. as part-time or temporary workers. According to time-series data from the period after 2000, the employment gap between persons with disabilities and nondisabled people has tended to grow after the age of 20 (Bø & Håland, 2016; Halvorsen & Hvinden, 2014). In 2013, only 25 per cent of persons with intellectual disabilities of expected working age were employed. Out of these, about 90 per cent were employed in sheltered employment. For this population group the most common way of spending time has been participation in day activities organised by the municipality (Norwegian Green Paper, 2016, p. 82).

For young people, participation in education is a socially recognised activity that gives social status. As they get older, the dominant expectation is that – at some point during their twenties – they ought to achieve paid work in the ordinary labour market. In Norway, persons with higher education are the most likely to be employed among all the population groups. Among persons with disabilities, the returns from education were twice those of non-disabled people (Molden, Wendelborg &Tøssebro, 2009). When controlling for a range of factors and adopting different operational definitions of disability, the most significant factors for predicting employment participation among Norwegians with disabilities were educational level and, next, severity of disability (Molden & Tøssebro, 2012).

Since the early 1990s, public disability policy has aimed to include disabled children and youth in the ordinary education system together with their non-disabled peers. However, Norwegians with disabilities have had lower education levels than non-disabled people (Molden et al., 2009). In 2010, as many as 64 per cent of youth with physical disabilities did not complete high school, compared to 17 per cent of their non-disabled peers (Finnvold, 2013). Longitudinal data from 1997–2012 demonstrate that the segregation and exclusion of disabled pupils and students increase, as they grow older. In kindergarten, almost all children with disabilities participated together with their non-disabled peers. However, at every transition point between kindergarten, primary school, lower secondary school and high school, the segregation increased, especially for youth with intellectual disabilities or complex needs. In high school, only one third of students with disabilities received education together with their non-disabled peers (Tøssebro & Wendelborg, 2014). Persons with intellectual disabilities more often had teachers without formal education, and the authorities reviewed the education they received less systematically (Bachmann, Haug & Nordahl, 2016).

Overall, earlier research provides a mixed picture of the opportunities for participation in education, employment and non-paid day activities in Norway.

The literature provides important insights into the reproduction of inequality, social exclusion and segregation in an affluent welfare state, despite stated goals of normalisation, community living and inclusion in the ordinary labour market (Magnus & Tøssebro, 2014; Söderström 2016; Tøssebro, 2016).

The literature focusing on the transition from education to employment has produced important insights about how youth with disabilities experience and cope with dominant social expectations to become active in the labour market. However, it is a risk that researchers interpret the lives of disabled youth only from an economic perspective and view youth primarily as the next generation of the labour force. Reviewing the transition literature in youth studies, Wyn and Woodman (2006) argue that an economistic model of youth has obscured other state policies of relevance to youth, such as health, and has ignored other life-priorities of youth, such as well-being, establishing one's own household and having a family. Others scholars have raised concerns that a one-sided focus on school-to-work transitions risks overshadowing other dimensions of young people's everyday practices, self-identity and belonging – such as interaction with peers (Larsen, Wulf-Andersen, Baagø Nielsen & Holger Mogensen, 2016). Both scholars in disability research (Beresford, 2004) and general youth studies (Wyn & Woodman, 2007) have criticised a one-sided focus on transitions from education to employment for masking other dimensions of young people's lives and misrecognising the contributions and lives of people not participating in the labour market.

Overall, we find that there is scope for more dynamic analyses of the transitions to adulthood for disabled youth. When we are focusing on these transitions, we are interested not only in generative processes that reproduce social inequalities, social exclusion and segregation of disabled youth. We are equally interested in processes that promote substantial freedom of choice, social inclusion and opportunities for community living. In our efforts to capture these processes, we will draw on the Capability Approach of Sen and Nussbaum.

Conceptualising transitions to Active Citizenship through the Capability Approach

The Capability Approach provides important conceptual tools for how one can better understand the agency/structure dynamics in transitions to adulthood. In brief, this approach distinguishes between capability inputs, the capability set, achieved functionings, conversion and agency. The capability inputs are the resources individuals can avail themselves of in their efforts to live the life they want for themselves (e.g. money, material resources and services). The potential transformation of capability inputs into capabilities is mediated by conversion factors, i.e. the structures constraining or facilitating conversion. Where functionings refer to what people actually do and are, the capability set denotes what people really 'can do and can be' if they want to. Functionings, then, are a subset of the capability set. They are the realised options or life chances of the individual. The relationship between the concepts can be illustrated in the following way (Figure 11.1):

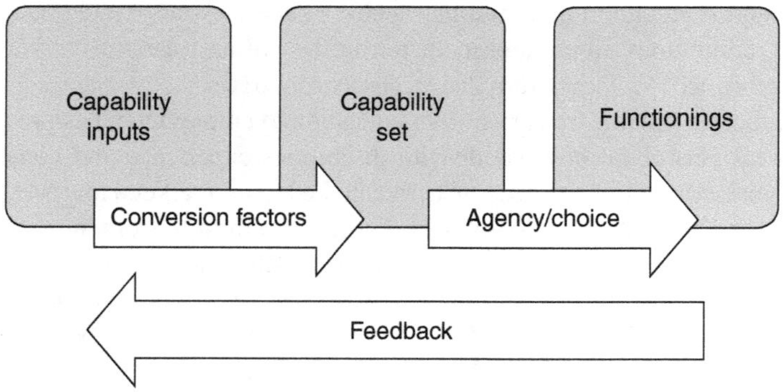

Figure 11.1 A dynamic model of capabilities and functionings.

Crocker and Robeyns (2010) argue that 'the ideal of individual and group agency plays an important role in Sen's … way of addressing capability selection, weighting, and sequencing' (p. 67). In his early writings, Sen (1985) argued that 'agency freedom is freedom to achieve, whatever the person, as a responsible agent, decides he or she should achieve' (p. 204). Later Sen (1999) has argued in favour of an 'agent-oriented view', in which individuals and groups should decide by themselves which capabilities and functionings are important to them, ' "effectively shape their own destiny and help each other" ' (Sen, 1999, 11), and be "active participant[s] in change, rather than … passive and docile recipient[s] of instructions or dispensed assistance" (Sen, 1999, 281)' (Crocker & Robeyns, 2010, p. 75).

A key concern for Amartya Sen is that, if we want a properly satisfactory analysis of social inequality, we cannot define it through the resources that are available alone. Rather we want 'to look directly at the quality of life that people are able to lead, and the freedom they enjoy to live the way they would like' (Sen, 2006, p. 34). According to Sen, the capability to function should be put at the centre stage of assessment. Because people's experience of access to capability inputs differs and their exposure to conversion factors varies, their abilities to convert resources into capabilities will also differ. By addressing conversion factors, the Capability Approach provides a conceptual tool to address human diversity and differences in needs between people (Sen, 1999, 2005, 2009). In her codification of the Capability Approach, Ingrid Robeyns (2005) distinguishes between three types of conversion factors (see also Crocker & Robeyns, 2010, p. 68):

- personal conversion factors (e.g. metabolism, physical condition, sex, reading skills or intelligence);
- social conversion factors (e.g. public policies, social norms, practices that unfairly discriminate, social hierarchies, power relations); and
- environmental conversion factors (e.g. the physical and built environment).

In this chapter, we are interested not only in how conversion factors influence the achievement of effective freedom (security, autonomy and influence) on the part of youth with disabilities. We are also interested in the extent to which people with disabilities can exercise active agency, including their capacity to modify their conditions for exercising Active Citizenship (the capability inputs and the diverse conversion factors). By drawing on longitudinal life-course data, we seek a better understanding of the processes where a disabled person, by being active possibly together with others in a similar situation, over time achieves more desirable functionings through subsequent cycles of change. Alternatively, focusing on conversion processes may help us conceptualise the mechanisms behind reproduction of social disadvantages among persons with disabilities (Hvinden & Halvorsen, 2017). We use the interview data to identify inductively positive and negative feedback loops that emerged in the life-course interviews (Figure 11.1).

Overview of the Norwegian life-course data

In this section, we provide an overview of the Norwegian life-course interviews collected in the DISCIT project (see Chapter 3 in this volume for details). Of the 28 disabled persons we interviewed in Norway, one third had higher education (Table 11.1). Among interviewees with psychosocial disabilities, several had not completed their higher education, while all interviewees with intellectual disabilities had gone to special school or special classes at an ordinary school.

Despite the above average level of education, only one person had full-time employment at the time of the interview. Although we aimed to recruit interviewees who had participated in the ordinary labour market, the interviewees with intellectual disabilities all had their experience from activities in day care

Table 11.1 Overview of sample: category of disability and education level

Disability	*Compulsory education (including high school)*	*Intermediary education* (x < *3 years)*	*Higher education* (x > *3 years)*
Visual	1970m, 1990w	1950m*, 1970w	1950w, 1990m
Mobility	1950w	1950w, 1970m**	1950m, 1970w, 1990w, 1990m
Intellectual	1950m*, 1950w*, 1970w*, 1970m*, 1990w*, 1990m*		
Psychosocial	1950m, 1990w	1990m**, 1970w1, 1970w3**, 1970m1, 1970m2**,	1950w, 1970w2

Notes
Born around 1950, 1970 or 1990. w = woman, m = man: N=28.
* Special school/special class in ordinary school.
** Incomplete.

centres or sheltered employment. Several of the interviewees in their twenties (born around 1990) had not managed to achieve an ordinary paid job at the time of the interview (Table 11.2).

The interviewees represented a broad variation in social background (socio-economic position, geographical region, parents and siblings with or without disabilities). Some interviewees had managed to complete higher education and achieve a full-time position but ended up working reduced hours due to deteriorating health or the extra time they needed before work and to recover after working hours. Others had managed to return to working life after a mental breakdown and reorientation. This was particularly the case in the two older age cohorts. In the youngest cohort, several were in the process of getting their first work experience or they had just recently achieved their first employment contract.

Analysis

Negotiating access to education – barriers and facilitators

What kind of barriers and facilitators did youth with disabilities experience in the transition from education to the labour market? Unsurprisingly, students with mobility and visual disabilities experienced lack of access to buildings and transport, inaccessible and unavailable books and inaccessible information technology (e.g. lack of voice-to-text in Norwegian).

For John (28 years old), access to buildings and transport had been recurrent issues throughout childhood and youth, and the expertise at the different schools varied. In class, he had assistants who wrote for him. However, he had not always participated in school trips or been invited to birthday parties of schoolmates in primary school. In high school, the teacher had adapted the homework

Table 11.2 Overview of sample: category of disability and employment

Disability	*Full time employment*	*Part-time employment*	*Former employment*	*Never in ordinary employment*
Visual		1970w, 1970m**	1950w, 1950m	1990w, 1990m
Mobility		1950w, 1970w	1950m, 1950w, 1970m, 1990w	1990m
Intellectual			1970m*	1950m*, 1950w*, 1970w*, 1990m*, 1990w*
Psychosocial	1970m1	1990m, 1990w, 1970w1, 1950w	1950m, 1970m2, 1970w2, 1970w3	

Notes

Born around 1950, 1970 or 1990. w = woman, m = man. N = 28.

* Day care centre and/or sheltered employment.

** Combined with sheltered employment.

to ensure that he could write it himself but it was only at university that he felt welcome:

> They had a dedicated employee with responsibility for the accommodation. I was contacted by the school before I had taken any initiative myself, and they ensured that everything was accommodated. And they called us and they invited me together with the caretaker and the one responsible for the accommodation. They asked which classroom I wanted and which toilet I wanted.... It was one of those moments when you do not represent a problem or a burden.
>
> (From an interview with John, 28 years old, male, mobility disability)

Others told similar stories of varying degree of accessible school buildings, inaccessible transport, information and communication technology and literature resources.

A second issue that emerged in the interviews was how much help and assistance they should accept from public authorities. During primary and secondary school, all students in the 1990 age group, except those with psychosocial disabilities, received personal assistance. As the service could be conceived of as both help and control, the interviewees sometimes expressed ambivalence to receiving help from others ('avoid feeling of surveillance', 'not had a good relationship to all my assistants'). In other cases, interviewees blamed themselves for having refused to accept help and assistance from others. Partly they wanted to participate on equal conditions with others. Partly they avoided using assistive technology or accepting help and assistance to avoid being conceived of as more 'disabled' than necessary.

> When I was younger I limited myself. I said I could not manage.... Using crutches was exhausting ... But when I accepted using a wheelchair I got much more energy.... The last three years I have had a personal assistant but I have too few hours. A friend persuaded me to apply. I wanted to be independent and a good girl. But then I applied. And look how much energy I have saved on returning home to a clean apartment and dinner being prepared by somebody else.
>
> (From an interview with Ann, 28 years old, female, mobility disability)

Ann (28) and others experienced repeated negotiations with the Norwegian welfare administration about how many hours of assistance they should receive and for which purposes. To negotiate access to services was associated with both potential benefits and costs. On the one hand, the social services represented resources in cash and in kind (capability inputs) for achieving desired functionings. For this, the interviewees sometimes expressed gratitude ('like winning in the lottery to live in Norway'). On the other hand, the same persons also told stories about experiences of humiliation and unwanted dependency ('you have to argue that you are sick', 'the previous officer called me a scrounger').

A third issue that emerged in the interviews was the need to use extra time to complete their studies. Due to hospitalisation, deteriorating health conditions or recurrent time spells of absence from school due to sickness, several interviewees had not been able to complete their education. Other students needed extra time to recover after classes and spent longer finishing school ('got too tough with so long hours', 'was a wise decision to postpone some classes to a fourth year'). Yet others had changed to a different education programme to adjust to capacity and activity restrictions. In the case of Ann (28), the rules in the social security system prevented her from pursuing the Master's degree she wanted in chemistry. As she needed more time than the standard norm and she had exhausted her time in the vocational rehabilitation programme, she had to apply for disability benefit. However, for the first year on disability benefit she was not allowed to study or have paid work.

Overall, in negotiations with public authorities the interviewees varied between presenting themselves as victims of circumstances outside their control, reminding authorities about their legal entitlements, and protesting against discrimination against persons with disabilities as an oppressed minority. This seemed especially to be the case for youth with mobility and visual disabilities. The youth with intellectual disabilities were less articulate and appeared to be more dependent on parents and care providers.

Self-identity and autonomy among youth with psychosocial disabilities

A general finding from the interviews with persons with psychosocial disabilities was the challenge of exercising autonomy and living 'the life they had reason to value' – as exemplified by the case of 'Thomas' (27 years old) and diagnosed with paranoid schizophrenia. While Thomas met regularly with physicians, psychiatrists and psychologists on a monthly basis, he described the lack of a clear self-identity and direction in his own life as the main reason for his mental health problems ('I have been very confused'). He lacked a clear idea of the life he wanted to live and what values and visions to believe in, and described how this culminated in emotional turbulence and suicidal thoughts in his early twenties. A turning point was when he was hospitalised:

> The mental health problems were the result of that. I withdrew very much because I had a horrible inner emotional life. So, I pulled out a lot, it was a lot of nature and I read books … and suddenly I started to behave in a horrible way. And then I felt I had to throw myself in front of the metro but I didn't do it. And then I was hospitalised at. … So it was a horrifying experience.
>
> (From an interview with Thomas, 27 years old, male, psychosocial disability)

Throughout the interview, he had difficulties in explaining the relationship between his positive and negative emotions when reconstructing past events.

Being carried away with strong emotional feelings made it difficult to formulate a clear plan for what he wanted for the future. When Thomas felt that life was not worth living anymore, the ideal of 'living the life you have reason to value' (autonomy) became irrelevant. If life itself, by default, is not worth living, it is impossible to live the life you have reason to value.

His story about the lack of a clear self-identity was also reflected in his difficulties in talking about his own sexuality. On several occasions during the interview, he hinted that he regretted his behaviour towards women at the time. The way he talked about it was rather cryptic during large parts of the interview ('girls I should not have slept with', 'mistakes I was not so conscious about'). Towards the very end of the interview, however, he mentioned in passing – as he was about to leave – that he now participated in a gay sports club and had made friends there. To discover his own sexuality and identify as 'gay' seemed to have been part of the efforts to define for himself what he wanted for his own life. The embarrassment or lack of pride in self hampered his ability to articulate his own wants and needs, and have a voice of his own.

In other parts of the conversation, Thomas explained how he had coped with the challenge of not knowing what he wanted. He described his difficulties in managing the dominant expectations about pursuing a higher education and achieving a well-paid job, and the wide range of opportunities that existed. Growing up in an upper-middle-class neighbourhood ('grandmother had a lot of money'), he had felt he had to 'take a degree and be something'. He embarked on various studies, including law school, teaching school and nursing school in different regions of the country but without finishing any degree:

> But I started at the wrong study. I should have started with something I really knew I could contribute with, but I did not have that perspective then. I studied what I did just because it sounded great but without having any more meaning to it. I completed two years (at law school) but I had no interest in it. I did not really know why I was studying it. I studied it perhaps because it looked impressive and it was prestigious – according to others.
>
> (From an interview with Thomas, 27 years old, male, psychosocial disability)

In his own view, it was only when he managed to disregard the social pressure that he was able to start defining a life of his own. As examples of facilitators that contributed to the process of redefining who he is and wanted to be, he mentioned reading philosophy, the outdoor life, and enjoying sports. During the summer he had mostly slept outdoors and in his car, or stayed over with different friends. After seven stays in psychiatric hospital, he now received a vocational rehabilitation allowance. While the significance of reading and doing sports could be criticised for being elusive, the activities helped Thomas in achieving a life that was pleasurable and worth living again, and exposed him to his sensory world and emotions in new ways. At the time of the interview, he was working 60 per cent in a vocational training programme, was coaching a boys and girls' sports team and participated in a self-help centre for persons with mental health problems. At this stage he had started considering a future job in the after-school programme for children in primary school. Overall, he had started building capacity, self-esteem and defining life-objectives for himself ('feel I have a good life now', 'feel more healthy than I did before I was hospitalised'). In other words, he had achieved experience of more security and autonomy. Overall, this was a story of a *virtuous cycle* of expansions in desired functionings after hospitalisation.

We found similar developments in desired functionings over time in the case of 'Vilde'. Her childhood was a story of bullying, deteriorating mental health and social isolation, suicidal thoughts, and forced hospitalisation at the age of 17. During this time period she experienced a *vicious cycle* of decreasing security, autonomy and influence.

> But then I got a supervisor. And to go straight into employment when you have been to an institution. It did not work. I was scared. She (the supervisor) understood and took me to (self-help centre) and now I have been here for four years.... It started to get better in 2013, so I have developed a lot. I could actually do something.... I have become very focused on exercising and nutrition, because I think that it is important for my mental health.... And then I got a job at the gym where I was exercising. So I got the training as a personal instructor in January this year, finishing in June. And now I am working as an instructor at the gym. I do not work 100 per cent and I do not know if that is a goal either, but it is a long way from where I was at high school.
>
> (From an interview with Vilde, 28 years old, female, psychosocial disability)

At the time of the interview Vilde lived with her parents. After six years of forced hospitalisation, Vilde had managed to achieve a part-time job and received a vocational rehabilitation allowance as a top up. She had given up finishing high school but had an active approach to her own physical and mental health ('try to use the people around me', 'I will always have pains in the shoulder but exercising helps'). After hospitalisation, she had gradually experienced a *virtuous* cycle of improved mental and physical health, a larger social network, more leisure activities, education and paid work.

In the cases of Thomas and Vilde, it was striking how their Active Citizenship depended on their self-identity and self-esteem. Different from the youth with mobility and visual disabilities, Thomas and Vilde did not experience any physical or material barriers. As the external reasons for their problems were less obvious, youth with psychosocial disabilities more easily blamed themselves for not having completed education, being employed, or having any friends. The interviewees with psychosocial disabilities were more inclined to present their experiences as the outcome of individual circumstances and conditions – not of discrimination or socially constructed barriers against participation.

Active citizen – inside or outside the labour market?

Among the young adults with mobility and visual disabilities, a repeating question was whether they eventually would manage to achieve paid work in the ordinary labour market. Many of the interviewees mentioned they had not been able to achieve any work experience so far. While students often have had paid work during the summer holidays and sometimes at the weekends, the lack of accommodation, the physical constraints often associated with typical unskilled work and/or the need to recover during the summer had prevented interviewees from gaining similar experiences ('hard manual work is impossible'). One exception was Ann (28 years old) who had been able to use crutches when she was younger. In this case, the employer had volunteered to accommodate the work tasks to her needs. Others, like 'Richard' (27 years old, visual disability), had unsuccessfully applied for a large number of positions.

Although the issue of self-identity was not as critical as in the case of the young adults with psychosocial disabilities, even the interviewees with physical disabilities had to reflect on alternative scenarios for their future and what they wanted for their lives, and whether it was realistic to achieve (full-time) paid work in the ordinary labour market. One example is the story of John. While he had managed to complete his MA degree, it was uncertain whether he would manage to find a 20–30 per cent position that would allow him to work 3–4 hours per day. The Norwegian Welfare Administration had provided him with a job coach:

> But it does not mean that I will give up. A completely different alternative I have been willing to or have considered if it turns out that there is not to be any paid work available is to work for a charity and use my expertise there. Where the money is coming from is not the most important thing. It would have been great with real paid work but it is not a disaster if I receive a disability benefit. The most important thing for me is to do something that is meaningful to me.
>
> (From an interview with John, 28 years old, male, mobility disability)

John had started to prepare mentally for the outcome that he might not be able to achieve paid work and might have to define other goals and ways of defining a meaningful life, being involved and of significance to others. According to John:

> Paid work is not everything, I have to use my resources, kind of, whether it is in paid work or non-paid work. There are a lot of care tasks and so on that are equally or more important than being able to work.
>
> (From an interview with John, 28 years old, male, mobility disability)

Confronted with the attitudinal, organisational and physical barriers to participation in the labour market, and in some cases deteriorating health, the interviewees were forced to actively reflect on what to make out of their lives. In our cases, the youth with the least prospects of achieving paid work were actively considering other options than participation in the labour market to achieve a meaningful life. Such adaptations manifested themselves not as adjustment of preferences per se – or 'adaptive preferences' (Elster, 1985) but rather as a change in perception of what it is realistic to achieve, when taking all personal, social and environmental conversion factors into account ('doing something meaningful'). These were cases of being aware of the limitations in their options and adjusting their projects so as to settle for activities they realistically could fulfil. This did not, however, mean that they adjusted their preferences to what they realistically could get (Nussbaum, 2001). Even if the adaptations implied that they adjusted to the fact they were likely to be excluded from or marginalised in the labour market, they did not do so without regret ('would prefer a regular job').

Exercising autonomy and influence – self-organised activities with peers

The last major issue that emerged in the interviews with the young adults was the biographical significance of active involvement with their peers. While they all were concerned to have an active life and belong to a social network, participation in leisure activities together with non-disabled persons was not always easy. Several of the interviewees expressed difficulties in making friends with non-disabled peers at school due to long-term sickness absence from school and/or experiences of social exclusion – e.g. not being invited to birthday parties of their class mates or not being able to attend school trips. For youth with mobility or visual disabilities, to meet people outdoors sometimes required extensive planning (find accessible routes, parking space and toilets) and it was sometimes easier to meet via social media and on Skype. While most of the interviewees reported physical and technical factors that hampered their functionings, some of the young adults also reported financial barriers. For instance, Richard (27 years old, visual disability) had grown up with a single mother who worked as a cleaner. For him, the financial barriers to participating in leisure activities had been equally or more important for his experience of social exclusion; as a child, summer holidays abroad, music school and down-hill skiing had been too expensive.

To a varying degree, social activities together with other disabled youth offered alternative opportunities for avoiding social isolation and for peer support. The self-organised activities provided opportunities for exercising both autonomy and influence. Several of the interviewees emphasised the mixed character of the organisations and networks of youth with disabilities as networks for both leisure activities and political discussions and activism. While the self-organised peer activities could be interpreted as a form of segregation, it also provided the youth with a sense of belonging, opportunities to share experiences about coping strategies, and information about welfare services.

> The summer camps with the Association for the Blind were a relief. There I was popular.... You feel more confident when you travel with others who are blind.
>
> (From an interview with Tina, 21 years old, female, visual disability)

> I did not have any friends after I came out (from psychiatric hospital) and I was very lonely. And then I came to the Club House and met people. After some time I could call them my friends. It was probably the most important for me.... Now I am not here that much anymore. But, when I am here, I talk to people I know here. Sometimes I join some meetings. And I attend the lunches some times.
>
> (From an interview with Vilde, 28 years old, psychosocial disability)

Tina (21 years old, visual disability) and Vilde (28 years old, psychosocial disability) emphasised especially the friends they had achieved through the self-organised activities. Others, like Richard (27 years old, visual disability), emphasised more the political activism. For certain purposes, persons with similar experiences, identity or background emerged as better and more relevant support than professional help providers. Several of the youth who were born with mobility and visual disabilities had been registered as members of organisations of persons with disabilities by their parents and been to summer camps or medical rehabilitation with other children with similar disabilities. Interviewees with mobility and visual disabilities particularly articulated a collective identity and pride ('we should not hide'). As the psychiatric diagnoses were vague or invisible, it was less obvious what the youth with psychosocial disabilities had in common. While the youth with psychosocial disabilities presented stories about their individual needs (especially health and social services), the youth with mobility and visual disabilities more often presented stories about societal barriers to participation.

Overall, youth with mobility and visual disabilities benefited from better conditions for identifying and giving voice to their collective needs and demands, and influencing their individual and societal conditions for exercising Active Citizenship. For those with mobility, visual and intellectual disabilities, their impairments were permanent conditions. For youth with psychosocial disabilities, the inclination to view their mental health problem as temporary had the effect that they to larger extent participated in the self-help organisation as a transition stage. As the interviewees experienced their mental health improving, some of them, like Vilde (28), visited the organisation less often. Yet, even in such cases, the self-organised activities represented opportunities for building capability to articulate their own needs and wants.

Concluding discussion: virtuous and vicious circles of achieved functionings

We started by asking under which conditions young adults with disabilities are most likely to achieve Active Citizenship. To answer the question, we first identified conversion factors facilitating and hampering the transition from education to employment. A striking feature was the complexity of conversion factors that influenced the transition process. Personal factors included differences in activity and capacity restrictions, self-identity and time perspective on their disability or health status. Social factors included experiences of power imbalance and unwanted dependency in negotiations with the social services. Environmental factors included resource depletion and exclusion due to inaccessible books, transport, buildings and information and communication technology.

Second, our data suggest that questions about self-identity are intrinsically linked to problems of achieving Active Citizenship. Some of the young adults with psychosocial disabilities in particular reported existential questions about self-identity. Issues of adjustment of life objectives and achieving a meaningful social life also emerged in interviews with young adults with mobility, visual and intellectual disabilities. Confronted with the various barriers to labour market participation, the interviewees actively reflected on alternative forms of valued participation and involvement in society, and avoiding other people perceiving of them only as persons in need of help and assistance from others.

While earlier research has identified many of the conversion factors that influence the Active Citizenship of youth with disabilities, this chapter has suggested how we might achieve better understandings of how agency/structure dynamic impinge on the life-courses of disabled youth. As a matter of paradox, we found the clearest examples of vicious and virtuous circles of functionings among the young adults with psychosocial disabilities. Although they in certain respects were more vulnerable than young adults with mobility and visual disabilities, we found the clearest examples of positive and negative feedback loops (see Figure 11.1) in this group. Several of the interviewees experienced fundamental insecurity about self-identity, future health and income. Yet, we identified how youth with disabilities – sometimes together with others in a similar situation – over time achieved more desirable functionings through subsequent cycles of change in health, social networks, participation in leisure activities, education and employment. These were stories of virtuous cycles of incremental change in desired functionings. In other cases, we identified stories of vicious cycles of change: deteriorating health conditions, resignation and/or social exclusion.

Initially we argued that youth are 'citizens in the making'. This is not to say that youth are 'waiting for citizenship to be bestowed upon them' (Miles, 2015, pp. 103–104). On the contrary, we have stressed the active agency of disabled youth in their endeavours to exercise Active Citizenship. For this purpose, we have pursued a wide conceptualisation of the transition. This has involved recognition of the complexity of the transition and that youth may have reasons to adjust and redefine the values and objectives for their lives – both in the immediate and the distant future.

All youth have to make active choices about their functionings or 'doings and beings'; i.e. who they want to be and what they want to do with their lives. For disabled youth, the transition from education to employment tends to take longer than expected. As they are likely to be exposed to different conversion factors – more barriers at the personal, social and environmental levels – the processes tend to be more complicated than for non-disabled people. Even in cases when the youth manage to achieve employment, it is less likely to be available with the same capability inputs or by following the standard trajectory or without any accommodation of the disability. The unfavourable social conditions required the active agency of the interviewees. In this sense, the experiences of disabled youth may serve as a magnifier of many of the processes young people go through today.

Several commentators have argued that contemporary processes of individualisation have dissolved old constraints that bound people to certain lifestyles and opened up many areas of life to personal choice. While the accounts of sociologists such as Beck and Beck-Gernsheim (2002, 2009) and Giddens (1991) differ, they share the idea that social life has been set free from traditional boundaries, structures and culture. If we are to believe Ulrich Beck, individual choices and decisions have become centre stage in contemporary society as tradition and the lives of past generations is no longer a common standard or reference point. According to the individualisation thesis, societal changes have resulted in more responsibility being placed on the individual for making active choices and justifying his or her choices (Beck, 1992; Beck & Willms, 2004). In this sense, disabled youth can be regarded as hyper-modern citizens. At the same time, given their structural disadvantages (both in terms of capability inputs and conversion factors) at the personal, social and environmental levels, the individualised responsibility can become a particularly heavy burden to carry for disabled youth.

References

Amanda, A. A. (2016). *Voices and visions from ethnoculturally diverse young people with disabilities: Diverse young people with disabilities.* Rotterdam: Sense Publisher.

Amsterdam, N., Knoppers, A. & Jongmans, M. (2015). It's actually very normal that I'm different. How physically disabled youth discursively construct and position their body/self. *Sport, Education and Society*, *20* (2), 152–170.

Bachmann, K., Haug, P. & Nordahl, T. (2016). *Kvalitet i opplæringen for personer med utviklingshemming [Quality in education for persons with intellectual disabilities].* Report no. 2. Volda, Norway: Volda University College.

Beck, U. (1992). *Risk society: Towards a new modernity.* London: Sage.

Beck, U. & Beck-Gernsheim, E. (2002). *Individualization.* London: Sage.

Beck, U. & Beck-Gernsheim, E. (2009). Global generations and the trap of methodological nationalism for a cosmopolitan turn in the sociology of youth and generation. *European Sociological Review*, *25*(1), 25–36.

Beck, U. & Willms, J. (Eds). (2004). *Conversations with Ulrich Beck.* Cambridge: Polity Press.

Beresford, B. (2004). On the road to nowhere? Young disabled people and transition, *Child: Care, Health and Development*, November, *30*(6), 581–587.

Bø, T. P. & Håland, I. (2016). *Funksjonshemma på arbeidsmarknaden i 2016 [Disabled people in the labour market in 2016].* Oslo: Statistics Norway.

Coleman-Fountain, E. (2016). Youthful stories of normality and difference. *Sociology*, 1–17.

Crocker, D. A. & Robeyns, I. (2010). Capability and agency. In C. W. Morris (Ed.), *Amartya Sen* (pp. 60–90). Cambridge: Cambridge University Press.

Elster, J. (1985). *Sour grapes: Studies in the subversion of rationality*. Cambridge: Cambridge University Press.

Finnvold, J. E. (2013). *Levekår og sosial inkludering hos mennesker med fysiske funksjonsnedsettelser*, NOVA Report, 12–13. Oslo: Oslo and Akershus University College.

Giddens, A. (1991). *Modernity and self-identity. Self and society in late modern age*. Stanford, CA: Stanford University Press.

Grue, L. & Heiberg, A. (2000). Do disabled adolescents view themselves differently from other young people? *Scandinavian Journal of Disability Research*, *2*(1), 39–57.

Hagestad, G. O. & Neugarten, B. L. (1985). Age and the life course. In B. Binstock & E. Shanas (Eds), *Handbook of aging and the social sciences* (pp. 35–61). New York: Van Nostrand Reinhold.

Halvorsen, R. & Hvinden, B. (2014). *New policies to promote youth inclusion. Accommodation of diversity in the Nordic welfare states*. TemaNord report 564, Copenhagen: Nordic Council of Ministers.

Halvorsen, R., Hvinden, B., Bickenbach, J., Ferri, D. & Guillén Rodriguez, A. M. (Eds). (2017). *The changing disability policy system. Active Citizenship and disability in Europe, volume 1*. London: Routledge.

Hvinden, B. & Halvorsen, R. (2017). Mediating agency and structure in sociology: What role for conversion factors? *Critical Sociology*, 1–7.

Larsen, L., Wulf-Andersen, T., Baagø Nielsen, S. & Holger Mogensen, K. (2016). Udsatte unges uddannelsesdeltagelse: tilhør og steder som teoretiske perspektiver, *Sosiologi i dag* 46, 3–4.

MacIntyre, G. (2014). The potential for inclusion: Young people with learning disabilities' experiences of social inclusion as they make the transition from childhood to adulthood. *Journal of Youth Studies*, *17*(7), 857–871.

Magnus, E. & Tøssebro, J. (2014). Negotiating individual accommodation in higher education. *Scandinavian Journal of Disability Research*, *16*(4), 316–332.

Marshall. T. H. (1950). *Citizenship and social class, and other essays*. Cambridge: University Press.

Merton, R. K. (1984). Socially expected durations: A case study of concept formation in sociology. In W. W. Powell & R. Robbins (Eds), *Conflict and consensus: In honor of Lewis A. Coser* (pp. 262–283). New York: Free Press.

Miles, S. 2015. Young people, consumer citizenship and protest: The problem with romanticizing the relationship to social change, *Young*, *23*(2), 101–115.

Molden, T. H. & Tøssebro, J. (2012). Disability measurements: Impact on research results. *Scandinavian Journal of Disability Research*, *14*(4), 340–357.

Molden, T. H., Wendelborg, C. & Tøssebro, J. (2009). *Levekår blant personer med nedsatt funksjonsevne. Analyse av levekårsundersøkelsen blant personer med nedsatt funksjonsevne 2007 [Living conditions among persons with disabilities in 2007]*. Report. Trondheim: NTNU Social Research.

Norwegian Green Paper. (2016). *På lik linje. Åtte løft for å realisere grunnleggende rettigheter for personer med utviklingshemming [On equal terms. Eight improvements to realize fundamental rights for persons with intellectual disabilities]*. Report from expert committee appointed by royal resolution. Oslo: Norwegian Ministry of Children and Equality.

Nussbaum, M. (2000). *Women and human development*. Cambridge: Cambridge University Press.

Nussbaum, M. (2001). Adaptive preferences and women's options. *Economics and Philosophy*, *17*, 67–88.

Robeyns, I. (2005). The capability approach: A theoretical survey. *Journal of Human Development*, *6*(1), 93–114.

Sen, A. (1985). Well-being, agency and freedom: The Dewey lectures 1984. *Journal of Philosophy*, *82*(4), 169–221.

Sen, A. (1992). *Inequality reexamined*. Oxford: Clarendon Press.

Sen, A. (1999). *Development as freedom*. Oxford: Oxford University Press.

Sen, A. (2005). Human rights and capabilities. *Journal of Human Development*, *6*(2), 151–166.

Sen, A. (2006). Conceptualizing and measuring poverty. In D. B. Grusky & R. Kanbur (Eds) *Poverty and inequality* (pp. 30–46). Stanford: Stanford University Press.

Sen, A. (2009). *The idea of justice*. London: Penguin.

Söderström, S. (2016). Socio-material practices in classrooms that lead to the social participation or social isolation of disabled pupils, *Scandinavian Journal of Disability Research*, *18*(2), 95–105.

Tuffrey, C., Bateman, B. J. & Colver, A. C. (2013). The questionnaire of young people's participation (QYPP): A new measure of participation frequency for disabled young people. *Child: Care, Health and Development*, *39*(4), 500–511.

Tøssebro, J. (2016). Scandinavian disability policy: From deinstitutionalisation to non-discrimination and beyond. *ALTER – European Journal of Disability Research/Revue Européenne de Recherche sur le Handicap*, *10*(2), 111–123.

Tøssebro, J. & Hvinden, B. (2017). Operational definitions of disability: Usable in comparative research on Active Citizenship? In R. Halvorsen, B. Hvinden, J. Bickenbach, D. Ferri & A. M. Guillén Rodriguez (Eds), *The changing disability policy system. Active Citizenship and disability in Europe volume 1* (pp. 55–71). London: Routledge.

Tøssebro, J. & Wendelborg, C. (Eds). (2014). *Oppvekst med funksjonshemming – Familie, livsløp og overganger*. Oslo: Gyldendal.

Waldschmidt, A. (2017). Disability goes cultural: The cultural model of disability as an analytic tool. In A. Waldschmidt, H. Berressem & M. Ingersen (Eds), *Culture – theory – disability. Encounters between disability studies and cultural studies* (pp. 19–28). Bielefeld: Transcript Verlag.

Worth, N. (2013). Visual impairment in the city: Young people's social strategies for independent mobility. *Urban Studies*, *50*(3), 574–586.

Wyn, J. & White, R. (1997). *Rethinking youth*. London: Sage.

Wyn, J. & Woodman, D. (2006). Generation, youth and social change in Australia, *Journal of Youth Studies*, *9*(5), 495–514.

Wyn, J. & Woodman, D. (2007). Researching youth in a context of social change: A reply to Roberts. *Journal of Youth Studies*, *10*(3), 373–381.

12 Technologies for Active Citizenship and the agency of objects

Kjetil Klette Bøhler and G. Anthony Giannoumis

This chapter investigates the role of technology in the exercise of Active Citizenship for persons with disabilities. By discussing how Active Citizenship is conditioned by technology, we draw attention to how people's ability to act is shaped by the technological environment in which they live. We examine how technology structures action choices and thus shapes opportunities for exercising Active Citizenship (see Chapter 1, this volume). Through a theoretical discussion of how technology and the action choices of persons with disabilities mutually influence each other, this chapter demonstrates how technology and the exercise of Active Citizenship work together in practice. The chapter takes as its point of departure theoretical perspectives on Active Citizenship and Structuration Theory and compares these with perspectives on agency in Actor-Network theory and Material Agency theory. We introduce these two theories – Actor-Network theory (Latour, 1999, 2007a) and Material Agency theory (Knappett & Malafouris, 2008) – and argue that these may enrich our understanding of the conditions for Active Citizenship. Finally, we conclude by discussing implications for theories on Active Citizenship.

Previous research has shown how accessible technology (both assistive technology and universally-designed mainstream technology), and in particular information and communication technology (ICT), may contribute to a more inclusive society for persons with disabilities (Berry, 1999; Blanck, 2008, 2014; Myhill, Cogburn, Samant, Addom & Blanck, 2008; Noble, 2002; Oudshoorn & Pinch, 2003; Schreuer, Keter & Sachs, 2014; Söderström, 2009, 2013). These findings suggest that ICT potentially contributes to social inclusion, especially for the younger age cohorts, by creating new arenas for and forms of social interaction. Other researchers on disability have suggested that accessible technology plays a key role for inclusion in education and the labour market (Parker & Banerjee, 2007), leading some to suggest that technological competence has become a precondition for communication and the exercise of Active Citizenship in contemporary society (Suchman, 1993). In addition, some have argued how new technologies change the relationship between people and the government (Barry, 2001; Dittrich, Ekelin, Elovaara, Eriksén & Hansson, 2003; Goggin & Newell, 2003; Rose & Novas, 2004). For instance, Sirkkunen and Kotilainen (2004) identify the various ways in which web technologies enable new forms of political participation, allowing users to influence decision-making in new ways.

Other research has focused on barriers – technological, financial, informational and procedural – regarding the use of new technology (see Chapter 7, this volume). For persons with disabilities to be able to benefit from new technologies, the technologies need not only to be *accessible* in technical terms; they must also be *usable* (fulfilling functions and meeting the needs of the end users without excessive training or education), *affordable* (for people to be able to purchase or borrow the products) and *available* without too many obstacles from bureaucracy. The prevalence of these four barriers varies significantly across European countries (Cullen & Kubitschke, 2007; Halvorsen, 2010; Kubitschke, Cullen, Dolphin, Laurin & Cederbom, 2013).

From the perspective of Structuration theory (see Chapter 2, this volume), new technology conditions human agency. Technology is, however, not considered to have agency in itself. Yet, properties inherent in technology enable and constrain the opportunities available to persons with disabilities. Several scholars have argued that it is not sufficient to conceptualise technologies as mere technical devices. Rather, researchers should pay attention 'to not only the new tools that come out but also the way these tools modify human action and, in particular, what new actions they make possible' (Toboso, 2011, p. 111).

Despite the importance earlier disability policy research has ascribed to technology, the research usually holds the view that technology has no agency in itself and presupposes the active agency of humans. This is reflected in both a common lack of in-depth accounts of how technology works and a preference for broader forms of social and political analysis in the social science literature. In practice, this literature views technology as a passive instrument that can only enable active participation in society through active human agency. With the notable exceptions of Moser (2003, 2005, 2006), Moser and Law (2003) and Roulstone (2016), few studies have addressed the potential agency of technology through processes that facilitate or prevent opportunities for full and effective participation by persons with disabilities.

Moser (2006) argued that Actor–Network theory reveals how 'positions, capacities and competences are enabled through the mobilization of technologies' (p. 374), creating new modes of acting and being and new forms of subjectivity. Inspired by Moser's (2006) argument that this conceptualisation can be used to examine 'the generative and transformative power of technologies in the lives of disabled people' (p. 374), we aim to contribute to a more robust understanding of the conditions for Active Citizenship. For this purpose, we draw on existing research in Actor–Network theory and Material Agency theory. However, we start by situating our arguments in relation to Structuration theory.

Technology for Active Citizenship

Recent developments in Structuration theory (e.g. Greenhalgh & Stones, 2010; Stones, 2005) have aimed to operationalise the dialectic relationship between external physical structures and internal structures (see Chapter 2, this volume) in empirical research. Stones (2005) argued that non-human objects can both be part of an external structural context of human agency *and* be part of the internal structures through which active agency is practised. In short, non-human objects such as 'land, weapons and food [may shape] … the particular phenomenological perspective or cultural schema of the agent(s) in focus, in the internal structures (the virtual) that can be drawn upon by the agents' (Stones, 2005). While material structures may influence the internal structures that are mobilised when exercising active agency, there also exists a challenge of theorising the agency of technology within this framework. By exclusively focusing on physical structures such as 'land, weapons and food', which in a sense are instrumental for human survival, Stones (2005) only presented external physical structures that serve as means to an end. However, much of a human's interaction with the physical environment is to a lesser extent defined instrumentally in advance. One example of this may be a person engaging with the physical structure of a computer and the virtual structure of the internet while simply 'Googling around' with no specific purpose.

In the last decade, scholarship has criticised Structuration theory for under-theorising the technical aspects of the social realm (Greenhalgh & Stones, 2010; Leonardi, 2011). Giddens and Pierson (1998), for instance, have rejected the agency of technology a priori and argued that 'technology does nothing, except as [being] implicated in the actions of human beings' (p. 22).

In short, these studies suggest that 'doings' of technical artefacts cannot merely be explained by social practice and that scholars should rather focus on more in-depth studies of how technology works in interaction with people. Greenhalgh and Stones (2010) developed this argument by scrutinising the role of non-human actors in Structuration theory. They argued that Strong Structuration theory needs to incorporate insights from Actor–Network theory to better account for the recursive relationship between humans and technology and to allow for the possibility that non-human technological objects may act in concert with people and not merely be a by-product of active human agency. Greenhalgh and Stones (2010) argued: 'we must also theorise the technology artefact – a task for which ATN [Actor–Network theory] offers some insights' (p. 1287). However, more theoretical work needs to be done to specify how agency operates in the dialectic between human subjects and non-human objects, and we will presently move to a discussion of agency informed by perspectives within Actor–Network theory and Material Agency theory. More importantly, we argue that a redefinition of agency has vital repercussions for the Active Citizenship of persons with disabilities and its interplay with technology.

Theorising agency within Material Agency theory and Actor–Network theory

Scholars within the fields of Actor–Network theory and Material Agency theory have suggested that agency is played out within a network influenced by three related factors: social structures, individual choices and the material environment. In other words, the material environment is singled out to a larger extent as a key component as opposed to its role within Structuration theory. Figure 12.1 provides a visualisation of the relationship between the three factors.

Authors working within this perspective have suggested that none of the three factors have the upper hand in an a priori sense and that one has to study in-depth the small-scale processes through which acts are made to reveal the dynamic interplay between them. Moreover, they have suggested that agency should be understood as 'the ability to act' (Giraudo & Martell, 2015, p. 484) and not as something exclusively governed by human intention and motivation (e.g. Giddens & Pierson, 1998).

Material Agency theorist Malafouris (2008) drew on the example of pottery making to describe how both objects, in this case the clay and the subject (e.g. the hands of the potter), influence each other. The potter may state, 'I made the pot out of the clay'. However, the issue becomes more difficult for the potter to address when confronted with precise questions like: '"How did you decide the force of the grip?" or "How did you decide the appropriate speed of the wheel?" or "When and how much water to add on the clay?"' (Malafouris, 2008, p. 19). The potter knows how to make a pot out of clay, but when asked about the process, can seldom explain it. Instead of taking the potter's answer, 'I made the pot', at face value, Knappett and Malafouris (2008) proposed an alternative explanation: 'The potter's fingers simply receive information from the clay and transmit it to the appropriate area inside the potter's brain' (p. 20). Based upon this information, the potter decides upon his grip of the clay. In short, both the clay and the potter himself are authors of the potter's actions as the clay provides information about how hard the potter can push and bend the material. This cuts to the heart of the issue of conceptualising agency. According to Malafouris (2008), there are reasons to ask, 'Who is the author of the act?' (p. 21). When

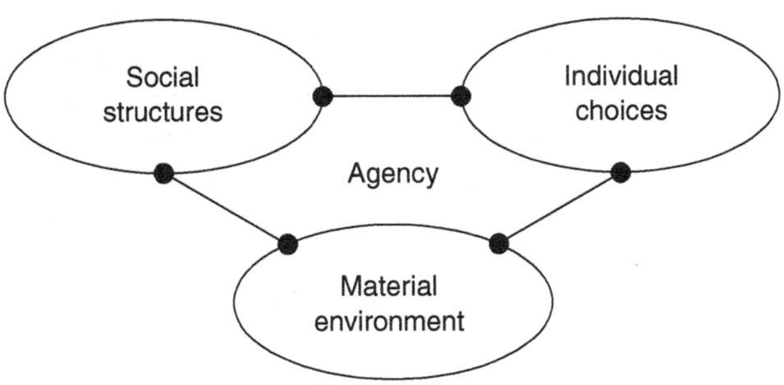

Figure 12.1 Agency conceptualised as the interaction between social structures, individual choice and the material environment.

confronted with the question of who made the pot, the potter may still reply, 'I did', because he may be totally unaware of how his brain is making all these small-scale decisions based upon information transmitted from the clay. He is partly right, because he interprets the information from the clay through his sensory systems and translates this information into future actions (e.g. grip, force and so forth on the clay). At the same time, these future actions are defined by prior experiences – that is, what actions the clay affords so that it does not break but instead becomes a pot. Agency, then, is divided partly in the hands of the potter and partly in the substance of the clay.

Many scholars have described the potter's answer as examples both of humans' tendency to overestimate their own ability to act and of how scholars of agency tend to neglect these small-scale processes and interactions between the subject and object(s) that constitute the act (e.g. Bateson, 1972; Malafouris, 2008). Malafouris (2008) argued that this judgement error is made up of two related errors: 'The first is an error of apparent mental causation and the second and correlated one is that of agency attribution' (p. 21). The first ties the notion of agency to theories of causality, which is already part of the question, 'Who is the author of the act?' This can be explained by people's tendency to think in retrospect that 'we are the authors of our actions' without realising that this causality is in part imaginary and is a result of downplaying the potential subject–object interactions that influenced the act. As a matter of common sense, humans ascribe agency to their own actions and downplay other factors (e.g. the role of objects, such as the clay in the potter case). Knappett and Malafouris (2008) summarised this relationship between causality and agency:

> And if we accept that agency is essentially about doing and that the problem of agency is essentially about who or what is the cause of the doing, then what we need to try first to understand is the relation between agency and causality.
>
> (p. 23)

Applied to research on the role of technology in the exercise of Active Citizenship for persons with disabilities, the presented arguments suggest a more careful analysis of 'what' or 'who' caused the act when people act on shared online platforms (e.g. Google and Facebook). If we start analysing this issue by understanding agency as a given, exclusive human property, then we are starting with what should, or could, have been the end of the analysis. Following the outlined arguments, we should instead look at the processes of interactions between substance and subject in experience. Implicitly, this underscores the obvious but important fact that temporality plays a crucial role in agency and causality, which is often glossed over when agency is understood as a series of independent acts. It is only by looking at the micro-acts as interactions and processes in time – that is, the hand–clay dynamics that feed into the larger macro-act of creating the pot – that we may understand how agency is played out through the mediated relationship between subject and object(s). Within this network of agency, Knappett and

Malafouris (2008) stated that it is crucial to examine the doing of the object, because whenever things are doing the work they tend to be 'sealed in a black box and sink below the surface of our conscious horizon' (p. 34), as witnessed in the Potter's statement, 'I made the pot'.

To summarise, a Material Agency-informed understanding of agency is grounded in: (1) a critique of 'agency attribution through mental causation' – that is, people's tendency to overestimate their ability and reason to act – and (2) a closer empirical emphasis on the temporal nature of acting and the various micro-acts that constitute an act. An important conceptual implication of these arguments is also to redefine the distinction between the micro- and macro-levels of actions in contrast to prevailing understandings within much social theory and the described Structuration theory. Rather than seeing the macro-level as a given social structure and the micro-level as played out through the subject's active agency, the Material Agency perspective consider the potter's statement, 'I made the pot', as a macro-act that can be examined by looking at the various micro-acts that went into producing the pot. Compared to Structuration theory, the presented perspective has a higher resolution that gives privilege to more in-depth descriptions of these interactions between subject and object and conversely invites us to rethink the relationship between the micro- and macro-levels.

Similar arguments have been made within Actor–Network theory (Callon & Latour, 1981). Latour introduced the analytic concept *actant*, which refers to how both humans and non-humans may have agency and act upon each other in various networks. Latour (2007a) underscored how these *actants* are connected in a network that includes both people and objects, and described these networks as anything that 'modify other actors through a series of…' actions (p. 75). He placed this within a semiotic tradition:

> An 'actor' in [Actor–Network theory] is a semiotic definition – an *actant*, that is, something that acts or to which activity is granted by others. It implies no special motivation of human individual actors, nor of humans in general. An actant can literally be anything provided it is granted to be the source of an action.
>
> (Latour, 1999)

Thus, rather than viewing objects as constituting a passive backdrop for human action, the notion of *actants* draws attention to how objects 'authorize, allow, afford, encourage, permit, suggest, influence, block, render possible, [and/or] forbid' (Latour, 2007a, p. 72) human action in conjunction with human motivation. According to Piekut (2014), Actor–Network theory attempts 'to register the effects of anything that acts in a given situation, regardless of whether that actor is human, technological, discursive or material' (p. 193). Understanding agency from the viewpoint of Actor–Network theory and Material Agency theory decouples the concept from intention and rather draws attention to the ability to act and the abovementioned micro-processes of subject–object interactions that make actions possible. According to Piekut (2014), this forces us to rethink agency empirically:

> The question of what an actor is in a given situation and how it might act belong properly to empirical investigation, not theoretical speculation. [...] For [Actor–Network theory], an actor need not realize, understand, or intend the difference it makes, but it nonetheless should be accounted for in the analysis.
>
> (pp. 195–196)

Applied to studies of accessible digital technology and Active Citizenship, the abovementioned arguments allow for interpretations that both hardware (e.g. computers, smartphones and so forth) and software (e.g. Google, Facebook and various smartphone applications) have agency as *actants* that enable people to act and think in new ways. More importantly, these understandings of technology enable us to examine the ways in which human motivation and thinking is the product of earlier micro-processes of human–technology interactions. Looking closely at these micro-processes and the many acts that constitute a social outcome, we illustrate how technology influences human choices, preferences and behaviours through for example the software provided by Google or Facebook. This is by no means a return to technological determinism, in which material objects exclusively define human action. Rather, Actor–Network theory assumes that all three factors mentioned in Figure 12.1 have agency and that these factors interact in a network that forms the basis of possible future actions. Thus, both the arguments presented by Material Agency scholar Malafouris and the perspectives within Actor–Network theory provide a more nuanced conceptual apparatus to address the role of the material environment in human actions compared to what is found in Structuration theory. Implementing the presented perspectives, together with the developments in Structuration theory in the 2000s, may provide a more robust conceptual framework to address the interplay between subjects and objects.

An example from the life-course interviews

To discuss the relevance of the presented arguments in relation to persons with disabilities' experience of Active Citizenship in practice, we now turn to an empirical analysis of a life-course interview with 'Vilde', a Norwegian person with mobility impairments born in the 1970s. The interview was taped and completed in Norwegian, in Norway, as part of the DISCIT project and was an in-depth interview lasting approximately two hours. It followed a semi-structured interview guide that included several questions relating to how technology enables or hampers Active Citizenship for persons with disabilities (see Chapter 3, this volume).

'Google is my best friend' (Vilde)

To address micro-interactions, we will provide an in-depth analysis based upon a life-course interview with Vilde. She has a university degree, works part-time and has her own apartment. Most of her friends are other people with disabilities. Vilde travels widely in other countries. She uses computers and a mobile phone to communicate and uses social media to maintain her international social network.

During the interview, Vilde extensively described how Google has enabled her to travel and enjoy culture and decide and think in new ways by providing relevant information with regards to, for example, the accessibility of different places she intends to travel to. After being asked if she had a favourite country, Vilde described the importance of Google:

> Yes, South Africa. I have been there two times, and it is a great place for wheelchair users if you do some research … beforehand … Google is my best friend when it comes to this. After the development of Google, and [the] internet in general, I have … better opportunities to find out about accessibility for wheelchair users like me. So, I have more opportunities to find suitable travel destination[s] and [information regarding] the accessibility of hotels, restaurants and so on.

Following the perspective of Latour (1999), we argue that Google functioned as an *actant*, providing Vilde with information about South Africa that caused her to travel there. In a Latourian sense, Vilde's statement, 'Google is my best friend', refers to Google's role as an important *actant* in her life that makes possible new actions that otherwise would not be possible. Still, Vilde's descriptions of her own actions above, such as the fact that she has been to South Africa two times, can be more fully understood if we understand her descriptions as macro-acts consisting of related micro-acts wherein Google and Vilde interacted. When Vilde begins to enter search terms such as 'accessibility wheelchair South Africa', Google automatically analyses Vilde's query, suggests relevant search terms based on analyses of Vilde's earlier behaviour(s) and the behaviour(s) of previous users, processes a query and returns relevant results as Vilde continues to type the query. Google uses an algorithm that not only infers what Vilde and other users have searched for but also includes what Google 'thinks' they intended to search for. Google tries to predict Vilde's search on a micro-level by suggesting the word(s) Vilde wants to type after she has written the first letters. Although we unfortunately did not have access to these micro-processes of Vilde's Google search in the interview, the sentence below may outline a possible scenario of how Google hypothetically could work as an *actant*, in this case by spelling out the words given a few indicators: '**acce**ssibility **wh**eelchair **south Af**rica'. (Letters in bold are letters that would be typed by Vilde, while the words would be suggested by Google.) Although the example is hypothetical, it cuts to the heart of the material agency that Google imparts upon Vilde by proposing words given a few indicators. What in a Latourian sense could be termed the 'Google–Vilde Network', or dialogue, illustrates the importance of understanding the micro-acts that make possible Vilde's macro-act of travelling to South Africa. The ways in which Google functions as an *actant*, together with Vilde, in this case is the result of complex information processing and algorithms beyond the scope of this article that underscore the material agency of Google.

Seen through the lens of Malafouris' description of how the clay moulds the hands of the pottery maker, we suggest that Google moulds Vilde's search enquiry. In addition, Google influences the results of Vilde's search by ranking their importance, drawing on coordinated big databases. In doing so, Google influences the knowledge from which she decides upon future search enquiries and which ultimately led to her act of travelling to South Africa. In fact, we argue that the agency of Google is even stronger than that of the clay described by Malafouris, because the pottery maker has a clear motivation of creating a pot whereas Vilde's web behaviour can be more open-ended. She may search the web for accessibility availability in various countries, before Google informs her that South Africa is the place to go. In short, the complex search engine system of Google (including page ranking systems, information retrieval systems, etc.) influences Vilde's actions on the web, as identified in the selected example above. What Vilde may conceive as her own intentions are informed by prior interactions between her brain, fingers, the computer and Google's search algorithms. When Vilde later in the interview stated, 'In the future I want to travel to South Africa', this intention was firmly rooted in the network of prior subject–object interactions between Vilde and Google, as well as her earlier experiences. Figure 12.2 may illustrate how the decision to go to South Africa was the product of multiple action choices.

Even though humans tend to overestimate their own ability to act based on the previously presented theoretical arguments (Bateson, 1972; Malafouris, 2008), Vilde clearly acknowledged during the interview how Google co-worked as an *actant* together with herself to inform her decision-making. Of course, she did not adopt that language to describe the mathematical basis for Google's various algorithms nor the vocabulary term *actant*, but she recognised Google's importance for her own actions.

When asked specifically about the importance of the internet and social media for opportunities to be an active citizen, she elaborated on how they had informed her actions:

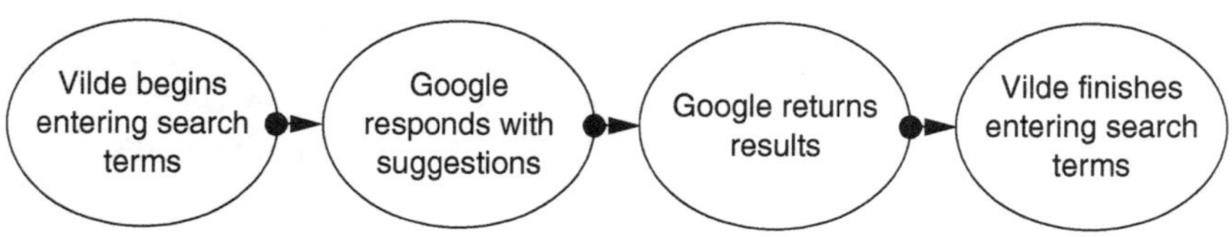

Figure 12.2 Vilde searches for wheelchair accessibility in South Africa.

> It [the internet] has lowered the threshold for how much contact you can have. It is much easier to access information and exchange information and engage in networks. It is, for example, much easier today to post something on your Facebook page than update your own web site. Also, Facebook has enabled me to have contact with other persons who are not disabled. Facebook has made it possible for me to keep in contact with family living in different places, and also with friends within disability organisations across the world. These points of connection were not possible before the internet and Facebook, and they have created vast arrays of opportunities.

Similar to Google, Facebook functioned as an *actant* that affords Vilde the opportunity to broaden her social network. Facebook also enables Vilde to access and exchange information by making it easy for her to interact with other people and even by proposing to her new friends. The software allows Vilde to communicate efficiently with friends, family, friends of friends, friends of family and larger social and political communities through Facebook groups. As illustrated in Figure 12.2, several of the statements Vilde made in the quote above can be illuminated by looking at the various acts that were part of them. All of Vilde's actions on Facebook are 'co-authored' by the algorithms and data banks that make up Facebook. Based upon earlier information Vilde gave Facebook, the information of other users and several programmes aligned with Facebook (e.g. Spotify), the technology influences Vilde's online behaviour. Of course, Facebook grants Vilde freedom to act within the programme by writing messages, searching for information and contacting friends. However, the technology also constantly provides Vilde with new information (e.g. in her news feed) and with recommendations to act. More importantly, Facebook directs Vilde's actions into a specific Facebook language of likes and dislikes, creating events and sharing information in a network. In addition, Facebook calculates the information in Vilde's social network by counting likes and dislikes, attendees at events and the number of participants in groups, as well as how these develop over time. When Vilde uses Facebook to 'post something' or 'to keep in contact with family', the Facebook technology – to a large extent – determines who receives that information and when, as well as how that information is stored and the procedures upon which that information is transmitted. Similar to both the clay example and the Google example, Vilde's actions on Facebook should be considered as part of a network shaped by various Facebook *actants*. Figure 12.3 illustrates this concept.

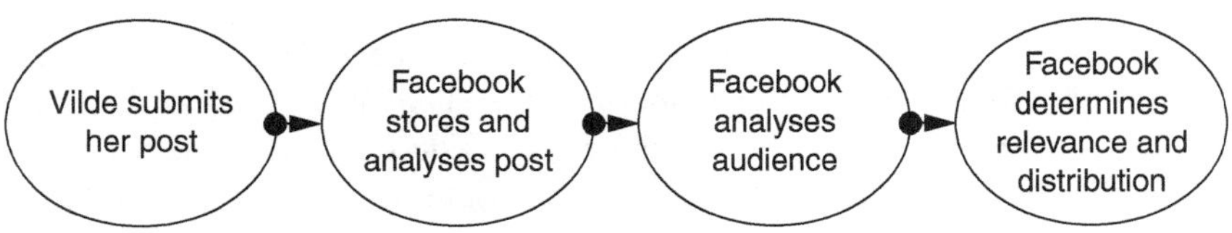

Figure 12.3 Micro-processes of Vilde's Facebook communication.

As in the other examples, Vilde is not the only author of the act. Rather, Vilde co-authors her acts together with Facebook. Each of Vilde's acts on Facebook can be considered macro-acts that consist of various related micro-acts, as illustrated in the figure.

Translated into theories of Active Citizenship, the Facebook *actant* enables her to exercise autonomy and influence as it shapes the life she wants to live and the people with whom she can form social and political networks. Thanks to social media, Vilde has been able to play a role in larger international networks related to disability politics. These networks have in turn consolidated and strengthened the organisations that work to improve the conditions for people with mobility impairments, and they have paved the way for making new policies. In fact, thanks to internet *actants* such as Facebook, Google and Skype, Vilde considered leaving work for a year to work internationally with this kind of disability politics and devote her time to improving policy development in the field. In various ways, the internet *actants* enabled Vilde to communicate and access this political influence and made it possible for her to travel and live in settings that had earlier been restricted for her. In what follows, we elaborate on how the analysis and theoretical discussions have implications for our understanding of Active Citizenship, while also summing up the main arguments of this chapter.

Concluding discussion

In this chapter, we have argued in favour of a broader notion of agency understood as 'the ability to act' (Giraudo & Martel, 2015, p. 484), in contrast to Giddens' (1984) notion of agency as exclusively linked to human intention and motivation. The theoretical discussion of agency and the empirical analysis underscored how technology and people act upon each other. Moreover, we showed how this interplay influences people's ability to exercise Active Citizenship, especially with regard to the dimensions of 'influence' and 'autonomy' (see Chapter 1, this volume). Starting with the latter, we found that the opportunity for persons with disabilities to live the life they have reason to value cannot be reduced exclusively to a question of active agency and broader social structures; this possibility is also shaped by the technological environment through which these intentions are made.

As illustrated by the case concerning Vilde, ICT substantially changed the conditions from which she made active choices by providing her with new information. By deciding upon the search results that Vilde received and ranking them in a specific order, Google's artificially intelligent systems and algorithms influenced Vilde's knowledge and thus her capacity to act. This then became a context for her future actions. In a Latourian sense, both Vilde and Google functioned as *actants* and mutually contributed to Vilde's goal by gathering and storing information, recognising patterns, processing information and performing actions in the 'Google–Vilde network'. Similar to how the clay shapes the movements of the pottery maker's fingers, the search results that Google allowed

Vilde to perform influenced her future actions. More importantly, what Vilde may consider as an independent act of 'autonomy' – 'travelling to South Africa' – can be understood as an outcome that is only possible thanks to various related forerunning action choices played out in the interaction between Vilde and Google. As illustrated in the analysis of how Google acts upon Vilde's typing on the keyboard, it also becomes clear that additional methods, such as in-depth analysis of how technology works, are crucial to address these mechanisms. The doings of Google and Facebook are difficult to verify through interviews, thus illustrating a potential bias present in the interview data. Similar to Malafouris' analysis of how the clay acted upon the pottery maker, the ways in which Google and Facebook acted upon Vilde were open-ended actions shaped by search algorithms and software design and not by discourse. Of course, Vilde's personal intentions and choices also influenced the search results. However, Vilde's intentions and choices could always be traced back to prior interactions between Vilde and the software technologies. Translated back to discussions concerning agency in sociology, and in particular within Structuration theory, the main argument of this chapter derived from the analysis is that established understandings of active agency as consisting of independent and intentional human actions (Giddens, 1984; Giddens & Pierson, 1998) should be complemented with a greater empirical sensitivity to how these actions are made based upon prior interactions between subjects and their technological environment. Active agency is not the product of a disconnected human body and purely mental constructs but of our engagement with the material world we live in. Of course, this argument is not new; it is reflected in both Material Agency theory and the Actor–Network theory's relationship to Marx's emphasis on materialism, as illustrated in Latour's (2007b) rhetorical article, 'Can we get our materialism back, please?' However, the presented arguments suggest that these interactions are open-ended and not necessarily directly governed by larger class struggles or broader social structures. Instead, the present discussion suggests that human actions should be grounded in analysis of their engagement with the physical environment in which they live.

If we accept the broader understanding of agency put forward in this chapter as 'the ability to act', it is clear that both technology and people act upon each other. Within disability studies, Moser (2006) summarises the importance of these arguments:

> There is no clear dividing line, at least in principle, between the technological, the social and indeed the human.... This is a material semiotics in which facts, artefacts, nature and objects are treated not as given categories lying outside culture or society, but as effects of interactions, relations and order building.
>
> (p. 376)

A three-fold understanding of the mutual interplay between social structures, individual actions and the physical environment, as illustrated throughout the case concerning Vilde, may enrich our understanding of how agency operates. Translated into the autonomy dimension of Active Citizenship (outlined in Chapter 1), these arguments enable a fruitful critique of humans' ability to make free and independent decisions. Many of our 'independent decisions' imply a wide array of material structures that inform and form our ability to make such acts. Still, as shown in the analysis of Vilde's situation, our interplay with these material structures may increase our opportunities for action when compared with available actions in the past. In short, our engagement with the material environment, such as technology, both constrains and increases our space for actions and is closely aligned with the sense of autonomy experienced by persons with disabilities today.

With regards to how this analysis shapes the concept of 'influence' and people's ability to participate socially and politically in society, we see how Google, Facebook and Skype provided Vilde with new arenas for political participation and engagement. The ways in which technology shapes what we termed the 'influence' dimension of Active Citizenship (see Chapter 1, this volume) resonates with the broad notion of politics of Latour (2005, 2007b, 2007c, 2007d), Barry (2001) and Alcadipani and Hassard (2010), inspired by Actor–Network theory. As Alcadipani and Hassard (2010) argued:

> Politics is not … exclusively about 'giving voice' by or in itself, but [it] can also be based, for instance, on how laboratory assemblies enact objects in order to give voice to them. The point here is to try to compare different techniques or re-presentation by arguing that there are many other ways of carrying out politics than usually considered.
>
> (p. 424)

By exposing Vilde to new information – either written, visual (Google) or sound-based (Skype) – and linking this information together in a network, Google, Facebook and Skype potentially served as *actants* that influenced Vilde's actions. Politics cannot be reduced to merely exercising 'a voice' but should also take into account the conditions that shape this voice and enable it to arise in the first place. Politics is concerned with the changing distribution of the sayable, audible and readable in a given community, and the present analysis clearly shows how Google increased these spaces for Vilde. The various *actants* in the Google–Vilde network provided new conditions for social and political participation and engagement that otherwise would not have existed. This aspect of politics is about representation and the ways in which voiceless persons and groups are given a voice through, for example, engagement with technology.

The present arguments echo Greenhalgh and Stone's (2010) arguments that Structuration theory has under-theorised how 'structurally relevant properties inscribed and embedded in technological artefacts constrain and enable human agency' (p. 1285). More than the political importance of considering citizens as subjects rather than objects, it is also crucial to critically examine the opportunities for exercising agency. The presented arguments suggest that both technology and humans act upon each other in the micro-processes that further or hamper Active Citizenship. If we are to investigate the conditions for Active Citizenship among persons with disabilities in today's Europe, we also have to take into account the pervasive impact of technology in an increasingly ICT-driven society. We should not treat common online software, such as Google and Facebook, as silent objects with no agency on their own; rather, they should be viewed as co-agents that may hamper or enable more active forms of citizenship.

References

Alcadipani, R. & Hassard, J. (2010). Actor–Network theory, organizations and critique: Towards a politics of organizing. *Organization, 17*(4), 419–435.

Barry, A. (2001). *Political machines: Governing a technological society*. London: Bloomsbury Academic.

Bateson, G. (1972). *Steps to an ecology of mind: Collected essays in anthropology, psychiatry, evolution, and epistemology*. Chicago: University of Chicago Press.

Berry, J. (1999). Apart or a part? Access to the Internet by visually impaired and blind people, with particular emphasis on assistive enabling technology and user perceptions. *Information Technology and Disabilities Journal*, *6*(3), 1–16.

Blanck, P. (2008). Flattening the (inaccessible) cyberworld for people with disabilities. *Assistive Technology*, *20*(3), 175–180.

Blanck, P. (2014). *eQuality: The struggle for web accessibility by persons with cognitive disabilities*. New York: Cambridge University Press.

Callon, M. & Latour, B. (1981). Unscrewing the big Leviathan: How actors macro-structure reality and how sociologists help them to do so. In K. Knorr-Cetina & A. V. Cicourel (Eds), *Advances in social theory and methodology: Toward an integration of micro-and macro-sociologies* (pp. 277–303). New York: Routledge.

Cullen, K. & Kubitschke, L. (2007). Assessment of the status of eAccessibility in Europe, Empirica Gesellschaft für Kommunikations-und Technologieforschung. Retrieved from https://ec.europa.eu/digital-single-market/en/news/final-report-study-measuring-progress-eaccessibility-europe. Brussels: European Commission.

Dittrich, Y., Ekelin, A., Elovaara, P., Eriksén, S. & Hansson, C. (2003). *Making e-Government happen: Everyday co-development of services, citizenship and technology*. Paper presented at the Proceedings of the 36th Annual Hawaii International Conference on System Sciences, Hawaii, US.

Giddens, A. (1984). *The constitution of society: Outline of the theory of structuration*. Berkeley, CA: University of California Press.

Giddens, A. & Pierson, C. (1998). *Conversations with Anthony Giddens: Making sense of modernity*. Stanford: Stanford University Press.

Giraudo, S. E. & Martel, A. R. (2015). Memory, identity, power. *Chinese Semiotic Studies*, *11*(4), 479–497.

Goggin, G. & Newell, C. (2003). *Digital disability: The social construction of disability in new media*. Oxford: Rowman & Littlefield.

Greenhalgh, T. & Stones, R. (2010). Theorising big IT programmes in healthcare: Strong structuration theory meets Actor–Network theory. *Social Science & Medicine, 70*(9).

Halvorsen, R. (2010). Digital freedom for persons with disabilities: Are policies to enhance e-Accessibility and e-Inclusion becoming more similar in the Nordic countries and the US? *European Yearbook of Disability Law*, *2*, 77–102.

Kubitschke, L., Cullen, K., Dolphin, C., Laurin, S. & Cederbom, A. (2013). *Study on assessing and promoting e-accessibility*. Final report. A study prepared for the European Commission DG Communications Networks, Content & Technology. Retrieved from https://ec.europa.eu/digital-single-market/en/news/study-assessing-and-promoting-e-accessibility. Brussels: European Commission.

Latour, B. (1999). On recalling ANT. In J. Law & J. Hassard (Eds), *Actor–Network theory and after*. Oxford: Wiley-Blackwell.

Latour, B. (2005). From realpolitik to dingpolitik: How to make things public. In B. Latour & P. Weibel (Eds), *Making things public: Atmospheres of democracy*. Cambridge, MA: MIT Press.

Latour, B. (2007a). *Reassembling the social*. Hampshire: Oxford University Press.

Latour, B. (2007b). Can we get our materialism back, please? *Isis*, *98*(1), 138–142.

Leonardi, P. M. (2011). When flexible routines meet flexible technologies: Affordance, constraint, and the imbrication of human and material agencies. *MIS Quarterly*, *35*(1), 147–167.

Malafouris, L. (2008). At the potter's wheel: An argument for material agency. In C. Knappett & L. Malafouris (Eds), *Material agency: Towards a non-anthropocentric approach* (pp. 19–36). New York: Springer Science & Business Media.

Moser, I. (2003). *Road traffic accidents: The ordering of subjects, bodies and disability*. Oslo: Unipub.

Moser, I. (2005). On becoming disabled and articulating alternatives: The multiple modes of ordering disability and their interferences. *Cultural Studies*, *19*(6), 667–700.

Moser, I. (2006). Disability and the promises of technology: Technology, subjectivity and embodiment within an order of the normal. *Information, Communication & Society*, *9*(3), 373–395.

Moser, I. & Law, J. (2003). 'Making voices': New media technologies, disabilities, and articulation. In G. Liestøl, T. Rasmussen & A. Morrison (Eds), *Innovation: Media, methods and theories* (pp. 491–520). Cambridge: MIT Press.

Myhill, W. N., Cogburn, D. L., Samant, D., Addom, B. K. & Blanck, P. (2008). Developing accessible cyberinfrastructure-enabled knowledge communities in the national disability community: Theory, practice, and policy. *Assistive Technology*, *20*(3), 157–174.

Noble, S. (2002). Web access and the law: A public policy framework. *Library Hi Tech*, *20*(4), 399–405. doi: 10.1108/07378830210452604.

Oudshoorn, N. & Pinch, T. (2003). *How users matter: The co-construction of users and technology (inside technology)*. Cambridge: MIT Press.

Parker, D. R. & Banerjee, M. (2007). Leveling the digital playing field: Assessing the learning technology needs of college-bound students with LD and/or ADHD. *Assessment for Effective Intervention*, *33*(1), 5–14.

Piekut, B. (2014). Actor–Networks in music history: Clarifications and critiques. *Twentieth-Century Music*, *11*(2), 191–215.

Rose, N. & Novas, C. (2004). *Biological citizenship*. London: Blackwell Publishing.

Roulstone, A. (2016). *Disability and technology: An interdisciplinary and international approach*. London: Springer.

Schreuer, N., Keter, A. & Sachs, D. (2014). Accessibility to information and communications technology for the social participation of youths with disabilities: A two-way street. *Behavioral Sciences & the Law*, *32*(1), 76–93.

Sirkkunen, E. & Kotilainen, S. (2004). *Towards active citizenship on the net: Possibilities of citizen oriented communication: Case studies from Finland*. Tampere: Tampereen yliopisto.

Stones, R. (2005). *Structuration theory*. Basingstoke: Palgrave-Macmillan.

Suchman, L. (1993). Working relations of technology production and use. *Computer Supported Cooperative Work, 2*(1–2), 21–39.

Söderström, S. (2009). Offline social ties and online use of computers: A study of disabled youth and their use of ICT advances. *New Media & Society*, *11*(5), 709–727.

Söderström, S. (2013). Digital differentiation in young people's Internet use – Eliminating or reproducing disability stereotypes. *Future Internet*, *5*(2), 190–204.

Toboso, M. (2011). Rethinking disability in Amartya Sen's approach: ICT and equality of opportunity. *Ethics and Information Technology*, *13*(2), 107–118.

13 Rethinking Active Citizenship

Lessons from life-course interviews in nine European countries

Rune Halvorsen, Bjørn Hvinden, Mario Biggeri, Julie Beadle-Brown, Jan Tøssebro and Anne Waldschmidt

In the introduction, we set ourselves the task to identify the conditions that are required for Active Citizenship to become an experienced reality for persons with disabilities. To undertake this endeavour, we have adopted a multidimensional concept of Active Citizenship, focusing on three dimensions: security, autonomy and influence. Drawing on findings from life-course interviews with women and men with mobility, visual, intellectual or psychosocial disabilities and belonging to three age cohorts (born around 1950, 1970 and 1990) in nine European countries (Czech Republic, Germany, Ireland, Italy, Norway, Serbia, Sweden, Switzerland and the United Kingdom), we have identified multiple possibilities and challenges that exist in terms of exercising Active Citizenship for persons with disabilities in Europe.

Based on our findings, we have examined the links between the *conditions* for exercising Active Citizenship, the *practices* of persons with disabilities and the *outcomes* achieved, as well as how such links develop over time. In this book, we have explored whether structuration theory (O'Reilly, 2012; Stones, 2005) provides a fruitful perspective, especially when used critically and in active dialogue with alternative theoretical perspectives. We have used structuration theory as a general framework for analysing how agency–structure dynamics influence the Active Citizenship of persons with disabilities, in particular the notions of external and internal structures, agency, and outcomes (Figure 2.1).

Additionally we have relied on the notion of 'conversion processes' in the Capability Approach (e.g. Bellanca et al., 2011; Nussbaum, 2011; Sen, 2009) to sensitise our analysis to factors, mechanisms and processes that may explain the linkages between external and internal structures, and the agency of persons with disabilities. Through several steps, Sen has developed the idea that the diverse characteristics and circumstances of a person may affect his or her prospects of being able to *convert* or transfer means into capability sets and functionings. We argue that the notion of conversion processes may sensitise our analysis to the diversity among persons with disabilities in needs and capabilities for participation (e.g. due to age, gender, health and impairment) and the conditions that need to be in place to enable them to exercise Active Citizenship.

In her codification of the Capability Approach, Robeyns (2005) has distinguished between *personal* (e.g. age, gender, health, impairment), *social* (e.g. social norms, disability policies, gendered division of labour, discriminatory practices) and *environmental* conversion factors (built and transport environment, accessible technology). We interpret conversion factors as 'consisting of a mix of patterns of some duration or stability, partly shaped by broader societal, economic and political structures, partly by the individual's background, circumstances and life course' (Hvinden & Halvorsen, 2017, p. 7). In other words, we consider that conversion factors and processes (interaction between factors over time) can be both external and internal to the agents.

In the next sections, we first summarise the overall patterns in the Active Citizenship of persons with disabilities in the nine DISCIT countries. Second, drawing on structuration theory, we present the main *external* structures or factors (social, environmental) we have identified in our data set and how their impact varied between persons with visual, mobility, intellectual and psychosocial disabilities. Third, we examine how *internal* structures or factors influenced the 'capability for voice' among persons with disabilities. Fourth, we discuss the relationship between changes in external and internal structures. Fifth, we conclude by identifying some implications of our findings for European disability policy.

To what extent do persons with disabilities exercise Active Citizenship in Europe?

Summarising the findings we have presented in this book, it is fair to say that all the nine DISCIT countries have moved towards making Active Citizenship a reality for all citizens with disabilities, although at somewhat different speed and emphasis on the three dimensions of Active Citizenship (security, autonomy and influence). The historical deinstitutionalisation process has played a key role here. More people than before receive the necessary support – for instance support for accommodation (housing) costs, access to personal assistants, personal budgets, or at least, home helps – to live their lives independently of institutional care or their parents.

Some countries have made considerable progress towards ensuring the conditions for persons with disabilities to exercise autonomy. Independent living has become a reality for a greater number of people through the granting of personal assistance or personal budgets, and making access to these a matter of individual right and not administrative or professional discretion. However, while a number of countries over some time have seen a process of deinstitutionalisation and a trend towards community living, in other countries, this process has stopped and to some extent even been reversed more recently. Despite a strong emphasis, both from the EU and national governments, on enhancing employment and economic independence among persons with disabilities, it is difficult to find a consistent and clear trend in this direction.

In general, the life-course interviews show that, despite the progress that has been made in disability policy since the 1990s, much work still remains in order to ensure that persons with disabilities have the opportunities to exercise Active

Citizenship on an equal basis with others. The life-course interviews have shown that many persons with disabilities still face specific barriers which prevent full and effective participation in the community, the labour market and in the education system (Chapters 4, 5, 8, 10). The constraints and barriers in the opportunities to make active contributions to society by raising children and providing care for family members were particularly evident in the interviews with disabled women (Chapter 10).

The data set we have reported from in this book demonstrates that women with disabilities are more at risk of poorer outcomes in terms of security, autonomy and influence than men with disabilities (see also Karačić & Waldschmidt, 2018). Experiences of legal, attitudinal, economic and organisational barriers to having children, and exercising Active Citizenship through domestic and care work, as well as difficulties in combining paid and unpaid work, were not uncommon among the women. Women with disabilities have sometimes been expected by service providers to manage with less home care service or personal assistance, to do more housework themselves or need fewer outdoor activities than men. Consistent with earlier research (e.g. Nosek, Clubb Foley, Hughes & Howland, 2001), risk and experience of domestic and sexual violence was associated with abuse of their physical vulnerability, low self-esteem, and dependency on help and assistance from others.

However, both disabled women and men described how participation in sports and cultural activities (e.g. music, theatre, computer games and watching movies) was important for their subjective well-being and sense of living a meaningful life. As such, several interviewees described these activities as ways in which to realise the life they wanted to live. Such activities clearly contributed to the experience of autonomy on the part of the interviewees. In addition, these cultural activities were also often arenas for social participation and achievement of a broader social network, which contributed to their experience of affiliation (the experience of security in a broad sense).

Others participated in political activities at local or national level in organisations of persons with disabilities, political parties and other civil society organisations. However, we find clear contrasts in the civil society and political engagement of persons with disabilities across the nine countries and between the four categories of persons with disabilities (Chapter 6 and 11). In several DISCIT countries, interviewees commented on the underrepresentation of persons with psychosocial and intellectual disabilities in terms of opportunities for political participation and self-representation. We assume that this indicates a general problem, as these population groups – particularly those persons lacking legal capacity – already face more discrimination as reported by Priestley et al. (2016) with regard to voting rights. Hence, we conclude that this group should be the touchstone to qualify the participation opportunities including influence and self-representation for all. According to Article 29 of the United Nations Convention on the Rights of Persons with Disabilities (CRPD), every human being, regardless of ascribed disability, shall have the 'political rights and the opportunity to enjoy them on an equal basis with others' (UN, 2006).

The longitudinal dimension of the life-course interviews has made it possible to demonstrate how the opportunities for exercising Active Citizenship changed in individual life courses (e.g. Chapters 8, 10 and 11). International, EU and national policies structured the conditions for participation. Yet, over time some interviewees – sometimes together with others in a similar situation – managed to achieve incremental change in their opportunities for exercising Active Citizenship ('virtuous cycles of functioning') (Chapter 11). Often such changes involved complex interactions or dynamics between personal, social and environmental factors. For instance, persons with psychosocial disabilities reported how improvement in mental health, self-confidence, expansion of social networks, participation in art and music therapy, culture, sports and employment depended on each other. In other cases, the interviewees experienced deteriorating opportunities for exercising Active Citizenship. There were stories about progressive diseases, downscaling of their aspirations and social exclusion ('vicious cycles of functioning') (Chapter 11).

By adopting a life-course perspective, we have been able to identify how persons with disabilities – against all odds – managed to expand and sustain their opportunities for exercising Active Citizenship. Similarly, the life-course perspective has provided insights about the risks of social exclusion and deteriorating opportunities for living a life as an active citizen at different life stages. If we had not adopted a life-course perspective in the DISCIT project, we would have had scarce data on the generative processes that may foster the Active Citizenship of persons with disabilities.

External factors enabling and constraining Active Citizenship

What were the main *external* factors enabling or constraining people with disabilities in exercising Active Citizenship and participating fully and effectively in society? In the following, we adopt our distinction between three types of external factors: meta-political factors, factors related to policy design and institutions, and factors related to take-up and use of disability-related policy measures (see Chapter 1).

Meta-political factors

The findings from the DISCIT research project indicate that there is a range of enabling as well as constraining factors that persons with disabilities face in exercising Active Citizenship. Many of these reflect broad societal processes, divisions and interactions far beyond what is directly within the remit of public authorities, policies and provisions. In all nine DISCIT countries, we see the impact of historical legacies of how dominant understandings and societal actors have tended to define or perceive persons with disabilities and particular groups of persons with disabilities (Schneider & Ingram, 1993). This includes the cultural classifications of persons with disabilities as deviants from the 'normal' bodily and mental functionings rather than as part of the normal variation and diversity in the population, or even as an oppressed minority group (Waldschmidt, 2017). For instance, there are many kinds of stereotypes and untested attributions about what persons with disabilities are able to do and achieve. In general, the surrounding society tends to underestimate the potential, knowledge, skills and capacities of persons with disabilities. Similarly, there is a broad tendency not to see or be aware of how one has designed the physical, social and organisational structures in which we all operate, or ways in which the characteristics of these structures may interact with different kinds of impairments.

Consequently, many people with disabilities face attitudinal barriers, for instance when they apply to study a particular subject, train for a particular occupation or obtain a particular position. An even more fundamental consequence of the underestimation of how persons with disabilities can contribute positively to society is the tendency to neglect them in the recruitment to political positions, to membership of boards or decision-making bodies or to stand as a candidate in public elections. Such exclusion does not only contribute to making persons with disabilities invisible in organisational and political processes; it is also likely that it adds to the frequent omission or neglect of the situation, well-being and interests of people with disabilities when political bodies make their decisions (Chapter 6).

Factors related to policy design and institutions

The life-course approach has allowed us to collect data on the interviewees' experiences of enabling and disabling social conditions. When relevant, we have situated the lived experiences of the interviews in the broader context of national and international disability policy at the macro level ('upper structural layers', O'Reilly, 2012, p. 24). Very few interviewees had, however, any substantial knowledge about the UN Convention on the Rights of Persons with Disabilities (UN, 2006) or EU disability policy. To the extent that they did report awareness about disability policy, it tended to be about national policy reforms and discussions. More often, the interviewees had practical knowledge about provisions and programmes of direct importance for their everyday lives.

We have identified a number of meso-level structures of direct importance for the active agency of persons with disabilities, such as stories about inaccessible transport systems and information and communication technology, and red tape in the social and health services or education system ('proximate structural layers', O'Reilly, 2012, p. 24). Such factors or mechanisms were reflected in stories about the (lack of) availability, affordability, accessibility and usability of goods and services.

First, access to free, relevant and high-quality education is an important enabling factor for Active Citizenship. There is a solid body of research showing that having a higher education especially has a strong impact on the employment prospects of persons with disabilities (e.g. Molden & Tøssebro, 2012). Among the DISCIT countries, some offer free education beyond upper secondary level to a greater extent than others. However, all education institutions need to build on universal design, full accessibility and necessary reasonable accommodation in order to be inclusive and prevent dropout from students with disabilities.

The life-course interviews reflected large variations in experiences with accessible school built environment and transport, and the receipt of personal assistance in the classroom, but also experiences of exclusion from after-school activities with peers. As many of the interviewees needed extra time to complete their education, a critical question is whether the educational programmes allow for and accommodate the extra time (Chapters 5, 8 and 11).

Because people with visual disabilities largely had to rely on audible information, many of the interviewees had taken various forms of music education, including studies at music conservatories, education in music therapy, and piano tuning. This was particularly striking in the interview data from the Czech Republic, which had a specific conservatory for the blind. In other countries, such as Norway, public authorities had left the idea that persons with disabilities were particularly suited for or fitted better in specific segments of the labour market. While Norwegians born around 1950 reported on efforts by the special services for the disabled at channelling them into particular professions in the 1960s and 1970s, such stories were absent in the 1970 and 1990 age cohorts.

Second, the availability of accessible technology is of great importance. This availability is safer to the extent that national authorities have introduced and enforced social regulations on accessibility of new technologies. Additionally we have touched upon the roles of public cash transfers and social services to make such availability a reality, although in some countries non-governmental organisations also have a role in such provision. Several interviewees in the Czech Republic, Ireland, Italy, and Serbia reported problems in getting access to up-to-date technology.

The historical changes in policies to enhance accessibility and reduce barriers to participation were particularly evident in the interviews with the 1950 age cohort. Those born around 1950 were able to look back at and reflect on a relatively long time period and describe the impact of the policy reforms since the 1960s and 1970s and the consequences of the disability policy systems for their opportunities to exercise Active Citizenship. The most consistent finding in this regard was the increased importance of barrier-free physical environments (e.g. elevators, ramps, absence of staircases) and more usable and affordable assistive technology (e.g. electric wheelchairs, speech-to-text technology, smart house technology). As a result of an increased focus on policies to promote universal design, persons with mobility disability reported how they can today live more autonomously, in contrast to the past.

Both persons with mobility and with visual disabilities described the importance of new information and communication technologies as devices which enabled the conversion of their resources into effective doings and beings. This included various mainstream computer software and hardware, as well as assistive technology such as speech-to-text, screen readers and eyeglass technology. New software such as Facebook and Skype made it easier for persons with visual and mobility disabilities to engage in paid work, culture and leisure activities, civil society organisations and political activities. The introduction of such technologies often represented a turning point in the lives of the interviewees and facilitated more Active Citizenship. However, new technology could also be a barrier if the user interface was not sensitive to the impairments of the end users (Chapters 7, 11 and 12). Such stories about the positive and negative impacts of new technology were almost absent among persons with intellectual and psychosocial disabilities, and they were more often disinterested in social media.

Third, income transfers linked with relevant social (or employment) services can enhance the employment prospects of persons with disabilities, for instance by securing work practice and temporary job placement and training for improving job skills and navigating in the labour market. Public cash transfers have a role in protecting persons with disabilities from poverty and material deprivation. However, it is also a risk that poorly designed systems for cash transfers can 'lock in' recipients through poverty or benefit traps, rather than strengthening the recipient's capacity for entering or returning to employment (Chapters 5, 8 and 11).

Fourth, situations of mental ill-health were more likely to happen during moments of 'transition', e.g. when individuals had to face increased demands of the environment due to changes in the workplace or in the family. Therefore, social services had a major role to play, not only to prevent the recurring apparition of such moments of mental ill-health and disability, but also to support the individual to regain a situation of health and capability. Helpful measures were among others mental health care settings where the individual can have a say in the treatments and medication, peer-support groups, various forms of access to art and art therapy, measures of support in the community, and flexible work arrangements which take into account the various needs of the individual.

While the deinstitutionalisation of the social services for this group had come far in some countries (Italy, Norway, Sweden and the UK), other countries had just started on this avenue (the Czech Republic and Serbia). Yet other countries were in an intermediary stage of deinstitutionalisation (Ireland, Germany and Switzerland) (Chapter 4). In parallel to an incomplete deinstitutionalisation process, we have seen in recent years the development of a decentralisation of the welfare state and the introduction of New Public Management, leading to a 'marketization' of care, meaning that different welfare provisions are delivered by a variety of public and private suppliers (Newman, 2005). This has also limited the involvement of persons with psychosocial disabilities, preventing them from exercising their influence in designing and planning the services that meet their needs (Chapter 8).

Fifth, equal treatment, non-discrimination and accessibility regulations are important for the employment opportunities of persons with disabilities, if governments ensure that employers are fully aware of such regulations and that there are low-barrier channels for filing complaints about employers' failure to comply with the regulations. Very few of the interviewees had, however, experience with filing complaints. Due to the social costs and risks associated with presenting oneself as a 'disabled' worker to an employer, most of them hesitated to file complaints (Chapters 5, 8 and 11). This suggests that the EU and the member governments should not rely entirely on individual complaint mechanisms but aim for a broader set of approaches to promote structural change to ensure non-discrimination and accessibility. The EU and the member states have already started on this avenue through the adoption of duties for employers and providers of goods and services to report and demonstrate compliance to social regulations to qualify as participants in public procurement (EU, 2000, 2016; Waddington, 2017).

Factors related to the take-up and use of disability-related cash benefits, services and social regulations

At the micro level, the life-course interviews have allowed us to examine how the active agency of persons with disabilities unfolds in 'communities of practices' (O'Reilly, 2012, p. 31) with other actors on the ground ('conjuncturally specific external structures', O'Reilly, 2012, p. 31). In several cases the facilitators of positive transformations processes were factors other than the type of resources the welfare state has been able to provide: active support and backing from one's family is an important enabling factor for Active Citizenship (Chapter 9).

The significance of the family environment was particularly evident in the case of persons with intellectual disabilities. At the best, the interviewees with intellectual disabilities managed to exercise choice, achieve education and work, and participate in leisure activities due to the support they received from family members. When the disabled person grew up and parents reach old age, other family members and friends became more important. Similarly, support from social networks, friends of the family, other acquaintances or contacts made in neighbourhoods and civil society have generally proved to be important for achieving employment, and this is also the case for persons with disabilities (Chapter 5).

Interdependencies between the external conversion factors

Our analyses demonstrate that conversion factors at macro, meso and micro level were interdependent. The findings further demonstrate that we find significant differences between the four categories of persons with disabilities (visual, mobile, intellectual and psychosocial) in how external conversion factors structure the opportunities for exercising Active Citizenship. For instance, accessible technology was more critical to persons with mobility and visual disabilities, while social services were more critical to persons with psychosocial disabilities. Often, however, the opportunities for exercising Active Citizenship depended on the combination and coordination of several conversion factors. Among those who were most active as parents, students, employees and politicians, we find people who benefited from a combination of a supportive family, accessible and affordable education, assistive technology and cash benefits to compensate for extra costs associated with the disability.

While participation in education and work was a possibility for many persons with mobility disabilities, they often paid a high price for their involvement. At a personal level, many interviewees needed extra time to prepare in the morning and to recover in the afternoon. Due to barriers in the environment, transport also took a longer time. Despite the increasing attention to universal design and reasonable accommodation requirements in national and EU regulations, many persons experienced difficulties going to concerts, pubs, and museums, and participating in interest organisations and political activism. However, increasing opportunities for online participation enabled younger persons with mobility and visual disabilities to participate in new ways socially (in networks of significant others), politically (in civil society organisations and political parties), and economically (in paid work).

Enabling and constraining internal factors in Active Citizenship – individual and collective self-representation

In addition to the varying external or objective conditions for exercising security, autonomy and influence, we find large variations in the capabilities of persons with disabilities to articulate their needs and express them individually – as individual persons – as well as collectively together with others in a similar situation. This was in part due to the cultural classifications and interpretations of disabilities and impairments, the attribution of meaning and perception of disabilities, varying significantly among mobility, visual, intellectual and psychosocial disabilities (Schneider & Ingram, 1993).

Mobility and visual impairments have often been associated with clear-cut medical diagnosis and the person is rarely blamed for the situation. Their linguistic and cognitive skills are usually not affected by the impairment. Such personal circumstances have made it somewhat difficult for others to conceive of them as 'immature', 'irresponsible' or 'incapacitated' from making sound decisions – although persons with mobility and visual disabilities do report such experiences (Chapters 6 and 11). Persons with mobility and visual disabilities have been able to present stories about being victims of circumstances outside their control, as worthy of help and assistance, or as an oppressed minority group. Drawing on such cultural narratives, these population groups have been able to appeal to the moral consciousness or solidarity of non-disabled people, to achieve sympathy and moral support, to present what have been recognised by others as legitimate demands, to establish relatively large organisations of persons with disabilities, and to succeed in political mobilisation and achieve important victories in disability policy reforms. In sum, persons with mobility and visual disabilities have largely succeeded in presenting themselves as 'worthy', 'unified', 'numerous' and 'committed' (WUNC). Charles Tilly (1998, pp. 212–217) has argued that framing of social movements constituencies as

WUNC has been central in presenting collective claims on public authorities and achieving support for their justice demands from people on the other side of the line.

For different reasons, such self-representations were more difficult for persons with intellectual and psychosocial disabilities. In some cases, the image of persons with intellectual disabilities as 'childish' and incompetent to make decisions has overshadowed their capabilities for expressing their views and needs. In the case of persons with intellectual disabilities, a key issue was how to accommodate their needs to ensure as much involvement as possible in decision-making processes of importance to themselves, and how to balance self-representation and representation by parents or guardians.

The issue of individual and collective self-representation was somewhat different in the case of persons with psychosocial disabilities. First, for several reasons the interviewees reported more individualised self-identities than among the three other categories of persons with disabilities. They often had unclear diagnosis and difficulties in articulating what they had in common (across problems and diagnosis such as eating disorders, attention deficits, hyperactivity disorders or bipolar disorders). This made it difficult for them to define a collective identity. Usually they focused on individual needs, including for health and social services, as well as individual accommodation in vocational rehabilitation and employment.

Second, in many cases the interviewees reported that it was difficult to point to external factors that hampered their opportunities for participation in society. Instead, they were inclined to blame themselves for their failures to live up to dominant life expectations. Largely their self-perceptions seemed to reflect the dominant characterisations of persons with psychosocial disabilities as 'unstable', 'erratic', 'unreliable' and 'fragile'. Although they did not necessarily share those views when we asked them directly, the negative characterisations influenced their self-representations.

A general insight in social science is that the dominant cultural characterisation and narratives about a group of people with a particular characteristic held in a community or society in general may affect adversely how members of the group see themselves and each other. The negative labelling by others may to a varying degree influence the person's self-conception and identity (e.g. Elias, 1994 [1977]). To the extent that persons with disabilities internalise others' negative perceptions, this may also function as a barrier to Active Citizenship. Particularly among persons with psychosocial disabilities we sometimes met persons who were somewhat victimised: persons who suffered from lack of self-confidence and a negative self-image (Chapters 8 and 11).

Differently from persons with mobility and visual disabilities, they were to lesser extent in a position to present themselves as an oppressed minority, demanding rights and blaming other people for the problems they experienced. In a few cases, the interviewees did, however, criticise the psychiatric services for wrong diagnoses and medication, or the use of forced hospitalisation. In other words, we found both stories of being victims of psychiatry and stories of self-blaming. In practice, the same persons sometimes switched between or combined the two types of self-presentations.

Third, many of them experienced psychosocial difficulties that were temporary or varied over time. The interviewees had experienced time spells without any psychosocial difficulties but also severe set-backs in their personal capacity to participate as an active citizen (e.g. psychoses, depression and suicidal thoughts). The experience of the psychosocial problems as temporary or fluctuating motivated several of the interviewees to contact self-help groups and organisations for and of persons with psychosocial disabilities in transition periods, but they pulled out when they felt they could manage on their own. Particularly in the older age cohorts, however, we also found persons who over the life course had experienced permanent or returning mental health issues.

Altogether, their experiences as a heterogeneous and stigmatised group and with temporary or varying mental health problems weakened their capability for collective voice, and participation on a regular basis in peer-support groups and organisations of persons with psychosocial disabilities (Chapters 6 and 11).

In the vocabulary of structuration theory, the three mechanisms (individualisation, stigmatisation and temporality) influenced the 'dispositions drawn upon by agents in producing performances' – i.e. their 'internal structure' (Stones, 2005, pp. 87–88). Similar to Pierre Bourdieu's (1977) conceptualisation of 'habitus' as the link between structure and agency, Stones' concept of internal structure refers to the 'transposable skills and dispositions, including worldviews and cultural schemas, classifications … habits of speech and gesture' (Stones, 2005, p. 88). Structuration theory emphasises that agents often conceptualise their problem understandings, interpretations and habits in a taken-for-granted manner and conceive of them as 'natural'.

In our cases, the individualisation, stigmatisation and temporality affecting the internal structures of persons with psychosocial disabilities were consequential for their social practice and their ways of coping with experiences of limitations in security, autonomy and/or influence. For instance, these factors affected their inclination to avoid or limit their involvement in collective actions such as peer-support and self-organisation together with other persons with psychosocial disabilities and constrained their opportunities to influence disability policy reforms and political decision-making processes of importance for society as a whole. Their self-concept and identity had consequences for their 'practical action horizon' (Stones, 2005, p. 83).

Self-organisation as link between external and internal structures

So far, our analysis might give the impression of rather static differences in the opportunities or conditions for self-presentation among persons with disabilities. In the section on internal structures, we have already suggested how the disability movement has used moral indignation as a weapon in their social struggles. Furthermore, we have suggested that the successful use of moral arguments in their struggles has varied between persons with visual, mobility, intellectual and psychosocial disabilities. However, by adopting a historical perspective and comparing three age cohorts of persons with disabilities, we have aimed to avoid a static representation of the opportunities for exercising Active Citizenship.

In addition to identifying generative processes which foster transformations in individual life courses, we have identified a number of victories and achievements by organisations of persons with disabilities. Such self-organisation or social mobilisation among persons with disabilities, we would argue, emerges as a link between – or a mechanism for – change in external *and* internal structures. Most people on their own are mainly able to influence their immediate environments ('conjuncturally specific external structures'), whereas under given circumstances collective actors may be able to influence larger structures at meso ('proximate structural layers') and macro ('upper structural layers') levels (O'Reilly, 2012, pp. 24, 31).

Since the 1990s, the disability movement has managed to reframe disability policy as human rights and a question of protection against discrimination rather than as a question of welfare dependent on the discretion, good will and charity of non-disabled people. We have witnessed the increasing social mobilisation of persons with disabilities, who no longer tolerate how they are treated. Persons with disabilities are still in the process of social recognition as subjects entitled to full and effective participation in society. However, with stronger and more substantive civil, political and social rights, the power imbalance between persons with disabilities and larger society is likely to diminish. From the literature, we would expect to find that, as the respect shown to persons with disabilities socially increases, their self-respect is likely to increase as well (Elias, 1994 [1977]; Stolk & Wouters, 1987). While recognising that other mechanisms or factors may influence the capacity for collective action among persons with disabilities, we have reasons to believe that the social recognition (reflected in a rights-based approach to disability policy), a positive self-image (high degree of self-respect) and social mobilisation among persons with disabilities are mutually reinforcing (Figure 13.1).

Our analysis suggest that a rights-based approach and opportunities for choice in the provision of social services may create an avenue for more active agency for persons with disabilities and reduce the power imbalance between service providers and beneficiaries. As the dependency on the discretionary provision of help and assistances diminishes, persons with disabilities will hold a stronger position to articulate their needs and interests and they will be less exposed to humiliating and degrading treatment. As the respect they receive increases, their sense of self-respect and sense of entitlement to non-discrimination and reasonable accommodation to ensure opportunities for participation is likely to increase as well. As Hobson (2017) has argued in her discussion of the capability approach, 'the sense of entitlement to make claims' is a key mechanism-enabling agent to profit from available resources and convert them into 'agency freedoms and achievements' (p. 12). When the stigma, shame or embarrassment attached to the disability decreases, development of a group identity and social mobilisation also become easier.

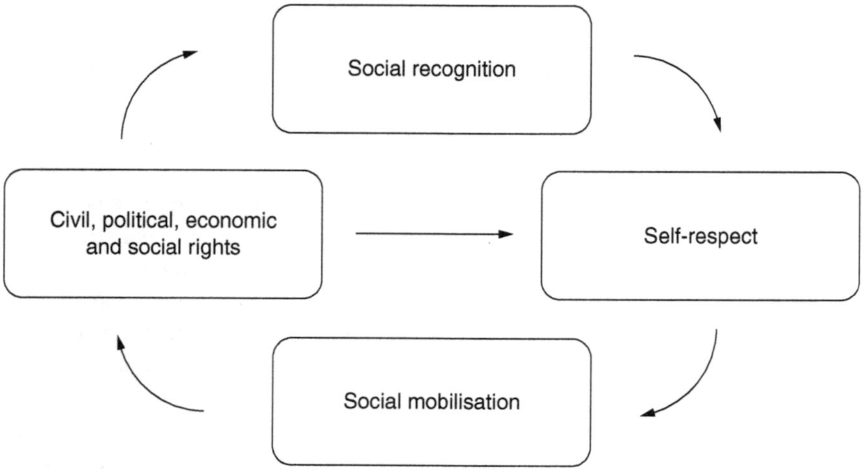

Figure 13.1 Ideal-typical cycle of social recognition and social mobilisation.

Conversely, we have reasons to assume that social misrecognition (reflected in discretionary provision of help and assistance), a negative self-image (low degree of self-respect, shame and embarrassment), individual coping strategies, and weak and ineffective civil, political, economic and social rights are mutually reinforcing (Figure 13.2). Such processes will be cases of social reproduction in social inequalities between disabled and non-disabled population groups.

Do we have any support for our hypotheses? In his theorisation about 'established-outsider relations', Norbert Elias (1994 [1977]) argued that we find an internal relation between developments in power relations and developments

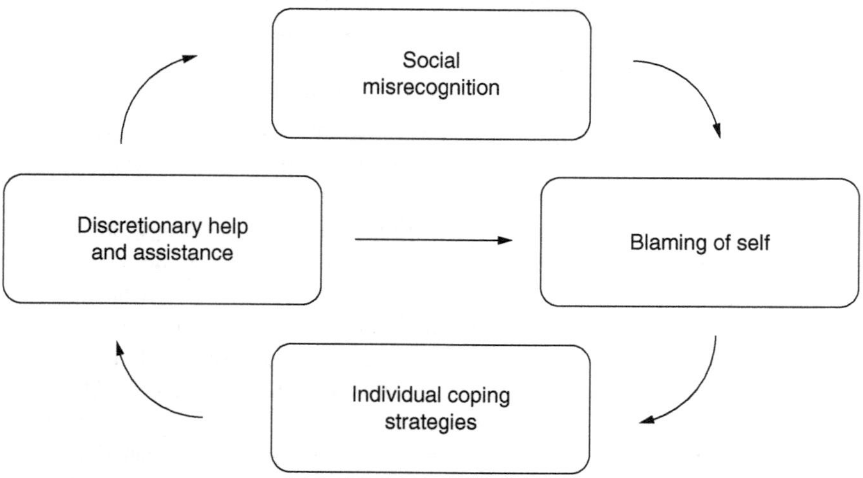

Figure 13.2 Ideal-typical cycle of social misrecognition and individual coping strategies.

in personality – or more specifically in self-image. Elias argues that powerful groups tend to look upon themselves as 'better' people. The more powerful groups also tend to manage to deprive the less powerful of a positive self-image or self-respect, i.e. to make less powerful people themselves feel they lack virtue – that they are inferior in human terms (p. xvi). Elias provides a wide range of examples of established–outsider figurations: e.g. 'whites' in relation to 'blacks', men in relation to women, and aristocracy in relation to working class. Although he does not mention disability specifically, his theorisation of the relationship between power relations and self-image has relevance for our own theorisation about the relationship between external and internal conditions for exercising Active Citizenship. According to Elias 'the established usually have an ally in an inner voice of their social inferior' (p. xxiv). He maintains that a feeling of inferiority usually has a paralysing effect on groups with a lower power ratio and disarms them (p. xxii, xxiv, xxviii).

While recognising that other resources are necessary to sustain the power to stigmatise, Elias argues that stigmatisation is in itself a weapon in maintaining a privileged position. However, when the unevenness of the power balance diminishes, he argues, the former outsiders tend on their part to retaliate (p. xxi). Elias refers to the labour movement and the civil rights movement as examples of such changes in power balances (see also Stolk & Wouters, 1987).

To what extent stigmatisation has a paralysing effect, Elias argues, depends on the overall situation. While the opportunities for group identity and collective action are weaker for stigmatised groups, he also identifies examples of individual protests and sporadic acts of revenge against the more powerful groups (p. xxviii). This later observation is important, as weak opportunities for collective action and self-organisation do not preclude opportunities for individual coping and resistance strategies. This is also consistent with the data we have reported from on the scope for agency at the individual level among persons with disabilities.

Our findings suggest that persons with visual and mobility disabilities were more likely to enjoy social recognition as subjects entitled to participation on a par with non-disabled persons, have a sense of entitlement to make claims, and mobilise together with others in a similar situation to pursue their justice demands. Conversely, persons with psychosocial and intellectual disabilities more often suffered from social misrecognition, and were more inclined to blame themselves for their situation and limit their contact with others in a similar situation.

In Europe, persons with disabilities are still struggling to be recognised as full citizens. Future change in the power balance between persons with and without disabilities can affect the self-image of less powerful groups such as persons with intellectual or psychosocial disabilities. In this book, we have only started identifying the generative processes that impact on the capability for voice, whether that is at the individual or at the collective level in and through organisations of persons with disabilities. Future research should examine these processes more systematically and in greater detail. Such endeavours should include a focus on how different age cohorts and impairment groups in different European countries position themselves in the disability movement.

In future examinations of social mobilisation processes among persons with disabilities, structuration theory may represent a promising starting point. One strength with strong structuration theory is that the conceptualisation of external and internal structures allows theorisation about the relationship between societal and individual change. To us, this seems to be one advantage in structuration theory compared to role theory (applied in Chapters 6 and 10 in this volume). In his development of structuration theory, Giddens (1984) criticises role theory for the tendency to 'emphasize the "given" character of roles, thereby serving to express the dualism of action and structure characteristic of so many areas of social theory' (p. 84). The Parsonian version of role theory especially has been criticised for an overly deterministic view of man (Wrong, 1961). From within role theory, we find different efforts to overcome this criticism and conceptualise the scope for individual agency, e.g. Merton (1957) on 'role set' and Goffman (1961) on 'role distance' (see Chapters 6 and 10, this volume) (see however West & Zimmerman, 1987). Such analytic concepts have contributed to a more dynamic view of structure–agency relationships but have to a lesser extent been able to conceptualise societal change, individual emancipation and social mobilisation, and the relationship between the three processes.

Self-representation as capability for voice – revisiting the capability approach

As we have demonstrated in this and earlier chapters, a special type of barrier to exercising Active Citizenship was related to the problem of articulating one's preferences. In general, if you do not see reason to value anything, do not know what you want to do or be, believe you are not entitled to assert your own preferences, or you are too embarrassed or ashamed to present your needs and wants, then exercising active agency becomes rather difficult. This mode of thinking was particularly striking in the case of some of the interviews with persons with psychosocial disabilities. Yet, even among persons with rather complex mental health issues, we have found cases of improvement in the ability to identify and express wants and desires, make decisions about what one wants and pursue those interests (Chapters 8 and 11). To what extent can the capability approach help us explain such transformations in capability to articulate one's preferences during the life course?

The capability approach holds that freedom of choice matters for evaluating a person's standard of living. Freedom of choice requires that more than one option is feasible. Also, the available options have to be desirable from the agent's point of view (Sen, 1999, pp. 24, 288). Although for a long time scholars working within the capability approach have focused on the choice between different options, they have given more attention to the procedural dimension of choice since the 2000s.

Sen recognises the role of the public debate for discussions and decisions about which values are worth pursuing. 'The exercise of freedom is mediated by values, but the values in turn are influenced by public discussions and social interactions, which are themselves influenced by participatory freedoms' (Sen, 1999, p. 15). To Sen, therefore, participation in the public debate about the public good is essential for the value-judgements and discussions about which values should inform collective decisions. Similarly, Alkire (2006, p. 135) observes that 'when judgements as to which capabilities are valuable must be made, and when these judgements affect wider groups of people, procedural considerations enter'.

What Bonvin and Thelen (2003, cited in Bifulco, 2013) have conceptualised as the 'capability for voice' touches on the capacity to articulate one's preferences and values, to discuss and critically examine those with other citizens, and to participate in and influence decision-making processes of importance to oneself and to society at large, taking into account the interdependencies of human lives. In light of this, 'the capacity to express one's opinions and thoughts and to make them count in the course of public discussion' is essential (Bonvin & Thelen, 2003, cited in Bifulco, 2013, p. 181). In this sense, the capability approach 'throws light on voice as an attribute of agency' (Bifulco, 2013, p. 181).

Scholars working within the capability approach have discussed preference formation in the public in relation to ideals about participatory or deliberative democracy (Crocker, 2008; De Leonardis & Negrelli, 2012; Salais, 2009). Sen (2009) has himself highlighted conversion factors at the institutional level, including which rights people are entitled to and whether institutions to safeguard these rights are in place. While conversion factors at the institutional level are clearly relevant for the 'capability for voice' among persons with disabilities, our findings suggest that future research should pay more attention to the interdependencies between external and internal factors or structures. At this point the capability approach could benefit from the conceptualisation of agency and social practices in structuration theory. So far, 'the interplay between social structure and individual agency' seems to be somewhat underdeveloped in the capability approach (Lessman, 2011, pp. 1, 14, 20).

Conclusion

In our theorisation of the conditions for the Active Citizenship of persons with disabilities, we have examined the fruitfulness of structuration theory (Stones, 2005; O'Reilly, 2012) and the capability approach (Sen 1992, 1999; Nussbaum, 2000, 2006). In this endeavour, we have explored how the two theoretical perspectives may inform each other, especially when taking the criticism of the two perspectives into account. In the discussion, we have made the strengths and weaknesses of the perspectives explicit. We have argued that the perspectives may enrich each other and help researchers improve their conceptualisation of actor–structure dynamics in the structuration of opportunities for exercising Active Citizenship. In particular, we have stressed the social embeddedness of choice/agency, the internal relationship between external and internal structures, the temporal aspect of agency–structure dynamics, and conversion factors as analytic tools to model the linkages between external/internal structures and the agency of persons with disabilities.

Rather than identifying a definitive list of capability inputs, conversion factors and capabilities, we have focused on generative processes that facilitate or constrain the Active Citizenship of persons with disabilities. Our findings demonstrate that internal conversion factors such as personal characteristics, world views, desires and self-identity convert capability inputs (or resources) into capabilities and eventually choice of functionings. Such conversions are also dependent on external conversion factors: i.e. social and environmental characteristics (Trani, Bakhshi, Bellanca, Biggeri & Marchetta, 2011, p. 145). The findings we have reported here demonstrate interdependencies between different 'external' (social and environmental) and 'internal' (personal) conversion factors.

Often researchers have only had statistical data on the achieved functionings. From a capability perspective, this has not been completely satisfactory as the capability set, rather than the actual functionings, is the ultimate proof of the scope persons with disabilities have for choosing the life they have reasons to value. In the absence of data on the capability set, gaps in achieved functionings between persons with disabilities and non-disabled people can be regarded as indicative of social inequalities in capabilities (Robeyns, 2003, p. 85) – there is no reason to believe that group-based inequalities in functionings between persons with disabilities and non-disabled people are due to differences in preferences between the two groups – the life-course interviews we have collected in the DISCIT project have, however, provided data on the capability sets as experienced and presented by the interviewees. This has provided us with subjective data on the substantial freedom and scope of agency among persons with disabilities in Europe. Additionally, we have gathered data on their achieved functionings. Together, the life-course interviews have provided rich data on mechanisms and processes which structure the Active Citizenship of persons with disabilities.

How have UN, EU-level and national disability policies influenced the scope for agency and capability on the part of persons with disabilities? Overall our findings demonstrated that public disability policies matter. UN, EU and national policies structure the opportunities for, but do not determine, the Active Citizenship of persons with disabilities. In Volume 1, we mapped not insignificant differences between European countries in what we have referred to as the national 'disability policy systems'. The countries have given different priorities to the cash benefit subsystem, services subsystem and regulatory subsystem (Halvorsen, Waldschmidt, Hvinden & Klette Bøhler, 2017). The cross-country comparisons of data from the life-course interviews have further demonstrated that access to resources in cash and in kind matters for the opportunities to participate in the community, education, the labour market, culture and sports, informal care for family members, civil society organisations and politics.

In this volume, we have demonstrated how one might apply our conceptualisation of Active Citizenship to specify the meaning of 'full and effective participation in society on an equal basis with others' in the CRPD (UN 2006, preamble, item e). The further process of implementing the CRPD in the EU, the member states and associated countries will offer enhanced opportunities for persons with disabilities and their organisations to *influence* the development towards Active Citizenship and push for the necessary reforms both at European and at national levels. Yet, for several reasons it is unlikely that this implementation will involve any clear trend towards convergence in this area. In the foreseeable future, we are likely to see notable and stable contrasts between the different combinations of strategies, policies and instruments that European governments pursue, albeit with variable success.

European countries have made significant progress since the 1990s in ensuring the Active Citizenship of persons with disabilities. Yet, many persons with disabilities still do not have the opportunities for full and effective participation in society, policymaking and the economy on an equal basis with others. In interpreting the findings presented in this book, one needs to bear in mind that the life-course interviews did not involve a representative sample of people with disabilities. They did not, among others, include persons with more complex disabilities, in particular those with severe communication impairments. However, given that even our sample of relatively able, well-resourced and, in many cases, politically active persons with disabilities still experienced difficulties and barriers to their ability to live full lives in the community, it is reasonable to assume that those with more severe and complex needs experience even greater difficulties in exercising Active Citizenship.

What are the implications of our findings for the disability policies in the EU and European governments? First, European governments need to adopt a broad approach to the promotion of more Active Citizenship among persons with disabilities. The life-course interviews have demonstrated that paid work continues to be the dominant path or avenue to Active Citizenship. A majority of the population, including a majority of persons with disabilities, wants to achieve and retain employment in the ordinary labour market. Opportunities to participate in the labour market continue to be one of if not the most important source of income, wealth accumulation and social respect. Having said that, it is important to acknowledge that not all people may realise Active Citizenship in the same way. How persons with and without disabilities engage with the labour market and the extent to which they are able to do so is also partly a matter of personal choice and preference. The assumption that being an active citizen necessarily includes having paid work within the mainstream labour market is challenged by the accounts of some of the persons with disabilities we have interviewed. Voluntary and caring roles or participation in other activities may equally give a person a sense of being an active citizen in ways that make participation in the labour market less important or even irrelevant.

The EU, member states and associated countries should continue to strengthen their efforts to improve the opportunities for men and women with disabilities to participate in the labour market. A great deal of thought goes into improving the skills and resources of disabled persons, and efforts are made to minimise exclusion and discrimination through anti-discrimination laws, notions of reasonable adjustment and quota systems. However, there are also the issues of the labour market structure, labour market demand and the nature of jobs, which might exclude and deny choice for persons with disabilities. The need is for long-term thinking about the kinds of work persons with disabilities can and hope to do. In the future, rethinking work with disability in mind may contribute as much, and possibly more, to enhancing Active Citizenship for persons with disabilities through mainstream labour market participation.

Second, the findings we have reported here suggest that the EU, member states and associated countries should continue their efforts to promote more gender sensitive disability policies and achieve better understanding of how differences in opportunities for exercising Active Citizenship between women and men with disabilities, and between women with and without disabilities, are socially reproduced.

Third, the life-course interviews have demonstrated the need not to focus only on the differences between persons with and without disabilities. Policy makers should also accommodate the needs of persons with different types of disabilities when designing and adopting policy measures to promote Active Citizenship. Particular attention should be given to the needs and interests of persons with intellectual disabilities and persons with mental health problems.

Fourth, the EU, the member states and associated countries may want to adopt a life-course perspective in their disability policies. Public authorities need to take into account that physical and mental health may vary over time, for instance by ensuring opportunities to combine paid work and receipt of social security benefits, by providing personalised and flexible services in cash and in kind, and by reasonable accommodation to ensure opportunities for Active Citizenship in all stages of life. Providers of social services in cash and in kind should design and adopt policy measures to minimise risks of disabling barriers at different life stages and associated with different transitions (from education to employment, establishing a separate household, etc.) and turning-points (unemployment, sickness, divorce, loss of parents, etc.) during the life course.

Fifth and finally, when governments formulate and adopt their disability policy measures, a procedural approach to the promotion of Active Citizenship will prove useful. Public authorities should be concerned not only with the substantial outcomes of disability policies but also the choice process, including the recognition and representation of persons with disabilities in those decision-making processes. This means involving persons with disabilities and their representative organisations in making the political priorities, and designing and evaluating the policy objectives and measures.

References

Alkire, S. (2006). Public debate and value construction in Sen's approach. In A. Kaufman (Ed.), *Capabilities equality: Basic issues and problems* (pp. 133–154). London: Routledge.

Bellanca, N., Biggeri, M. & Marchetta, F. (2011). An extension of the capability approach: Towards a theory of dis-capability, ALTER. *European Journal of Disability Research*, 5(3), 158–176.

Bifulco, L. (2013). Citizen participation, agency and voice. *European Journal of Social Theory*, *16*(2), 174–187.

Bourdieu, P. (1977). *Outline of a theory of practice*. Cambridge: Cambridge University Press.

Crocker, D. A. (2008). The capability approach and deliberative democracy. In *Ethics of global development: Agency, capability and deliberative democracy* (Chapter 9). Cambridge: Cambridge University Press.

De Leonardis, O. & Negrelli, S. (2009). A new perspective on welfare policies. Why and how the capability for voice matters. In O. De Leonardis, S. Negrelli & R. Salais (Eds), *Democracy and capabilities for voice. Welfare, work and public deliberation in Europe* (pp. 11–33). Frankfurt/Main: Peter Lang Verlag.

Elias, N. (1994 [1977]). Introduction. A theoretical essay on established and outsider relations. In N. Elias & J. L. Scotson (Eds), *The established and the outsiders. A sociological enquiry into community problems* (pp. xv–lii). London: Sage.

EU. (2000). Council directive 2000/78/EC of 27 November 2000 establishing a general framework for equal treatment in employment and occupation. *Official Journal* L 303, 02/12/2000, 0016–0022.

EU. (2016). Directive (EU) 2016/2102 of the European Parliament and of the Council of 26 October 2016 on the accessibility of the websites and mobile applications of public sector bodies. *Official Journal* L 327, 2.12.2016, 1–15.

Giddens, A. (1984). *The constitution of society. Outline of the theory of structuration*, Berkeley, CA: University of California Press.

Goffman, E. (1961). Role distance. In *Encounters: Two studies in the sociology of interaction*, Indianapolis, IN: Bobbs-Merrill.

Halvorsen, R., Waldschmidt, A., Hvinden, B. & Klette Bøhler, K. (2017). Diversity and dynamics of disability policy in Europe: An analytic framework. In R. Halvorsen, B. Hvinden, J. Bickenbach, D. Ferri & A. M. Guillén Rodriguez (Eds), *The changing disability policy system. Active Citizenship and disability in Europe Volume 1* (pp. 12–33). London: Routledge.

Hobson, B. (2017). Gendered dimensions and capabilities: Opportunities, dilemmas and challenges. *Critical Sociology* 1–16. doi: 10.1177/0896920516683232.

Hvinden, B. & Halvorsen, R. (2017). What role for conversion factors? *Critical Sociology*, 1–17. doi: 10.1177/0896920516684541.

Karačić, A. & Waldschmidt, A. (2018). Biographie und Behinderung. In H. Lutz, M. Schiebel & E. Tuider (Eds), *Handbuch Biographieforschung* (pp. 415–425). Wiesbaden: Springer VS. doi: 10.1007/978-3-658-18171-0_35.

Lessman, O. (2011). Freedom of choice and poverty alleviation. *Review of Social Economy*, *69*(4), 439–463.

Merton, R. (1957). *Social structure and social theory*. New York: Free Press.

Molden, T. H. & Tøssebro, J. (2012). Disability measurements: Impact on research results. *Scandinavian Journal of Disability Research*, *14*(4), 340–357.

Newman, J. (Ed.). (2005). *Remaking governance: Peoples, politics and the public sphere*. Bristol: Policy Press.

Nosek, M. A., Clubb Foley, C., Hughes, R. B. & Howland, C. A. (2001). Vulnerabilities for abuse among women with disabilities. *Sexuality and Disability*, *19*(3), 177–189.

Nussbaum, M. (2000). *Women and human development*. Cambridge: Cambridge University Press.

Nussbaum, M. (2006). *Frontiers of justice: Disability, nationality, species membership*. Cambridge, MA: Harvard University Press.

Nussbaum, M. (2011). *Capabilities: The human development approach*. Cambridge, MA: Harvard University Press.

O'Reilly, K. (2012). *International migration and social theory*. Houndmills, Basingstoke: Palgrave.

Priestley, M., Stickings, M., Loja, E., Grammenos, S., Lawson, A., Waddington, L. & Fridriksdottir, B. (2016). The political participation of disabled people in Europe: Rights, accessibility and activism. *Electoral Studies*, *42*, 1–9.

Robeyns, I. (2003). Sen's capability approach and gender inequality: Selecting relevant capabilities. *Feminist Economics*, *9*(2–3), 61–92.

Robeyns, I. (2005). The capability approach. A theoretical survey. *Journal of Human Development*, *1*, 93–114.

Salais, R. (2009). Conclusions: Labour and the politics of freedoms. In O. De Leonardis, S. Negrelli & R. Salais (Eds), *Democracy and capabilities for voice. Welfare, work and public deliberation in Europe* (pp. 227–244). Frankfurt/ Main: Peter Lang Verlag.

Schneider, A. & Ingram, H. (1993). Social construction of target populations: Implications for politics and policy. *American Political Science Review*, *87*, 334–347.

Sen, A. (1992). *Inequality reexamined.* Oxford: Oxford University Press.

Sen, A. (1999). *Development as freedom*. Oxford: Oxford University Press.

Sen, A. (2009). *The idea of justice*. Cambridge, MA: Harvard University Press.

Stolk, B. van & Wouters, C. (1987). Power changes and self-respect: A comparison of two cases of established outsider relations. *Theory, Culture and Society*, *4*, 477–88.

Stones, R. (2005). *Structuration theory*. Houndmills, Basingstoke: Palgrave Macmillan.

Tilly, C. (1998). *Durable inequality*. Berkeley, CA: University of California Press.

Trani, J. F., Bakhshi, P., Bellanca, N., Biggeri, M. & Marchetta, F. (2011). Disabilities through the capability approach lens: Implications for public policies. *Alter*, *5*, 143–157.

UN. (2006). *Convention on the rights of persons with disabilities* (A/RES/61/106). Resolution adopted by the General Assembly, 13 December. New York: United Nations.

Waddington, L. (2017). The potential for, and barriers to, the exercise of Active EU Citizenship by persons with disabilities: The right to free movement. In R. Halvorsen, B. Hvinden, J. Bickenbach, D. Ferri & A. M. Guillén Rodriguez (Eds), *The changing disability policy system. Active Citizenship and disability in Europe volume 1* (pp. 196–214). London: Routledge.

Waldschmidt, A. (2017). Disability goes cultural: The cultural model of disability as an analytical tool. In A. Waldschmidt, H. Berressem & M. Ingwersen (Eds), *Culture – theory – disability: Encounters between disability studies and cultural studies* (pp. 19–28). Bielefeld: Transcript.

West, C. & Zimmerman, D. H. (1987). Doing gender. *Gender & Society*, *1*(2), 125–151.

Wrong, D. H. (1961). The oversocialized conception of man in modern sociology. *American Sociological Review*, *26*, 183–193.

Index

Kolibri 360 GmbH
Ferdinand-Jühlke-Straße 7
99095 Erfurt, Deutschland
produktsicherheit@kolibri360.de